HEALTHCARE TECHNOLOGIES SERIES 2

Machine Learning for Healthcare Technologies

Other volumes in this series:

Volume 1	**Nanobiosensors for Personalized and Onsite Biomedical Diagnosis** Dr. P. Chandra (Editor)
Volume 3	**Portable Biosensors and Point-of-Care Systems** Prof. Spyridon E. Kintzios (Editor)
Volume 4	**Biomedical Nanomaterials: From Design To Implementation** Dr. Thomas J. Webster & Dr. Hilal Yazici (Editors)

Machine Learning for Healthcare Technologies

Edited by David A. Clifton

The Institution of Engineering and Technology

Published by The Institution of Engineering and Technology, London, United Kingdom

The Institution of Engineering and Technology is registered as a Charity in England & Wales (no. 211014) and Scotland (no. SC038698).

First published 2016

The Institution of Engineering and Technology
Michael Faraday House
Six Hills Way, Stevenage
Herts, SG1 2AY, United Kingdom

www.theiet.org

British Library Cataloguing in Publication Data
A catalogue record for this product is available from the British Library

ISBN 978-1-84919-978-0 (hardback)
ISBN 978-1-84919-979-7 (PDF)

Typeset in India by MPS Limited

Contents

Chapter 1

Machine learning for healthcare technologies – an introduction

David A. Clifton

1.1 The changing needs of healthcare

Much has been written concerning the manner in which healthcare is changing, with a particular emphasis on how very large quantities of data are now being routinely collected during the routine care of patients. The use of machine learning methods to turn these ever-growing quantities of data into interventions that can improve patient outcomes seems as if it should be an obvious path to take. However, the field of machine learning in healthcare is still in its infancy. This book, kindly supported by the Institution of Engineering and Technology, aims to provide a "snapshot" of the state of current research at the interface between machine learning and healthcare.

Necessarily, this is a partial and biased sampling of the state of current research, and yet we have aimed to provide a wide-ranging introduction to the depth and scale of work that is being undertaken worldwide. In selecting material for this edited volume, we have placed special emphasis on machine learning projects that are (or are close to) achieving improvement in patient outcomes. For many reasons, uncovered variously in some of the chapters that follow, it is a truism that "healthcare is hard"; there are unique constraints that exist, and considerations that must be taken, when working with healthcare data. However, for all its difficulties, working with healthcare data is exceptionally rewarding, both in terms of the computational challenges that exist and in terms of the outputs of research being able to affect the way in which healthcare is delivered. There are few application areas of machine learning that have such promise to benefit society as does that of healthcare.

1.2 Online resources

The remainder of this chapter seeks to survey the various research programmes described in this book, and draws the readers' attention to the fact that many of the projects described were presented by the authors in person, at a workshop held at

Balliol College, Oxford, during the summer of 2015. The Institution of Engineering and Technology (IET) video-recorded the event, and has made the resulting recordings available for free via its IET.tv online resource. There is seldom a better introduction to a research programme than to hear it described by its originators, and so we hope that the reader finds the online resources to be a useful and accessible complement to the more comprehensive descriptions provided in this volume.

Balliol College celebrated its 750th anniversary a little while before the "Machine Learning in Healthcare" workshop took place, and it has a good claim to being the oldest college, in what is the oldest university of the English-speaking world. Since coming to Balliol from a series of other colleges in the university, I have been greatly impressed by the open spirit of enquiry that exists in the place, and the substantive and very real manner in which it supports its fellows to do the same. The workshop combined the extensive efforts of both Balliol and the IET, in which the old buildings were repurposed for professional video-filming and audio recording, and where attendees came from both academia and (healthcare) industry to discuss the work presented in this volume. As a "snapshot" of some of the best work at the interface between machine learning and healthcare, it struck me as being fitting that this should be recorded against the backdrop of an institution that remains both ancient and modern, in the best of ways. It is our hope that some of this spirit is apparent in both the videos maintained on the IET.tv website, and the volume before us.[1]

1.3 Survey of contents

Chapter 2: The team led by Prof. Chris Williams at the University of Edinburgh, UK, has long been at the forefront of various aspects of machine learning, and an important theme of their work is the application of time-series analysis methods to healthcare applications – most notably, those pertaining to the intensive care unit (ICU) in the hospital. The ICU is a data-rich environment, in which patients are typically monitored continuously for the duration of their stay, and where the nurse-to-patient ratio is typically 1:1 in many healthcare systems. Entering an ICU is to be deluged by data in all its forms: various machines, which may or may not be interoperable, report measurements to the clinician almost constantly; there is typically a great deal of "alarm noise" from the various devices, and one receives the impression that there is far more data being generated than can be meaningfully interpreted by a human – even a highly trained expert as is typically the case with ICU clinicians. On seeing such an environment, one almost immediately concludes that machine learning has a key role to play in aiding the clinician, by guiding their attention to those components of the data that are most pertinent. Chapter 2 describes one such approach, in which a factorial switched linear dynamical system (FSLDS) is used to make sense of the data,

[1](https://tv.theiet.org/?event=3534)

with the goal of understanding what within a signal can be described as artefact, and what is clinically important information. It seems fitting to encounter this material first in the book, given the themes of signal understanding and subsequent modelling that Prof. Williams and colleagues describe.

Chapter 3: We noted previously the old adage that "healthcare is hard," and a contributing factor to this is that biomedical devices typically operate independently, without knowledge of other aspects of the patient's physiology other than that which it is measuring. Prof. Gari Clifford of Emory University, USA, is a long-standing contributor to the field of computational approaches to cardiology, and in performing analysis in the presence of the substantial noise that typically exists when patients are monitored while ambulatory. The latter is an important factor in the limited impact that "mobile health" (or m-health) has had in clinical practice, due to the fact that most ambulatory monitoring systems are typically insufficiently robust due to an inability to cope with such data uncertainty. Chapter 3 combines these two themes, by developing methods that permit the identification of atrial fibrillation from the electrocardiogram (ECG) under the most testing of circumstances. Again, these themes appear early in the book, due to the commonality that it shares with most chapters subsequently described.

Chapter 4: Continuing the topic of handling noisy biomedical waveform data, Dr. Julien Oster of the University of Oxford describes advances in the development of Bayesian filters for detecting important features of clinical relevance in the ECG. Dr. Oster's research career has focussed on the interface between cardiology and machine learning, where the goal is to improve upon human annotations and analysis of the ECG – as is appropriate when one is, for example, faced with screening very large quantities of cardiac data. This chapter provides a helpful tutorial in how the framework of Bayesian filtering may be applied to cardiology, and how one can use a generative model to understand the ECG waveform.

Chapter 5: Readers will probably be familiar with the traditional decompositions often used to summarise high-dimensional data by using a lower-dimensional version that can be used for parsimonious inference. For example, the likes of principal components analysis and its derivatives are becoming popular in many branches of genomic analysis. However, such representations of data are typically simplistic, and fail to capture much of the structure that may be present – Prof. Maarten de Vos and his team at the University of Oxford present a tutorial for using methods based on tensor decompositions for better understanding the structure in EEG (and other biomedical) time-series. Chapter 5 provides a helpful introduction to how and why tensor decomposition can be used in such situations, with illustrations of the method in the application area of detecting epileptic seizures.

Chapter 6: With earlier chapters concerning themselves with the understanding and modelling of biomedical waveform data, this chapter looks at methods by which data may be compared across patients. Based on some of the work from the Computational Health Informatics (CHI) Lab at Oxford, Dr. Marco Pimentel describes the development of principled, probabilistic methods for performing inference across entire time-series of patient data. We undertook a study of over 300 post-operative patients at Oxford University Hospitals, and present the results of how such methods might be used to provide risk stratification – the ultimate goal is to understand, as early as possible, which patients are at the highest risk of deterioration – a problem that is critical, because the mortality rate in this patient group approaches 1 in 6.

Chapter 7: In the second chapter from the CHI Lab at Oxford, Dr. Tingting Zhu presents the means by which the outputs of multiple algorithms may be fused to improve accuracy of classification for biomedical tasks. She focuses her attention on a cardiology application, similar to that addressed in Chapters 3 and 4, but where a panel of algorithms exist. She describes a fully Bayesian methodology for assuming that the outputs of each of these algorithms (which may be automated computational algorithms or, in the case of cardiology, human experts) are "noisy" with respect to the correct output; the noise distribution for each algorithm is then learned in an *unsupervised* manner. Dr. Zhu shows that the resulting estimates, across all algorithms, typically outperform even the single-best algorithm. This is especially appealing for the use of machine learning systems, whereby we may have multiple algorithms that have been created for a single task, the results of which may be fused to produce robust outputs.

Chapter 8: Prof. Suchi Saria and her team at Johns Hopkins University, USA, take a novel look at the case of competing models: the dollar-value associated with acquiring individual data-points for a patient in a healthcare setting is incorporated into a regulariser. This recognises the fact that acquiring different data may be associated with more costly measurement procedures; for example, ordering blood tests for an ICU patient may be more expensive (in terms of dollar-value) that acquiring another heart-rate estimate from a bedside monitoring. By taking this information into account within the regularisation framework, an estimate is provided of how the predictive accuracy of risk assessment (here, for risk of developing septic shock) varies as available dollar-value increases. While the "true" costs of estimating various data types is notoriously difficult to quantify (especially in centralised healthcare systems, such as the UK National Health Service), Prof. Saria's approach helps us make informed choices concerning which risk assessment system should be used, for example – where such decisions are typically made using predictive accuracy alone, without any information of the costs of data acquisition.

Chapter 9: Dr. James Hensman of the University of Lancaster and Prof. Theodore Kypraios of the University of Nottingham have an ongoing collaboration in which they have developed Bayesian non-parametric models for understanding the outbreak and spread of infectious disease. This chapter explores the log Gaussian Cox process, which is an interesting extension of the much-used Cox process, with its relationship to the traditional *Susceptible-Infective-Removed* epidemic model. This chapter provides, among other contributions, a helpful tutorial on the use of variational inference methods for estimating the values of the hyperparameters of a Gaussian process, used within the log Gaussian Cox process. There are many applications in which "arrival times" or rates are of interest, to which the methods described in this chapter are directly applicable.

Chapter 10: Perhaps one of the most troubling recent developments in healthcare is that of increasing antibiotic resistance, whereby bacteria are developing (via accelerated natural selection) resistance to the various classes of antibiotics with which we treat infection. As resistance increases, our ability to combat infectious disease becomes more limited, and we must turn to treatments that are potentially harmful for the patient. This problem is compounded by the fact that assessing resistance to antibiotics involves taking a biological sample from a patient, isolating the bacteria that are causing infection, and then growing those bacteria in a microbiological lab such that various antibiotics can be tested on those bacteria. For some strains, such as *Mycobacterium tuberculosis*, this process can take over one month. In Chapter 10, Dr. Yang Yang describes work from the CHI Lab at Oxford concerning the use of near-same-day genetic sequencing, in which the bacterium itself is sequenced. Machine learning methods are then applied to the results to estimate antibiotic resistance – in a fraction of the time taken by conventional methods, thereby allowing us to treat infectious disease in a timely manner, which timely treatment of the patient is especially important.

Chapter 11: Chronic disease is one of the greatest burdens on most healthcare systems, and, in this chapter, Katherine Niehaus introduces work from the Oxford CHI Lab on improving our understanding of various classes of immune disease. This work involves close collaboration with medical colleagues from Oxford University Hospitals, in which we have acquired genomic, time-series and other data for a large cohort of patients suffering from these types of disease. The challenge for machine learning is to determine how best one should link these very different classes of data; this chapter includes a description of methods from extreme value theory that are being used to assess "beyond normal" data – as are often acquired from patients with immune disease.

Chapter 12: Representing contributions from MIT and Harvard, Prof. Shamim Nemati describes "big data" approaches to a number of exemplar applications within healthcare, including the estimation of the dose of medication that should be provided to a patient. Conventional clinical methods of performing this estimation typically derive from simplistic factors, such as using initial measurements of the weight of the patient followed by a laboratory test performed some hours later. With the wide range of data available via the electronic medical record, this chapter describes how data-driven approaches can be used to improve upon standard clinical practice. Shamim's work includes analysis of the MIMIC-2 open-source dataset, created and curated by the Laboratory for Computational Physiology at MIT of which he is a member. Readers may be familiar with this resource as being a great asset to global critical-care research; it is no exaggeration to report that the editor alone knows at least 25 young data scientists from across the world who obtained their doctoral degrees thanks to the availability of MIMIC.

Chapter 13: Few application areas for healthcare are more testing than that of monitoring patients in their own homes. Such is the focus of the research of Prof. Bart Vanrumste and his team at KU Leuven, Belgium, in which sensors are embedded throughout a subject's home and where systems based on machine learning seek to identify patterns in the activities of daily living. A *novelty detection* approach can be taken, whereby deviation from a previously established model of normality can be used to highlight significant changes in mental- or physical-health status for a patient. Chapter 13 describes a number of approaches to this problem, including one based on extreme value theory using point processes, which is a branch of statistics typically employed to identify extremal observations – often from finance, meteorology or climate data.

Acknowledgement

DAC gratefully acknowledges the support of the Royal Academy of Engineering, the UK Engineering and Physical Sciences Research Council, the Wellcome Trust, the UK National Institute of Health Research, UNICEF, the UK Natural Environment Research Council, the UK Department for International Development, the Bill & Melinda Gates Foundation and Balliol College.

Balliol College, Oxford

Chapter 2

Detecting artifactual events in vital signs monitoring data

Partha Lal, Christopher K. I. Williams, Konstantinos Georgatzis, Christopher Hawthorne, Paul McMonagle, Ian Piper and Martin Shaw

2.1 Introduction

The presence of artifact in intensive care monitoring data is a major problem. For example, maintaining blood pressure in critically ill patients is a key management goal, and yet it is the physiological variable most prone to error. In addition to real-time monitoring, artifact detection is necessary for the proper audit or trial of therapies.

In this study we collect and annotate data from 27 intensive care unit (ICU) patients from the Southern General Hospital (SGH) in Glasgow. Two models are compared for the detection, removal and cleaning of artifact in the vital signs data, namely, the Factorial Switching Linear Dynamical System (FSLDS) and the Discriminative Switching Linear Dynamical System (DSLDS). We also consider a combination of the two, called the α-mixture (as described in Section 2.7.3). Three types of artifactual events are considered: blood sample, damped trace (in the arterial line) and suction events. The area under ROC curve (AUC) scores for the detection of these events are: blood sample 0.95, damped trace: 0.79, suction 0.64 (α-mixture), with similar results for the FSLDS and DSLDS. The system is able run in real time, and we discuss issues that had to be addressed to achieve this.

The structure of the rest of the paper is as follows: we describe the data collection, data preprocessing and data annotation processes in Sections 2.2–2.4. Section 2.5 evaluates what effect data cleaning can have on data summaries. In Sections 2.6 and 2.7 we describe the FSLDS and DSLDS models that are used to make predictions of artifactual events in the data. In order to use these models we need to identify a period of stability, when no artifact is present; the resulting stability detector is presented in Section 2.8. Section 2.9 describes the issues that needed to be addressed to make a real-time system, and Section 2.10 gives details of the software produced for the project. Experimental results are given in Section 2.11, and conclusions and future work are discussed in Section 2.12.

2.2 Data collection

Data was captured in the Neuro ICU of the SGH in Glasgow. Signals collected were arterial blood pressure (ABP), electrocardiogram (ECG), pulse oximetry pulse (Pleth), intracranial pressure (ICP), end tidal CO_2 ($EtCO_2$) and the respiratory signal (Resp) from the patient bedside monitor. Data sampling rates are signal dependent; the ECG signal is sampled at 500 Hz and all other channels sampled at 125 Hz. This raw waveform data was captured from the bedside ICU Philips Intellivue Monitors.

The data were captured in two different ways. For the first set of eight patients (labelled BioTBI), the waveform data was recorded onto a laptop computer connected into the bedside monitor. This system had some reliability problems, so that the data for a patient can be broken into a number of intervals, with gaps in between. So, for example, patient BioTBI001 has two records BioTBI001_1 and BioTBI001_2 in our database. In total there were 17 data intervals recorded for the 8 BioTBI patients.

Due to the unreliability of the above system, the waveform capture software ixTrend was purchased from Reference 1. Their "Netserver" software sits as a service on each of the Intellivue Monitor's embedded PCs and captures data from the monitor via the Medical Interface Bus (MIB) serial interface. Each minute, raw waveform data from all waveform channels is captured, compressed and sent via the local area network to an SQL Server database hosted on a local ICU server. Waveform data from each of the eight SGH Neuro ICU beds is continuously captured from the moment a patient is admitted to an ICU bed space and a valid patient identifier is entered onto the local bedside electronic record system (Philips ICCA). A system batch file running as an ixellence service detects when new patients are admitted into an ICU bed. Data collected in this fashion is labelled CSO_0001 onwards in our dataset.

Data for 84 patients were captured between December 2012 and January 2015. Of these, 27 patients were selected as suitable for analysis. The remaining 57 patients were excluded for the following reasons: (i) Inappropriate admission pathology: $N = 23$ (as study admission criteria were focused upon patients with TBI or SAH), (ii) Insufficient data or channel type within first 48 hours of admission: $N = 16$ (some patients that are admitted over weekend or at unsociable hours can have several days before annotation can begin), (iii) Network Hardware failure: $N = 10$ or Software down-sampling failures: $N = 2$, (iv) TBI patients excluded to ensure study design balance between SAH/TBI cohorts: $N = 3$, (v) Noisy data or no Events of Interest: $N = 2$ and (vi) Patient refused study consent: $N = 1$. Of the 27 patients, 15 were traumatic brain injury (TBI) and 12 subarachnoid hemorrhage (SAH) patients.

In addition to the raw waveform data capture, additional clinical data useful for event interpretation was captured and reviewed as required from the Philips Medical ICU eRecord system (ICCA) to supplement the waveform data. This included TBI/SAH status, age, gender, etc.

2.3 Data preprocessing

Although the waveform data is recorded at 125 or 500 Hz, second-by-second summary data is more than adequate for condition monitoring of patient status, as has been shown e.g. by the neo-natal ICU work of Reference 2.

C++ code was written to down sample the waveform quality data to second-by-second summary measures. The approach used is fully described in Reference 3. In brief, for each signal mentioned in Section 2.2, an *index* channel is identified (as specified in table 2 of Reference 3). The purpose of the index signal is to identify a physiologically meaningful interval over which to measure the signal. For example, ECG is used as the index for the ABP signal, and the ECG is processed to identify the R-R interval (the interval between ventricle depolarizations in the heart). Once an interval has been identified the signal is processed as appropriate, and the results are then interpolated to 1 Hz. For example, for the ABP signal, the mean, diastolic (minimum pressure) and systolic (maximum pressure) channels are obtained per interval and then interpolated.

2.4 Data annotation

The BioTBI patients plus CSO_0001 and CSO_0002 were annotated by CH. The aim was to annotate specific types of events that can affect the data quality and interpretation of the channels. Later, an experienced ICU nurse (PMc) was hired for a six-month period to carry out annotation of further data collected under the CSO project. To gain experience, PMc annotated patients CSO_0001 and CSO_0002 independently, and then CH and PMc discussed the annotations together to produce a consensus annotation.

Where possible PMc carried out "live" annotation of patients admitted to the Neuro ICU of the SGH. A total of eight patients in the study were annotated in this manner (CSO_0083, CSO_0099, CSO_0107, CSO_0112, CSO_0113, CSO_0115, CSO_0129, CSO_0158). However, as the annotator cannot be present 24/7 and to ensure consistency, these patients were re-annotated using recorded data to produce the dataset.

Forty six different annotation labels were used, as can be seen on the column headings of Table 2.1. Each event was annotated with a date, a start and end time, the event type, an indication of which signals are affected by the event and a field for free text comments. These events include taking blood samples, damped traces, patient turning and suctioning. Table 2.1 shows the number of events of each type for each patient, along with summary statistics at the bottom. Table 2.2 shows the total duration (in seconds) for each event type for each patient.

In Figure 2.1, for each patient-annotation combination, the area of the rectangle indicates the fraction of recorded time that the particular annotation was present for that patient. The most notable feature is that the damped trace events occupy a large fraction of time, particularly for the CSO patients. We see from Table 2.2 that the

Table 2.1 Table showing the number of events of each type for each patient, along with summary statistics at the bottom. The total column excludes dysrhythmia, since it is not an artifact

Patient	admission to ICU	aspiration ngt	blood sample - abp	blood sample - cvp	central line insertion	change closed suction system	coughing	damped trace - abp	dysrhythmia	extubation	fluid bolus	fluid/drugs bolus via cvc	flush - abp	flush - cvp	flush - ngt	intubation	medical examination	medication administration - iv bolus	medication administration - iv infusion	medication administration - topical	minor - eye care	minor - mouth care	minor - other	neuro obs	noisy - abp	noisy - cvp	noisy - ecg	noisy - pleth	noisy - resp	other	physiotherapy - chest	physiotherapy - other	position change - log rolling	position change - other	position change - turning	preparation for transfer	ramp - abp	return from transfer	suction - endo-tracheal	suction - oral	ventilation mode change	ventilator change - circuit	ventilator change - machine	zero - abp	zero - co2	zero - cvp	Total
BioTBI001.1	0	0	2	0	0	0	0	0	0	0	0	0	0	0	0	0	0	0	0	0	0	0	0	0	0	0	0	0	0	9	0	0	0	0	0	0	0	0	0	0	0	0	0	0	0	0	11
BioTBI001.2	0	0	4	0	0	0	2	2	0	0	0	0	0	0	0	0	0	0	0	0	0	0	1	0	0	0	0	0	0	13	0	0	0	0	5	0	0	0	9	0	0	0	0	2	0	0	38
BioTBI003.1	0	0	2	0	0	0	0	1	1	0	0	0	3	0	0	0	0	0	0	0	0	0	10	0	0	0	0	0	0	15	0	0	0	0	0	0	0	0	2	0	0	0	0	0	0	0	33
BioTBI003.2	0	0	3	0	0	0	3	0	0	0	0	0	0	0	0	0	0	0	0	0	0	0	1	0	0	0	0	0	0	3	0	0	0	0	0	0	0	0	4	0	0	0	0	0	0	0	14
BioTBI003.3	0	0	0	0	0	0	9	0	0	0	0	0	0	0	0	0	0	0	0	0	0	0	0	0	0	0	0	0	0	1	0	0	0	0	2	0	0	0	4	0	0	0	0	0	0	0	16
BioTBI004.1	0	0	4	0	0	0	0	0	1	0	0	0	0	0	0	0	1	0	0	0	0	0	9	2	0	0	0	0	1	11	0	0	0	0	4	0	0	0	5	0	0	1	0	3	0	0	41
BioTBI004.2	0	0	3	0	0	0	0	1	1	0	3	0	0	0	0	0	0	0	0	0	0	0	2	0	0	0	0	0	0	2	0	0	0	0	0	0	0	0	2	0	0	0	0	0	0	0	13
BioTBI005.1	0	0	3	0	0	0	0	0	0	0	0	0	1	1	0	0	0	0	0	0	0	0	2	0	0	0	0	0	0	8	0	0	0	0	0	0	0	0	4	0	0	0	0	2	0	2	23
BioTBI005.2	0	0	1	0	0	0	0	0	0	0	0	0	0	0	0	0	0	0	0	0	0	0	0	0	0	0	0	0	0	8	0	0	0	0	0	0	0	0	2	0	0	0	0	0	0	0	11
BioTBI007	0	0	1	0	0	0	2	3	0	0	0	0	0	0	0	0	0	0	0	0	0	0	2	0	0	0	0	0	0	8	0	0	0	0	1	0	0	0	11	0	0	0	0	2	0	0	30
BioTBI009.1	0	0	0	0	0	0	0	0	1	0	0	0	0	0	0	0	0	0	0	0	0	0	3	0	0	0	0	0	0	5	0	0	0	0	0	0	0	0	0	0	0	0	0	0	0	0	8
BioTBI009.2	0	0	2	0	0	0	7	20	0	0	0	0	1	0	0	0	0	0	0	0	0	0	1	0	0	0	0	0	0	1	0	0	0	0	0	0	0	0	1	0	0	0	0	0	0	0	33
BioTBI009.3	0	0	1	0	0	0	0	0	1	0	0	0	0	0	0	0	0	0	0	0	0	0	0	0	0	0	0	0	0	0	0	0	0	0	0	0	0	0	0	0	0	0	0	0	0	0	1
BioTBI010.1	0	0	5	0	1	0	1	2	0	0	0	0	0	0	0	0	0	0	0	0	0	1	2	0	0	0	1	0	0	11	0	0	0	0	2	0	0	0	5	0	0	1	0	2	2	1	37
BioTBI010.2	0	0	4	0	0	0	0	0	0	0	1	0	0	0	0	0	0	0	0	0	1	0	1	0	0	0	0	0	0	2	0	0	0	0	0	1	0	0	5	0	0	0	0	1	5	2	23
BioTBI010.3	0	0	0	0	0	0	0	0	0	0	0	0	0	0	0	0	0	0	0	0	0	0	0	0	0	0	0	0	0	1	0	0	0	0	0	0	0	0	0	0	0	0	0	0	0	0	1
BioTBI018	0	0	15	1	0	0	0	15	0	0	0	0	0	0	0	0	0	0	0	0	0	0	12	1	0	0	1	0	0	27	0	0	2	0	0	1	0	0	15	0	1	0	0	0	2	0	93
cso.0001	0	0	6	0	0	0	0	7	0	0	0	0	0	0	0	0	1	0	0	0	0	0	5	0	0	0	0	0	0	33	0	0	0	0	4	3	0	0	7	0	1	0	0	3	3	0	73
cso.0007	0	0	15	0	0	0	0	27	1	0	0	0	20	0	0	0	1	0	0	0	0	0	22	0	0	0	0	0	0	29	1	0	0	4	8	1	0	2	12	0	1	0	0	6	8	0	157
cso.0008	0	0	11	0	0	0	17	6	2	1	0	0	5	0	0	0	0	0	0	0	0	1	18	3	0	0	5	0	3	31	2	0	0	6	13	1	0	1	10	0	0	0	0	2	2	0	138
cso.0020	0	0	6	0	0	0	4	7	1	0	0	0	6	0	0	0	0	0	0	0	0	0	0	0	4	0	1	0	5	0	0	0	0	0	4	1	1	0	17	0	0	0	0	2	4	0	62
cso.0021	1	0	1	0	0	0	1	0	0	0	0	0	1	0	0	0	0	0	0	0	0	0	1	0	0	0	1	0	0	2	0	0	0	0	0	0	3	0	3	0	0	0	0	1	0	0	15
cso.0027	0	0	3	0	0	0	0	16	3	0	0	0	30	0	0	0	0	0	0	0	0	0	13	0	12	0	3	46	1	18	3	0	0	1	7	5	15	7	24	0	0	0	0	18	4	0	256
cso.0029	1	0	4	0	0	0	4	8	1	0	0	0	25	0	0	0	0	0	0	0	4	3	0	0	36	0	11	45	0	1	1	0	0	0	11	1	25	1	11	0	0	0	0	20	5	0	217
cso.0036	1	0	4	0	0	0	0	1	0	0	0	0	4	0	0	0	0	0	0	0	0	0	0	0	10	0	5	0	4	0	0	0	0	0	2	2	0	1	12	0	0	0	0	2	2	0	50
cso.0041	0	0	12	0	0	0	0	2	0	0	0	0	7	0	0	0	0	0	0	0	0	0	2	0	3	0	1	3	13	4	1	0	0	0	0	2	1	2	14	0	0	0	0	4	4	0	75
cso.0064	0	0	3	0	0	0	0	12	1	0	0	0	3	1	0	0	1	0	0	0	0	0	0	2	2	7	7	38	0	2	0	0	0	1	4	1	0	0	0	0	0	0	0	3	0	2	89
cso.0083	0	0	7	0	0	0	2	25	0	2	0	0	14	0	0	1	3	0	0	0	0	0	2	3	23	0	11	83	57	11	0	0	0	4	8	2	4	2	1	0	0	0	0	8	1	0	274
cso.0086	0	0	1	0	0	0	1	1	1	0	0	0	0	0	0	0	1	0	0	0	0	0	0	0	1	0	0	1	2	4	1	0	0	1	2	1	0	1	6	0	0	0	0	2	0	0	29
cso.0099	0	0	7	0	0	0	4	10	0	0	0	0	8	0	0	0	4	0	0	0	0	0	3	1	6	0	3	1	3	10	0	1	0	2	4	0	1	0	6	0	0	0	0	0	0	0	74
cso.0107	0	0	3	0	0	0	2	7	0	1	0	0	2	0	0	0	3	0	0	0	0	1	2	4	3	0	0	6	11	18	2	0	0	6	2	0	0	0	1	0	0	0	0	1	0	0	75
cso.0112	1	0	2	0	0	0	0	4	0	0	0	0	1	0	0	0	0	0	0	0	0	0	0	0	18	0	2	4	3	0	0	0	0	0	1	1	1	1	1	0	0	0	1	1	0	0	15
cso.0113	0	0	8	0	0	0	2	19	0	0	0	0	6	0	0	0	2	0	0	2	2	1	0	3	5	0	3	0	6	23	1	0	0	3	2	2	0	2	25	1	0	0	0	5	0	0	123
cso.0115	1	3	14	0	1	3	8	6	0	0	1	1	2	1	0	0	13	3	1	0	6	8	6	13	15	5	3	4	2	68	3	0	4	10	7	1	0	1	28	6	0	0	0	4	2	1	255
cso.0123	1	0	10	0	0	0	0	46	1	1	0	0	9	0	0	2	0	0	0	0	0	0	2	0	39	0	12	19	12	3	0	0	0	1	5	2	4	2	9	0	0	0	0	9	2	0	190
cso.0129	0	0	9	0	0	1	9	8	0	1	1	0	3	0	0	0	8	0	0	0	6	5	1	8	17	0	15	11	2	20	3	1	0	5	10	2	0	2	27	5	1	0	0	4	3	0	188
cso.0158	0	3	13	0	0	0	0	9	0	0	0	0	5	0	1	0	5	0	3	2	1	1	1	6	10	0	0	19	0	18	1	0	1	1	0	3	0	2	0	1	0	0	0	6	2	0	114
cso.0172	0	0	4	0	0	0	40	23	0	0	0	0	13	0	0	0	0	0	0	0	0	1	0	0	14	0	1	12	0	4	1	0	0	1	10	2	0	2	25	0	0	0	0	4	3	0	160
min	0	0	0	0	0	0	0	0	0	0	0	0	0	0	0	0	0	0	0	0	0	0	0	0	0	0	0	0	0	0	0	0	0	0	0	0	0	0	0	0	0	0	0	0	0	0	1
mean	0.2	0.2	5.1	0.0	0.1	0.1	3.2	7.6	0.4	0.2	0.2	0.0	4.5	0.1	0.0	0.1	1.1	0.1	0.1	0.1	0.5	0.6	3.3	1.2	6.5	0.3	2.3	7.7	3.3	11.2	0.5	0.1	0.2	1.2	3.1	0.9	1.4	0.8	8.1	0.3	0.1	0.1	0.0	3.1	1.4	0.2	81.2
median	0.0	0.0	4.0	0.0	0.0	0.0	0.0	3.5	0.0	0.0	0.0	0.0	1.5	0.0	0.0	0.0	0.0	0.0	0.0	0.0	0.0	0.0	1.0	0.0	0.0	0.0	0.0	0.0	0.0	8.0	0.0	0.0	0.0	0.0	2.0	1.0	0.0	0.0	5.0	0.0	0.0	0.0	0.0	2.0	0.0	0.0	47.5
max	1	3	15	1	1	3	40	46	3	2	3	1	30	1	1	2	13	3	3	2	6	8	22	13	42	7	15	83	57	68	3	1	4	10	13	5	25	7	28	6	1	1	1	20	8	2	274
std.dev.	0.4	0.7	4.1	0.2	0.2	0.5	7.1	10.1	0.7	0.4	0.5	0.2	7.2	0.3	0.2	0.4	2.6	0.5	0.5	0.5	1.5	1.6	5.2	2.7	11.4	1.4	3.9	17.5	9.6	13.4	0.9	0.2	0.7	2.3	3.7	1.1	4.7	1.3	8.4	1.3	0.3	0.2	0.2	4.5	2.0	0.6	78.6

Table 2.2 *Table showing the total duration in seconds for each event type for each patient, along with summary statistics at the bottom. The total column indicates the percentage of the patient stay affected by artifact, excluding dysrhythmia as it is not an artifact*

Patient	admission to ICU	blood sample - abp	blood sample - cvp	central line insertion	change closed suction system	coughing	damped trace - abp	dysrhythmia	extubation	fluid bolus	fluid/drugs bolus via cvc	flush - abp	flush - cvp	intubation	medical examination	medication administration - topical	minor - eye care	minor - mouth care	minor - other	neuro obs	noisy - abp	noisy - cvp	noisy - ecg	noisy - pleth	noisy - resp	other	physiotherapy - chest	physiotherapy - other	position change - log rolling	position change - other	position change - turning	preparation for transfer	ramp - abp	return from transfer	suction - endo-tracheal	suction - oral	ventilation mode change	ventilator change - circuit	ventilator change - machine	zero - abp	zero - co2	zero - cvp	Total
BioTBI001.1	0	96	0	0	0	0	0	0	0	0	0	0	0	0	0	0	0	0	0	0	0	0	0	0	0	1116	0	0	0	0	0	0	0	0	0	0	0	0	0	0	0	0	1.4
BioTBI001.2	0	510	0	0	0	53	765	0	0	0	0	0	0	0	0	0	0	0	29	0	0	0	0	0	0	555	0	0	0	0	196	0	0	0	277	0	0	0	0	150	0	0	0.0
BioTBI003.1	0	110	0	0	0	0	3202	6	0	0	0	60	0	0	0	0	0	0	1008	0	0	0	0	0	0	1790	0	0	0	0	0	0	0	0	231	0	0	0	0	0	0	0	23.2
BioTBI003.2	0	202	0	0	0	71	0	0	0	0	0	0	0	0	0	0	0	0	61	0	0	0	0	0	0	91	0	0	0	0	0	0	0	0	310	0	0	0	0	0	0	0	1.6
BioTBI003.3	0	0	0	0	0	371	0	0	0	0	0	0	0	0	0	0	0	0	0	0	0	0	0	0	0	25	0	0	0	0	178	0	0	0	273	0	0	0	0	0	0	0	3.2
BioTBI004.1	0	275	0	0	0	0	0	3	0	0	0	0	0	0	362	0	0	0	805	1604	0	0	0	0	985	3598	0	0	0	0	1819	0	0	0	580	0	0	16	0	155	0	0	19.4
BioTBI004.2	0	244	0	0	0	0	29	16	0	1022	0	0	0	0	0	0	0	0	776	0	0	0	0	0	0	776	0	0	0	0	0	0	0	0	98	0	0	0	0	0	0	0	6.1
BioTBI005.1	0	238	0	0	0	0	0	0	0	0	0	70	70	0	0	0	0	0	93	0	0	0	0	0	0	577	0	0	0	0	0	0	0	0	156	0	0	0	0	87	0	87	1.9
BioTBI005.2	0	100	0	0	0	0	0	0	0	0	0	0	0	0	0	0	0	0	0	0	0	0	0	0	0	615	0	0	0	0	0	0	0	0	349	0	0	0	0	0	0	0	2.8
BioTBI007	0	253	0	0	0	90	501	0	0	0	0	0	0	0	0	0	0	0	1666	0	0	0	0	0	0	9867	0	0	0	0	499	0	0	0	3857	0	0	0	0	39	0	0	21.6
BioTBI009.1	0	0	0	0	0	0	0	6144	0	0	0	0	0	0	0	0	0	0	67	0	0	0	0	0	0	74	0	0	0	0	0	0	0	0	0	0	0	0	0	0	0	0	0.0
BioTBI009.2	0	117	0	0	0	1501	2836	0	0	0	0	12	0	0	0	0	0	0	79	0	0	0	0	0	0	79	0	0	0	0	0	0	0	0	721	0	0	0	0	0	0	0	30.8
BioTBI009.3	0	42	0	0	0	0	0	2311	0	0	0	0	0	0	0	0	0	0	0	0	0	0	0	0	0	0	0	0	0	0	0	0	0	0	0	0	0	0	0	0	0	0	0.0
BioTBI010.1	0	706	0	1982	0	69	326	0	0	0	0	0	0	0	0	0	0	143	145	0	0	0	1195	0	0	3379	0	0	0	0	1544	0	0	0	2467	0	0	272	0	52	62	34	15.5
BioTBI010.2	0	110	0	0	0	0	0	0	0	380	0	0	0	0	0	0	35	0	232	0	0	0	0	0	0	393	0	0	0	0	0	4935	0	0	1308	0	0	0	0	38	16	77	45.5
BioTBI010.3	0	0	0	0	0	0	0	0	0	0	0	0	0	0	0	0	0	0	0	0	0	0	0	0	0	9	0	0	0	0	0	0	0	0	0	0	0	0	0	0	0	0	0.9
BioTBI018	0	1090	214	0	0	0	15169	0	0	0	0	0	0	0	0	0	0	0	13890	356	0	0	12080	0	0	24227	0	0	1887	0	0	2410	0	0	8190	0	0	0	0	0	23	0	32.7
cso.0001	0	613	0	0	0	0	7912	0	0	0	0	0	0	0	37	0	0	0	1361	0	0	0	0	0	0	7676	0	0	0	0	1625	16326	0	0	2280	0	1347	0	0	628	56	0	47.5
cso.0007	0	991	0	0	0	0	62909	17	0	0	0	532	0	0	211	0	0	0	1737	0	0	0	0	0	0	12298	850	0	0	2162	2165	5250	0	244	197	0	10	0	0	101	84	0	48.9
cso.0008	0	739	0	0	0	1331	2406	8	66	0	0	121	0	0	0	0	0	14	3826	193	0	0	2593	0	3210	7434	1019	0	0	2348	3565	12758	0	1209	2116	0	0	0	0	42	21	0	73.5
cso.0020	0	866	0	0	0	29	73925	8	0	0	0	15	0	0	0	0	0	0	0	0	1051	0	696	0	815	0	0	0	0	0	1023	34	98	0	1412	0	0	0	0	65	49	0	77.7
cso.0021	0	141	0	0	0	10	0	0	0	0	0	7	0	0	0	0	0	0	5	0	0	0	3039	0	0	330	0	0	0	0	0	0	57	0	130	0	0	0	0	2	0	0	44.1
cso.0027	0	125	0	0	0	0	8727	21	0	0	0	160	0	0	0	0	0	0	326	0	2530	0	241	2091	285	1472	919	0	0	150	764	2733	212	25888	1539	0	0	0	0	2017	115	0	75.9
cso.0029	0	333	0	0	0	83	126384	184	0	0	0	90	0	0	0	0	1163	1207	0	0	1799	0	11038	6531	0	286	286	0	0	0	3764	2564	327	641	1386	0	0	0	0	202	80	0	86.0
cso.0036	0	300	0	0	0	0	100	0	0	0	0	29	0	0	0	0	0	0	0	0	1007	0	494	0	541	0	0	0	0	0	394	138	0	729	582	0	0	0	0	56	54	0	64.8
cso.0041	0	878	0	0	0	0	171976	0	0	0	0	20	0	0	0	0	0	0	73	0	308	0	14	190	1157	710	569	0	0	0	0	926	97	1841	1098	0	0	0	0	107	3825	0	99.6
cso.0064	0	288	0	0	0	0	50621	4	0	0	0	9	8	0	183	0	0	0	0	203	50	24711	253	4897	0	3056	0	0	0	56	1072	5	0	0	0	0	0	0	0	45	0	43	75.7
cso.0083	0	728	0	0	0	50	161923	0	6	0	0	54	0	180	120	0	0	0	0	85	2983	0	1090	5946	16390	3178	0	0	0	3178	1527	0	280	0	72	0	0	0	0	995	20	0	98.4
cso.0086	0	87	0	0	0	368	6600	204	0	0	0	0	0	0	235	0	0	0	0	0	33	0	0	44	82	7260	897	0	0	1167	830	19	0	291	188	0	0	0	0	57	0	0	62.9
cso.0099	0	883	0	0	0	70	104705	0	0	0	0	38	0	0	240	0	0	0	0	0	365	0	637	175	678	3920	0	0	0	173	1284	0	1	0	267	0	0	0	0	0	0	0	89.9
cso.0107	0	200	0	0	0	373	3760	0	0	0	0	28	0	0	60	0	0	33	38	228	22	0	0	348	1170	2148	1895	0	0	150	476	0	0	0	39	0	0	0	0	14	0	0	25.1
cso.0112	0	166	0	0	0	0	2037	0	0	0	0	25	0	0	0	0	0	0	0	0	600	0	30	243	173	0	0	0	0	0	522	13	23	0	50	0	0	0	14	9	0	0	57.5
cso.0113	0	913	0	0	0	70	12186	0	0	0	0	103	0	0	120	47	0	0	0	62	355	0	94	0	1559	3271	480	0	0	1391	156	1037	0	0	1241	0	0	0	0	118	0	0	33.9
cso.0115	0	964	0	660	57	175	3139	0	0	0	237	15	27	0	1920	0	71	71	14	0	680	1677	18	197	44	10373	2760	0	120	95	2218	306	0	0	4332	34	0	0	0	58	161	6	13.9
cso.0123	30	950	0	0	0	0	27229	21	275	0	0	61	0	1830	0	0	0	0	251	0	1553	0	1875	2913	2382	1830	0	0	0	1579	1469	6538	281	336	1146	0	0	0	0	282	2493	0	38.4
cso.0129	0	927	0	0	15	111	107340	0	0	0	0	58	0	0	1080	0	0	0	0	127	787	0	395	549	217	10172	1260	16	0	571	2568	22	0	0	1409	133	123	0	0	111	240	0	55.8
cso.0158	0	1194	0	0	0	0	13230	0	0	0	0	32	0	0	0	0	0	0	0	0	510	0	0	994	0	37362	720	0	600	1080	0	44	0	0	0	120	0	0	0	148	68	0	86.1
cso.0172	0	155	0	0	0	2093	125308	0	0	0	0	133	0	0	0	0	0	73	0	0	783	0	35	755	0	796	212	0	0	12	2684	0	0	0	2128	0	0	0	0	82	559	0	80.3
min	0	0	0	0	0	0	0	0	0	0	0	0	0	0	0	0	0	0	0	0	0	0	0	0	0	0	0	0	0	0	0	0	0	0	0	0	0	0	0	0	0	0	0
mean	0.8	458.8	5.6	69.5	1.9	190.1	29616.4	235.6	9.1	36.9	6.2	14.0	2.8	52.9	136.0	1.2	33.4	40.6	696.9	156.5	484.6	694.1	943.3	704.6	781.3	1230.1	313.1	0.4	68.6	387.2	866.9	1475.2	37.1	820.5	1071.9	7.6	38.9	8.4	0.1	148.9	209.4	6.5	40.6
median	0.0	316.5	0.0	0.0	0.0	0.0	2987.5	0.0	0.0	0.0	0.0	13.5	0.0	0.0	0.0	0.0	0.0	0.0	21.5	0.0	0.0	0.0	0.0	0.0	0.0	1294.0	0.0	0.0	0.0	0.0	487.0	0.0	0.0	0.0	402.5	0.0	0.0	0.0	0.0	48.5	0.0	0.0	36.1
max	30	1194	214	1982	57	2093	171976	6144	275	1022	237	532	70	1830	1920	47	1163	1207	13890	1604	1553	24711	12080	6531	16390	37362	2760	16	1887	3178	3764	16326	327	25888	8190	133	1347	272	14	2017	3825	87	99.6
std.dev.	1.9	364.3	34.7	336.1	9.5	456.0	49802.6	1053.6	15.6	175.3	38.4	91.6	12.1	297.5	362.7	7.6	188.6	196.3	2320.9	760.3	974.4	1010.5	2637.9	1666.1	2696.9	7383.1	608.4	2.6	318.6	787.5	1053.5	3538.1	89.1	1193.5	1588.8	29.0	218.8	44.6	2.3	363.3	728.3	20.1	32.7

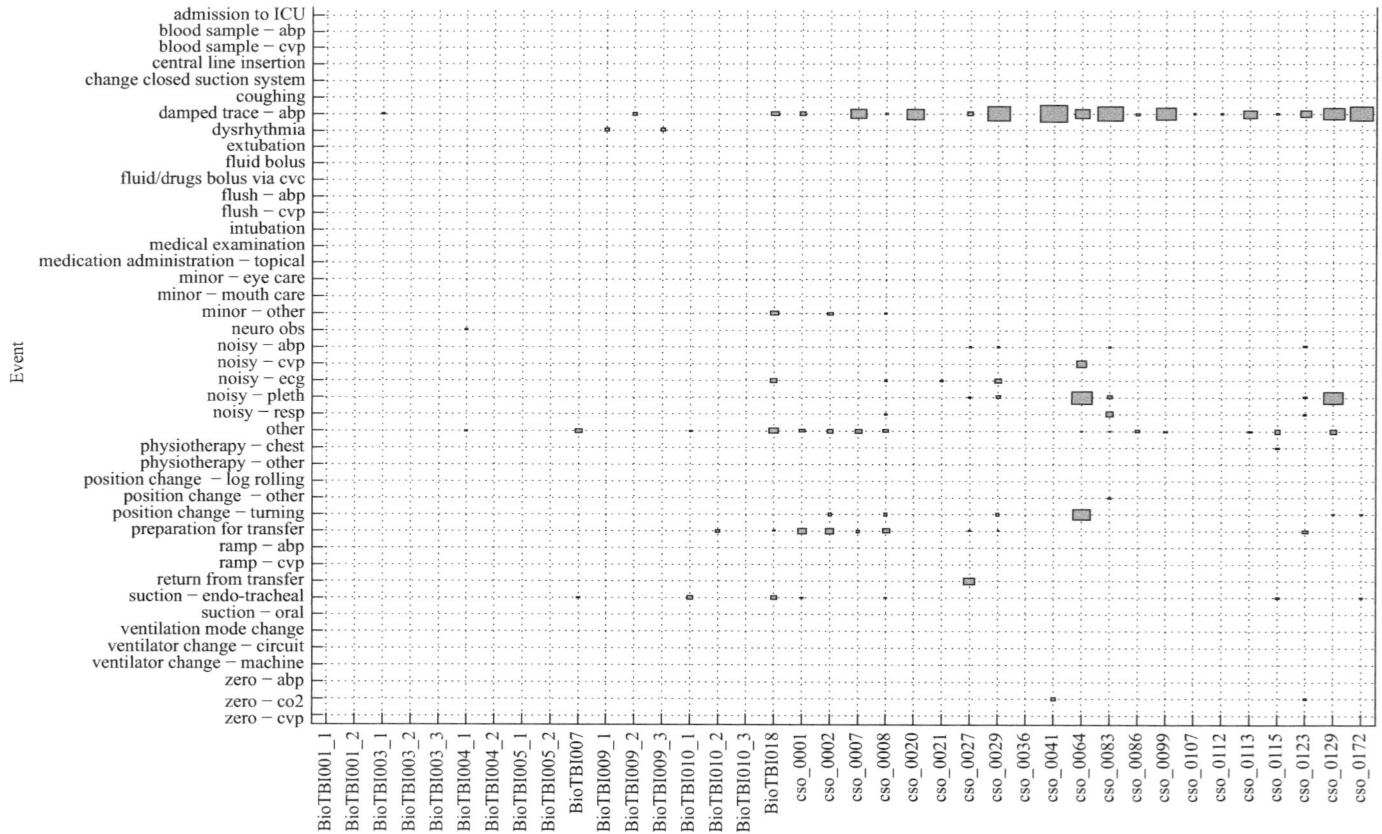

Figure 2.1 *Graphical representations of annotation durations per patient. For each patient-annotation combination, the size of the rectangle indicates the fraction of recorded time that the particular annotation was present for that patient*

mean duration of damped trace events is almost 30,000 seconds (over 8 hours). In contrast, the average duration of blood sampling is around 450 seconds per patient which is a very small fraction of the total duration, and so is not distinguishable from the dotted grid points in Figure 2.1.

Figures 2.5 and 2.6 show examples of damped trace and blood sample events.

2.5 The effect of data cleaning on data summary measures

Given the annotations described earlier, we can assess what effect cleaning the raw data will have on summary measures. Say for example we wish to compute the average of the systolic blood pressure (BP.sys) over 30-minute intervals (which could be useful for assessing trends in the blood pressure of the patient). If there are periods labelled as artifact during the 30-minute period, these are removed, and the average is computed only over the "clean" data in the interval.

The results of doing this can be visualized with a Bland-Altman plot [4], where the clean value is plotted on the x-axis, and the difference between the clean and raw values on the y-axis. The results for the various channels are shown in Figure 2.2 for all 27 available patients. The fraction of entries for which the differences are non-zero are as follows: Heart Rate (HR) 55%, Respiratory Rate 59%, Blood Pressure (diastolic) 59%, Blood Pressure (systolic) 70%, Blood Pressure (mean) 84%, ICP (diastolic) 56%, ICP (systolic) 75%, ICP (mean) 75%, End Tidal CO2 75%, Pleth 64%, Central Venous Pressure 64%. Hence for all channels well over 50% of the 30-minute summaries are affected in some way by artifact. Of course in many cases the difference may be small, although e.g. for BP.sys we observe the extreme differences can be more than $+20$ and -10 mmHg, which would certainly be clinically significant.

2.6 Factorial switching linear dynamical system

We have used two different models to make inferences from the time-series data, the FSLDS, and a newer variant called the DSLDS. The FSLDS is described in the following text, and the DSLDS in Section 2.7.

The FSLDS is a latent variable model for time-series data, where each time step represents an observation that covers one second of patient observations. At time step t the model has a hidden discrete state variable s_t, a hidden continuous state variable x_t and continuous observations y_t, as illustrated in Figure 2.3(a). The discrete state is factorial in nature – it is the cross-product of the factors. For each time step t, given M factors $f_t^{(1)} \dots f_t^{(M)}$ the state s_t is $f_t^{(1)} \otimes \dots \otimes f_t^{(M)}$. Factors are assumed to be independent of each other in the prior and to have Markovian dependence, i.e.

$$p(s_t|s_{t-1}) = \prod_{m=1}^{M} p(f_t^{(m)}|f_{t-1}^{(m)}) \tag{2.1}$$

If each factor $f^{(m)}$ can adopt one of $L^{(m)}$ values then there are K possible states, where $K = \Pi_{m=1}^{M} L^{(m)}$.

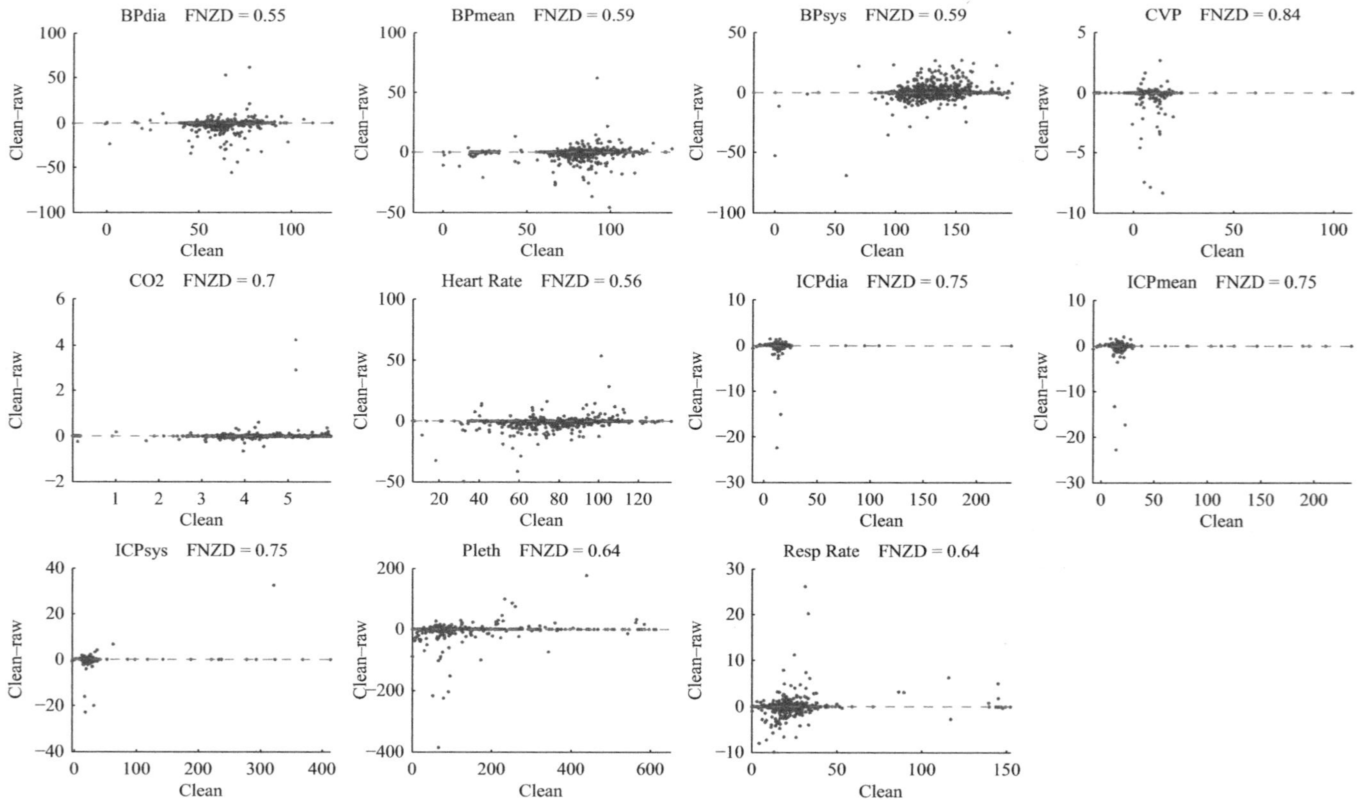

Figure 2.2 *Bland-Altman plots for various channels computed over 30 minutes. The* x*-axis shows the clean value, and the* y*-axis the difference between the clean and raw values. FNZD denotes the fraction of non-zero differences*

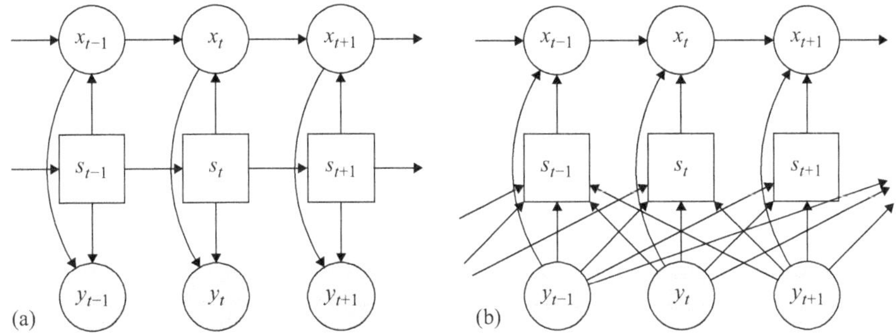

Figure 2.3 A graphical model representation of the FSLDS (a) and DSLDS (b)

The model is Markovian, so that s_t is independent of $s_{t-2}, s_{t-3}...$ given s_{t-1}, and the transition probabilities are specified by a matrix where the element (i,j) equals $P(s_t = j|s_{t-1} = i)$.

The continuous state x_t evolves in a linear Gaussian fashion so that

$$p(x_t|x_{t-1}, s_t) \sim \mathcal{N}(A^{s_t}(x_{t-1} - \mu^{s_t}) + \mu^{s_t} + d^{s_t}, Q^{s_t}) \tag{2.2}$$

where A^s is the system matrix for state s, μ^s is the mean value for the latent state, d^s is the drift term and Q^s is the corresponding system noise covariance matrix.

The observations y_t are derived from the continuous state with some additive Gaussian noise so

$$p(y_t|x_t, s_t) \sim \mathcal{N}(H^{s_t}x_t + o^{s_t}, R^{s_t}) \tag{2.3}$$

where H^s is the observation matrix, o^s is an offset term and R^s is the corresponding observation noise covariance matrix.

The joint distribution of the model is therefore

$$p(s_{1:T}, x_{1:T}, y_{1:T}) = p(s_1)p(x_1)p(y_1|x_1, s_1)\prod_{t=2}^{T} p(s_t|s_{t-1})p(x_t|x_{t-1}, s_t)p(y_t|x_t, s_t) \tag{2.4}$$

2.6.1 Factors

Each of the discrete variables (or factors) represents an event that can affect the observations. In the domain of interest here, this could include taking blood samples, endo-tracheal suctioning or a damped trace. A factor variable can either be inactive or in one of a number of possible discrete states. The discrete state of the system is obtained from the full specification of the values of all factor variables. Each factor affects a specific subset of channels. There is one further factor, the X-factor, which is there to catch all unusual events that aren't modeled by any of the other factors. The X-factor can be either active or inactive.

Each factor affects a specified set of channels and leaves others unaffected – for instance the blood sample factor *only* affects the ABP channels. When two factors both affect the same channel, one takes precedence over the other. The precedence rules are set using prior knowledge about how factors interact.

Details of the models used for each factor and the precedence rules are given in Appendix 2.13.

2.6.2 Channels

The continuous observation space in this work consists of the values of several physiological variables of interest such as HR, respiration rate, systolic and diastolic ABP and mean ICP.

Data on any channel can be missing, perhaps because of a disconnected sensor. If a channel has not been present up to a given point in time (e.g. if a sensor has not yet been attached), then it is ignored. This is done by setting the appropriate rows of all H matrices to zero. In addition, those parts of the output are set to `NaN`, overwriting the value that was inferred. If the channel *was* present at some time before but is currently missing (e.g. the sensor has been disconnected) then it is ignored in the same way but the estimated values are outputted.

2.6.3 Inference

The inference module performs filtering (rather than smoothing or prediction). Thus at each time step t it infers the latent state (s_t and x_t) given the observation history up to and including t ($y_{1:t}$).

In a model with no discrete state, Kalman filtering would consist simply of alternating prediction and correction steps (as described e.g. in appendix A.1 of Reference 5 or section 18.3.1 of Reference 6). However, there is also a discrete latent state. Exact inference in this case scales exponentially in t [7]. This problem is dealt with in the code by applying the Gaussian Sum Approximation, referred to in Reference 5 as the Generalized Pseudo Bayesian algorithm of order 1, or GBP(1). It works by collapsing the K different Gaussians at a given time down to a single Gaussian using moment matching, as detailed in Reference 5.

2.7 Discriminative switching linear dynamical system

The DSLDS was developed by Georgatzis and Williams [8]. The key idea is to make the prediction of discrete state s_t be a *discriminative* task based on the observations, and then to make the inference of continuous state x_t be dependent on the observations and the inferred discrete state.

We start by modeling $p(s_t|y_{t-l:t+r})$ with a discriminative classifier, where (features of) observations from the previous l and future r time steps affect the belief of the model about s_t. The inclusion of r frames of future context is analogous to fixed-lag smoothing in an FSLDS (see e.g. Reference 9, section 10.5). Inclusion of future observations in the conditioning set means that the DSLDS will operate with a delay of r seconds, since an output of the model at time t can be produced only after time $t + r$. However, provided that r is small enough ($r \leq 10$ seconds in experiments), this delay is negligible compared to the increase in performance. The LDS component can also be regarded from a similar discriminative viewpoint which allows us to model $p(x_t|x_{t-1}, y_t)$. The main advantage of this discriminative view is that it allows for a rich number of (potentially highly correlated) features to be used without having to explicitly model their distribution or the interactions between them, as is the case in a generative model. A combination of these two discriminative viewpoints gives rise to the DSLDS graphical model in Figure 2.3(b).

The DSLDS is summarized by the equation

$$p(s, x | y) = p(s_1 | y_1)p(x_1 | s_1, y_1) \prod_{t=2}^{T} p(s_t | y_{t-l:t+r})p(x_t | x_{t-1}, s_t, y_t) \tag{2.5}$$

We have used the simplest assumption for $p(s_t | y_{t-l:t+r})$ that it factorizes, so that $p(s_t | y_{t-l:t+r}) = \prod_{m=1}^{M} p(f_t^{(m)} | y_{t-l:t+r})$.

2.7.1 Predicting s_t

We model the conditional probability of each factor being active at time t given the observations with a probabilistic discriminative binary classifier, so that $p(f_t^{(i)} = 1 | y_{t-l:t+r}) = G(\phi(y_{t-l:t+r}))$, where $G(\cdot)$ is a classifier-specific function, and $\phi(y_{t-l:t+r})$ is the feature vector that acts as input to our model at each time step. Following Reference 8 we use a random forest classifier [10]. The output of the random forest for a new test point is an average of the predictions produced by each tree, where the prediction of each tree is the proportion of the observations that belong to the positive class in the leaf node in which the test point belongs to.

We use a variety of features to capture interesting temporal structure between successive observations. At each time step, a sliding window of length $l + r + 1$ is computed. For some features we also divide the window into further sub-windows and extract additional features from them. More precisely, the full set of features that are being used are: (i) the observed, raw values of the previous l and future r time steps ($y_{t-l:t+r}$); (ii) the slopes (calculated by least squares fitting) of segments of that sliding window that are obtained by dividing it in segments of length $(l + r + 1)/k$; (iii) an exponentially weighted moving average of this window of raw values (with a kernel of width smaller than $l + r + 1$); (iv) the minimum, median and maximum of the same segments; (v) the first-order differences of the original window; and (vi) differences of the raw values between different channels. The hyperparameters of the method (number of trees in the forest, l and r) were set by nested cross-validation, as described in section 2.4 of Reference 8.

2.7.2 Predicting x_t

The form of $p(x_t|x_{t-1}, s_t, y_t)$ is chosen as

$$p(x_t|x_{t-1}, s_t, y_t) \propto \exp\left\{-\frac{1}{2}((x_t - \mu^{s_t}) - (A^{s_t}(x_{t-1} - \mu^{s_t}) + d^{s_t}))^T \right.$$
$$\left. \times (Q^{s_t})^{-1}((x_t - \mu^{s_t}) - (A^{s_t}(x_{t-1} - \mu^{s_t}) + d^{s_t}))\right\}$$
$$\times \exp\left\{-\frac{1}{2}(C^{s_t}x_t + o^{s_t} - y_t)^T (R^{s_t})^{-1}(C^{s_t}x_t + o^{s_t} - y_t)\right\} \quad (2.6)$$

This closely mimics the structure of the FSLDS, but there are differences in C^{s_t}. In the DSLDS, C^{s_t} consists of 0/1 entries, which are set based on our knowledge of whether the observations y_t are artifactual or not under state s_t. In the FSLDS, the corresponding observation model encodes the belief that the generated y_t should be normally distributed around $x_t + o^{s_t}$ with covariance R^{s_t}, whereas in our discriminative version, the observation model encodes our belief that $x_t + o^{s_t}$ should be normally distributed around y_t with covariance R^{s_t}. The idea behind this model is that at each time step we update our belief about x_t conditioned on its previous value, x_{t-1}, and the current observation, y_t, under the current regime s_t. For example, under an artifactual process, the observed signals do not convey useful information about the underlying physiology of a patient. In that case, we drop the connection between y_t and x_t (for the artifact-affected channels) which translates into setting the respective entries of C^{s_t} to zero. Then, the latent state x_t evolves only under the influence of the appropriate system dynamics parameters $(A^{s_t}, Q^{s_t}, \mu^{s_t}, d^{s_t})$. Conversely, operation under a non-artifactual regime incorporates the information from the observed signals, effectively transforming the inferential process for x_t into a product of two "experts," one propagating probabilities from x_{t-1} and one from the current observations. The A^s, Q^s, μ^s, d^s, o^{s_t} and R^s parameters are estimated as in the FSLDS.

For inference, similarly to the FSLDS we wish to compute $p(s_t, x_t | y_{1:t+r})$. According to our proposed model, $p(s_t | y_{t-l:t+r})$ can be inferred at each time step via a classifier as described in Section 2.7.1. However, exact inference for x_t is still intractable; as with the FSLDS we make use of the Gaussian Sum Approximation.

2.7.3 Combining the FSLDS and DSLDS predictions for s_t

The FSLDS and DSLDS can be run independently and in parallel. One way to combine their predictions for s_t is via an α-mixture (see Reference 11), with

$$p_\alpha(s_t) = c\left(p_g(s_t)^{(1-\alpha)/2} + p_d(s_t)^{(1-\alpha)/2}\right)^{2/(1-\alpha)} \quad (2.7)$$

where $p_g(s_t)$ and $p_d(s_t)$ are the outputs for the switch variable at time t from FSLDS and the DSLDS respectively, and c is a normalization constant. For $\alpha = -1$ we obtain a mixture of experts (with equally weighted experts), while for $\alpha \to 1$, the formula yields a product of experts. $\alpha \to \infty$ yields the minimum of the two probabilities, while $\alpha \to -\infty$ gives the maximum.

2.8 Stability detection

One of the main purposes of the FSLDS is to detect artifact in observed data. For this to work we need some idea of what non-artifactual data looks like – the stability detector is trained to automatically label periods of non-artifactual data. This idea was introduced in Reference 12.

We first need to separate the idea of a channel and a signal – systolic ABP (ABP.sys) and HR are examples of channels, ABP and HR are examples of signals. Thus a number of channels can be derived from the same underlying signal measurement. It is signals that are labelled as stable or not, using a selection of channels to make that decision.

This problem is set up as an artifact/non-artifact classification task, where an interval is labelled as artifactual if it overlaps with any artifactual event. Williams and Stanculescu [12] found that a logistic regression model operating on a number of hand-crafted features was effective for this task, and this is the model used here. In the current work the mean, median, standard deviation, minimum and maximum of each signal channel in the interval are extracted for use as features.

The classifier is trained to minimize log loss, and its performance can be assessed with a ROC curve. However, the real mode of operation is rather different – intervals are considered one by one as they come in, and once a non-artifactual interval is identified it is used to train the stability model for the patient.[1]

The operation of this process given a trained detector depends on the threshold applied on the classifier; if it is too low one would expect that artifactual intervals would be accepted as "clean" ones, and if it is too high then the system waits forever and has no notion of stability, and therefore cannot produce useful output. To address this issue the accuracy and waiting times were assessed as a function of the threshold in a cross-validation procedure on the training data, and thresholds were chosen on a per signal basis to be as high as possible while minimizing the waiting time and obtaining good classification accuracy. The ultimate evaluation would be to ask about the quality of the inferences made by the FSLDS depending on the stability interval selected, but this is too hard to optimize directly.

In the experiments reported below the stability detector is trained in a leave-one-patient-out (LOPO) fashion – predictions for the stability of one patient make use of the data for all of the other patients in the dataset for training.

The work by Fawcett and Provost [13] on the Activity Monitoring Operating Characteristic (AMOC) curve is somewhat related to this problem. However, in their work one is considering a rare event which may occur zero or one time for a particular patient in their monitoring record. In contrast, our data show that over 75% of intervals are classified as non-artifactual for at least one of the signals, so we are not in this rare-event regime.

[1]To account for the changing condition of a patient in intensive care, a stability model expires after a certain period (the reset interval). At this point the model behaves as if no stability period is defined – this continues until a new stable period is received from the stability detector. The reset interval can be configured according to the problem domain or in light of expert clinical input.

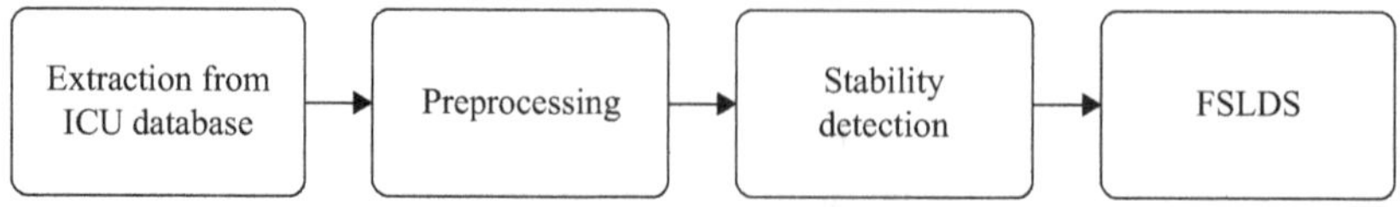

Figure 2.4 The real-time pipeline

2.9 Real-time implementation

To run the system in real time, the four stages of (i) data extraction from the Neuro ICU database, (ii) data pre-processing, (iii) stability detection and (iv) FSLDS[2] operation all need to connect up and work together in real time. See Figure 2.4 for a graphic of this pipeline.

Operating on live data introduces new issues that weren't present in prior work, which used historical data. We briefly discuss those issues below.

2.9.1 Computational efficiency

For the system to use live, inference needs to be performed at least as fast as real time. Given that there will be other concurrent demands on the server, e.g. database access and signal preprocessing, the inference implementation needs to ideally be several times faster than real time. The final implementation ran at approximately 10× real-time. In addition to common methods for speeding up code (minimizing disc access, passing by reference to avoid copying large amounts of data) this was achieved using:

Parallelization Elements of the inference are performed in parallel (using OpenMP). This was used wherever possible but most notably in the Gaussian Sum Approximation. Here the latent state is inferred in light of a new observation. The previous state is required for predicting the new current state but unknown, and so we perform the inference for all possible previous states and collapse the resulting Gaussian states together [5]. Those inferences can be performed independently and so were done in parallel, distributed across multiple cores.

Fast matrix libraries We perform a large number of matrix operations and so rather than implement them from scratch we used an existing library `eigen`.[3] This has been shown to compare favorably in performance benchmarks to other matrix libraries, see http://eigen.tuxfamily.org/index.php?title=Benchmark.

2.9.2 Stability model estimation

When using historical data, the period of stability can be selected from the entire patient stay and then used to train a model that is used from the start of the stay. If, however, the system is used in a live setting we can only select from the data we have seen so far. The FSLDS model cannot be used until a stability model has been learnt and so one should be found as soon as possible, as discussed in Section 2.8.

[2] Currently the DSLDS is only implemented in MATLAB® and is not available for real-time use.
[3] See http://eigen.tuxfamily.org/.

The stability model differs from artifactual models in that its parameters are estimated from the patient upon which we are performing inference; in contrast the parameters of the artifactual models are estimated from the training data. In a live scenario we are provided with artifactual models that were trained offline and a stability model that has been trained on-the-fly. Combining the two models requires care since for some artifactual models, parameters from the stability models should be used when a given channel is unaffected by the artifact – for instance HR channels are unaffected during a blood sample event.

Since a patient's condition changes over the course of their stay, the system allows for the stability model to be re-estimated periodically. Once a stability period has been identified then it is used until a given period of time has passed.[4] Once that period has passed, the system invalidates the existing stability period and starts detecting a new one.

2.10 Software

Software implementing the methods described here is available via http://dx.doi.org/10.7488/ds/300.

MATLAB code

MATLAB FSLDS MATLAB code for training and inference using the FLSDS model, as well as some utility scripts for examining data and inference outputs.

Stability detection MATLAB code for training a logistic regression classifier for stability detection, as well as methods to extract model parameters for use in the real-time system.

Demos Scripts are included that demonstrate the application of the FSLDS on example blood sample, damped trace and suction events. This provides any easy entry point to using the codebase.

Real-time code

Preprocessing A tool for extracting a 1 Hz signal from high-frequency clinical waveform data. C++ source code and documentation are available

Stability detection This component accepts the 1 Hz signal provided by the preprocessor and, for each channel, determines whether the signal on that channel is free from artifact or not. It uses the model trained on the MATLAB side above.

FSLDS C++ code for performing inference in the FSLDS model.

Tests The code is covered by a suite of unit tests, which are included with the code.

Data storage Once the waveform data has left the database all derived data is stored on the filesystem as CSV files. This has the advantage of making the files portable and easy to understand but is inefficient in terms of disk space.

[4]This is configurable and defaults to 12 hours.

Communication The various components of the system need to communicate with each other, passing on information about, for example, new observations or detected stability periods. This is done using the filesystem – a file is shared between the source and target process of any message and serialized JSON objects are appended to that file.

The above methods may be sufficient for a prototype but a more robust system would use a database instance for storing data and not rely on the filesystem for inter-process communication.

2.11 Experiments

We ran the FSLDS and DSLDS models on the data collected from the 27 patients. They were set up with factors to model blood sample, damped trace, suction and X. Ground truth for the X-factor is obtained from the full annotations – if there are annotations present at a given time which do not correspond to blood sample, damped trace or suction, then the X-factor is deemed to be active at that time. The evaluation was done in a leave-one-patient-out (LOPO) fashion, so predictions for a given patient can make use of the data for all of the other patients as training data.

At each second the models output posterior probabilities for each factor $p(f_t^{(m)}|y_{1:t})$, $m = 1, \ldots, M$, and the estimate of the state $p(x_t|y_{1:t})$. $p(x_t|y_{1:t})$ is a mixture of Gaussians – when visualizing outputs we show the weighted mean of the components and the overall variance of the mixture, which can be easily displayed with, for example, a line graph and error bars.

Examples of inferences are shown in Figures 2.5 and 2.6 for damped trace and blood sample events, respectively. On the damped trace example the FSLDS nicely detects the first part of the event (where the systolic and diastolic blood pressures are very close), but erroneously detects a blood sample (instead of a damped trace) in the latter part of the event. It also erroneously detects a suction event throughout the trace. The X-factor fires correctly at the end of the trace, but also erroneously at the beginning. Notice how beliefs about the systolic and diastolic BP are maintained during the time that the damped trace and blood sample factors are active, as shown by the lighter colored traces. In contrast the DSLDS correctly detects a damped trace throughout the event. The blood sample factor is correctly off the whole time, and the suction factor is correctly near to zero. The X-factor is quite active correctly near the end of the trace, but also erroneously at the beginning.

Looking at the blood sample example in Figure 2.6 we see that the FSLDS model divides this event up between the blood sample and damped trace factors being active. In addition the X-factor is active for most of the time. Again notice how inference for the continuous variables (channels) works in the artifactual ramp, zeroing and flushing stages of the blood sample. For the DSLDS, the blood sample factor is active for the majority of the time the event is happening, but we also see that the X-factor is incorrectly active for most of the time.

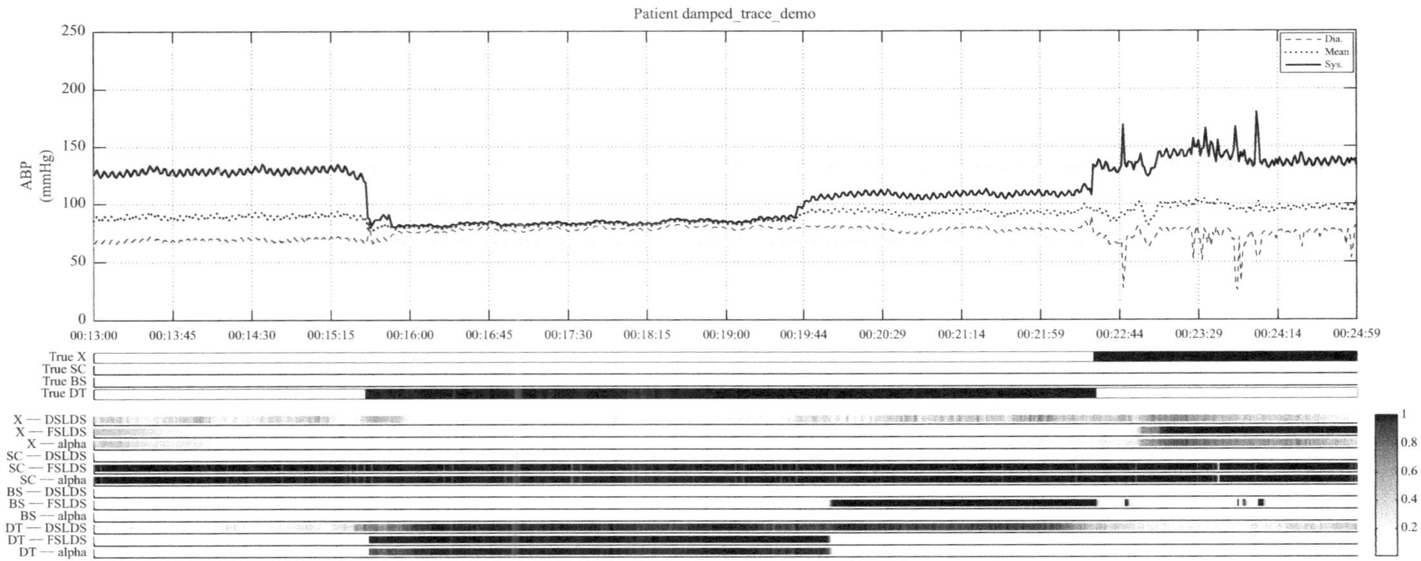

Figure 2.5 *An example of FSLDS and DSLDS inferences for a damped trace event. Note that the active X-factor at the end of the plot is due to a "noisy ABP" annotation. The data (diastolic, mean and systolic BP) is plotted with a darker colour, and the FSLDS inferences are shown as a lighter colour with a one standard deviation confidence interval. For each factor the DSLDS, FSLDS and α-mixture inferences are shown. Posterior and ground truth probabilities are denoted by grayscale intensity as shown in the vertical bar*

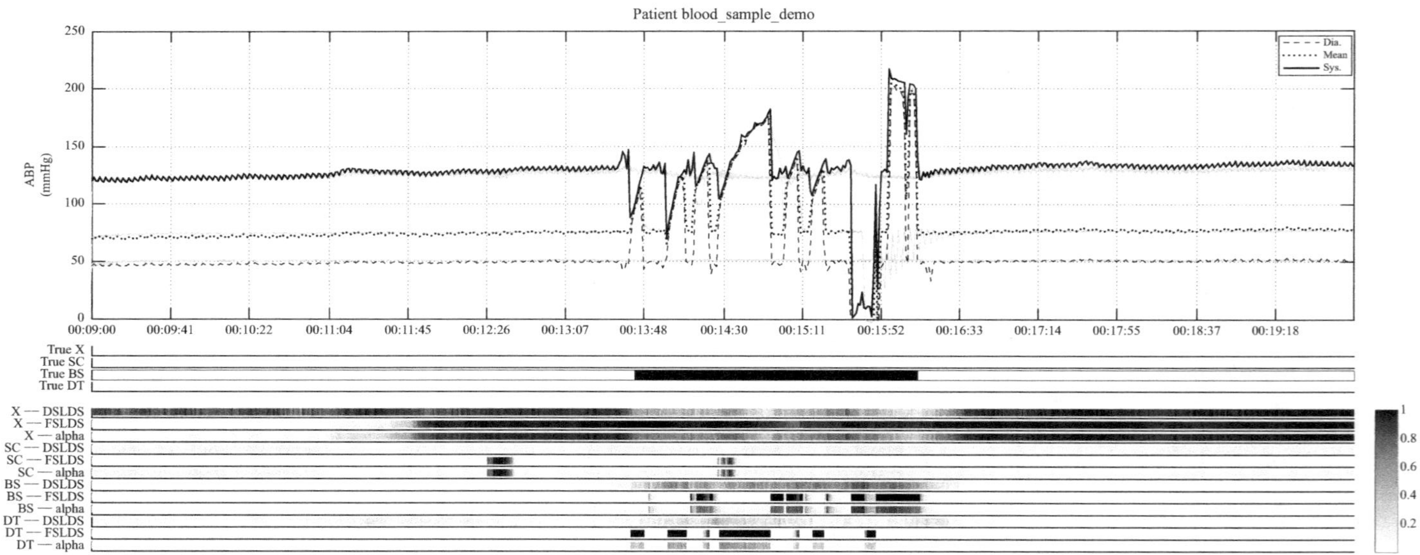

Figure 2.6 *An example of FSLDS and DSLDS inferences for a blood sample event. The data (diastolic, mean and systolic BP) is plotted with a darker colour, and the FSLDS inferences are shown as a lighter colour with a one standard deviation confidence interval. For each factor the DSLDS, FSLDS and α-mixture inferences are shown. Posterior and ground truth probabilities are denoted by grayscale intensity as shown in the vertical bar*

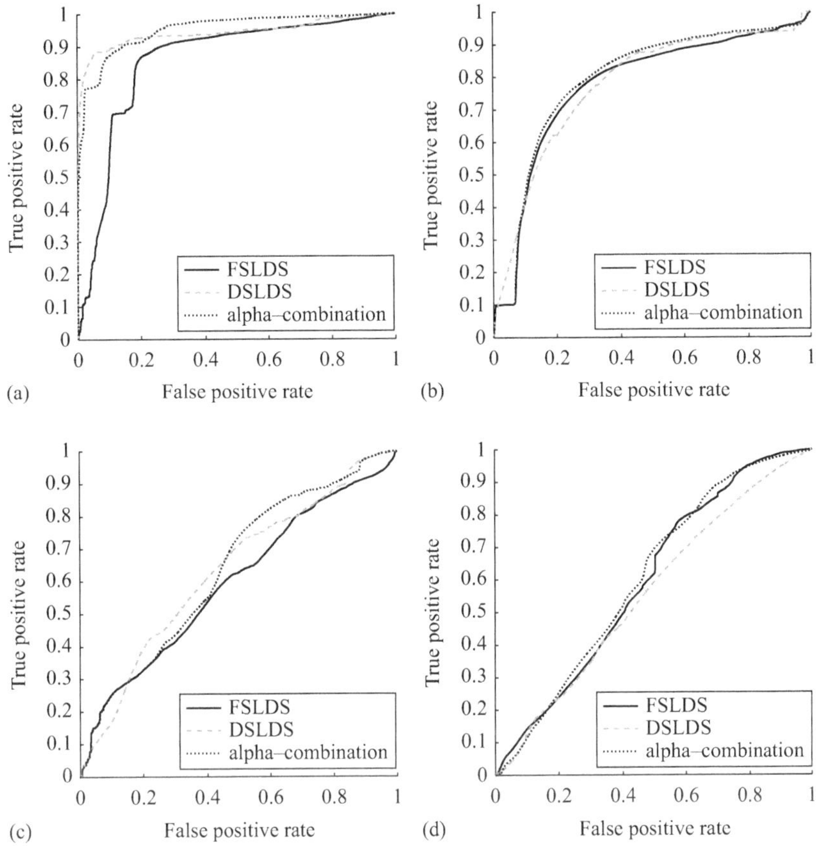

Figure 2.7 *ROC curves for the (a) blood sample, (b) damped trace, (c) suction and (d) X-factor computed from the FSLDS, DSLDS and α-mixture outputs*

As well as example inferences, we can also produce summaries of the performance. We plot a Receiver Operating Characteristic (ROC) curve for each factor, aggregating information over all times and all patients. Each ROC curve can be summarized by the AUC. Figure 2.7 shows the ROC curves for the FSLDS, DSLDS and α-mixture for each of the four factors. Table 2.5 shows overall results for each factor. The best results (obtained from the α-mixture) are AUC scores are 0.95 for blood sample, 0.79 for damped trace, 0.64 for suction and 0.61 for the X-factor.

The performance obtained for blood sample is very good, suggesting that this can be detected with high confidence. This is potentially useful for silencing false alarms. Even though the nurse is present at the bedside during a blood sample procedure and hence knows that the alarm is false, reducing unnecessary alarms would help reduce "alarm fatigue."

Table 2.3 Table showing the AUC scores per factor per patient-interval for the FSLDS. NA indicates that the AUC score is not available because no events of the specified type occurred for the given patient

AUC	BS	DT	SC	X
BioTBI001	0.90	0.99	0.74	0.64
BioTBI003	0.90	0.98	0.77	0.81
BioTBI004	0.73	0.83	0.65	0.61
BioTBI005	1.00	*NA*	0.81	0.44
BioTBI007	0.99	0.82	0.49	0.60
BioTBI009	0.69	0.21	0.28	0.25
BioTBI010	0.98	0.97	0.68	0.60
BioTBI018	0.96	0.90	0.54	0.61
CSO_0002	0.96	0.24	0.32	0.73
CSO_0007	0.47	0.89	0.47	0.57
CSO_0008	0.91	0.83	0.50	0.84
CSO_0020	0.84	0.70	0.53	0.74
CSO_0027	0.62	0.70	0.70	0.46
CSO_0029	0.69	0.90	0.51	0.80
CSO_0036	0.85	0.90	0.73	0.77
CSO_0041	0.95	0.64	0.58	0.35
CSO_0064	0.96	0.72	*NA*	0.33
CSO_0083	0.60	0.82	0.41	0.60
CSO_0099	0.98	0.87	0.57	0.75
CSO_0107	0.92	0.88	0.35	0.55
CSO_0112	0.43	0.80	0.41	0.65
CSO_0113	0.89	0.46	0.69	0.36
CSO_0115	0.97	0.71	0.13	0.33
CSO_0123	0.91	0.70	0.66	0.51
CSO_0129	0.91	0.96	0.77	0.39
CSO_0158	0.87	0.76	*NA*	0.58
CSO_0172	0.98	0.71	0.61	0.73
Overall	0.86	0.77	0.60	0.60

The damped trace performance is good. This is a particularly interesting case, as it is not an event caused by nursing interventions, and therefore it is particularly helpful to flag up. It would be very useful to identify such events automatically in order to prompt the nursing staff to correct the problem. Also, assessing the quality of the blood pressure data being recorded would be very important if automatic charting is in use.

For suction and X-factor the performance is not much better than random (which has an AUC of 0.5). Suction events are complex and have a variable time course, which may explain the difficulty in predicting them. Also note that suction and position change events can have similar effects on the patient, due to movement of the

Table 2.4 Table showing the AUC scores per factor per patient-interval for the DSLDS. NA indicates that the AUC score is not available because no events of the specified type occurred for the given patient

AUC	BS	DT	SC	X
BioTBI001	0.97	0.95	0.68	0.37
BioTBI003	0.98	0.99	0.48	0.44
BioTBI004	1.00	0.96	0.59	0.65
BioTBI005	1.00	*NA*	0.85	0.36
BioTBI007	1.00	1.00	0.44	0.41
BioTBI009	1.00	0.90	0.49	0.22
BioTBI010	0.96	1.00	0.83	0.56
BioTBI018	0.98	0.83	0.64	0.45
CSO_0002	0.96	0.76	0.64	0.48
CSO_0007	0.95	0.55	0.38	0.87
CSO_0008	0.99	0.88	0.73	0.61
CSO_0020	0.94	0.75	0.61	0.69
CSO_0027	0.97	0.75	0.56	0.63
CSO_0029	0.98	0.47	0.59	0.53
CSO_0036	0.96	0.72	0.47	0.48
CSO_0041	0.98	0.41	0.53	0.48
CSO_0064	1.00	0.66	*NA*	0.57
CSO_0083	0.85	0.76	0.38	0.46
CSO_0099	0.97	0.87	0.60	0.62
CSO_0107	0.94	0.73	0.62	0.61
CSO_0112	0.92	0.71	0.14	0.60
CSO_0113	0.83	0.34	0.64	0.44
CSO_0115	0.94	0.67	0.84	0.44
CSO_0123	0.98	0.69	0.72	0.33
CSO_0129	0.94	0.86	0.68	0.57
CSO_0158	0.99	0.62	*NA*	0.75
CSO_0172	1.00	0.75	0.46	0.64
Overall	0.94	0.78	0.64	0.56

endotracheal tube, and that position change was not modeled with a factor in our experiments. Thus it may not be surprising if these two event types are confused, which may explain the poorer performance for suction events.

As well as looking at the results aggregated over patients, we can also perform a more detailed analysis, as shown in Tables 2.3 and 2.4 for the FSLDS and DSLDS, respectively. For the blood sample event by comparing the tables line by line we see that the DSLDS performance is generally much better, giving a higher AUC on 21 out of 27 of the cases, and avoiding the low scores obtained with the FSLDS. For the other factors the results are generally quite similar between the two, in line with Table 2.5.

Table 2.5 Table showing the overall AUC scores per factor for the FSLDS, DSLDS and α-mixture. The optimal value of the α parameter per factor is shown inside parentheses

AUC	BS	DT	SC	X
DSLDS	0.94	0.78	0.64	0.56
FSLDS	0.86	0.77	0.60	0.60
α-mixture	$0.95^{(0.9)}$	$0.79^{(0.9)}$	$0.64^{(-\infty)}$	$0.61^{(1.4)}$

2.12 Conclusions and future work

In this project we have collected and annotated a valuable dataset of neuro ICU data, which can be made available to *bona fide* researchers on request, subject to regulatory approval. We were successful in implementing a real-time system carrying out FSLDS analysis on the raw data coming from the ICU, as described in Section 2.9. We have also made available the code for stability detection and the FSLDS in MATLAB and C++, and the preprocessing code in C++.

The Bland-Altman plots in Section 2.5 show that for all channels in over 50% of the time there is a difference between the raw and cleaned averages obtained over a 30-minute interval. This illustrates that artifact contamination is an important problem.

We have evaluated the FSLDS and DSLDS models for the task of predicting blood sample, damped trace, suction and X-factor events. The AUC scores for the α-mixture are very high for blood samples (0.95), good for damped trace (0.79), and poor for suction (0.64) and X-factor (0.61) events. This combination method slightly outperforms the individual DSLDS or FSLDS models. The damped trace is a particularly interesting case, as this is not an event caused by nursing interventions, and therefore it is particularly helpful to flag up. We have also seen that it is the event class that dominates in terms of time (on average over 8 hours per patient).

Of course these results have been obtained from one specific ICU, and it will be important to assess the model's performance in other patient populations and different centers to determine its robustness.

In terms of displaying the results to clinicians, we believe that plots like Figures 2.5 and 2.6 will be useful. It would be very dangerous to delete the raw data, but we can display the imputed data with error bars during artifactual periods, and show in grayscale the probability of artifactual factors being active.

In this chapter we have evaluated the performance on a second-by-second basis using ROC curves. However, it would be useful to look at evaluation in an episode-based fashion (how well did we pick up a given event that lasted say 5 minutes?), as has been studied in section IV.c of Reference 14.

We have focused on using the FSLDS/DSLDS for detecting artifact, but note that it can be used more generally; for example [14] used an extended FSLDS model to detect sepsis in neonates, and more generally one can model changes in the patient's state of health.

2.13 Appendix: Models for each factor

In this section we provide further details of the models used for stability, and for the blood sample, damped trace, suction, patient handling and X-factor events.

2.13.1 Stability

When none of the factors are active we are in a period of stability. Pulsatile channels are modeled with a relative AR model (as described in section 9.4.1 of Reference 15) consisting of an $AR(2)$ baseline and an $AR(2)$ signal. The filter that separates the baseline and signal components is a moving average filter with a window of width 3. Respiration rate, pleth rate and end-tidal CO_2 are instead modeled with a simple $AR(2)$ process.

Model parameters for each channel are estimated from the annotated stability period. Initial values are derived using the Yule-Walker equations and then updated using three iterations of expectation-maximization [16]. If EM results in a value for the system matrix A which is non-stationary,[5] then we revert to the initial value. Observation noise variance is an exception here, it set to a fixed value of 10.

2.13.2 Blood sample events

The blood sample factor consists of four stages: ramp, zero, flush and a fourth stage for periods within a blood sample event that appear the same as stability. A 5×5 transition matrix between these four stages and stability is estimated from training data.

The ramp model is detailed in section 9.4.2 of Reference 15.

During the zeroing stage the pressure transducer is being recalibrated through exposure to air. ABP drops to approximately zero and no trace of the patient's true ABP is visible. This is implemented by decoupling the state from the observations with H set to zero for the rows corresponding to the ABP channel, and setting the offset term to be the mean value observed during zeros. System noise covariance is unchanged but observation noise variance for each channel is set to the observed variance of the channel, as measured during zeroing events (this is multiplied by a scaling factor of 0.05). Since the boundaries of zeroing events aren't precise, the initial and final 20% of the event is excluded, both for observation variance and offset estimation purposes.

Typically towards the end of a blood sample, the arterial line is flushed. ABP rises to approximately 250–300 mmHg and no trace of the patient's true ABP is visible. This is implemented by decoupling the state from the observations with H set to

[5]The system matrix A is non-stationary if the absolute value of any of its eigenvalues is greater than or equal to 1.

zero for the rows corresponding to the ABP channel and setting the offset term to be the mean value observed during flushes. System noise covariance is unchanged but observation noise variance for each channel is set to the scaled variance of the channel, as measured during flush events (this is multiplied by a scaling factor of 0.05). Since the boundaries of flush events aren't precise, the initial and final 20% of the event is excluded, both for observation variance and offset estimation purposes.

For the "stability within a blood sample" stage the parameters are simply copied from the stability model. Transitions to that stage from stability are prohibited by setting zeros in the transition matrix.

2.13.3 Damped trace events

During a damped trace event there is an occlusion in the arterial line, typically causing the pulse pressure (the difference between the systolic and diastolic pressures) to drop to near zero. The systolic and diastolic pressures converge to the value that the mean pressure held before the event. The mean ABP signal is also somewhat damped in comparison to stability, and so the parameters of the AR model are re-estimated.

The $AR(2)$ model for mean ABP is estimated from the labelled damped trace events. The observation noise variance R for systolic ABP is the median variance of the difference between systolic and mean ABP – the diastolic value is computed similarly. The observation model H is such that elements for systolic and diastolic ABP are set to zero and only mean ABP is taken from the continuous state variable. The system model A for mean ABP is as learnt from the labelled events (using the Yule-Walker equations and EM) but remains unchanged for systolic and diastolic ABP channels.

2.13.4 Suction events

For these purposes "suction – endo-tracheal" and "coughing" are both treated as suction events. Based on an analysis of the annotation files, only HR, respiration rate, pleth rate and end tidal CO_2 are understood to be affected during suction events.

Model parameters are re-estimated using the labelled suction events, Yule-Walker equations are used to produce an initial value for three iterations of EM. If EM results in a system matrix A that is non-stationary then we revert to the initial value. Observation noise variance is, as for stability, fixed to the value of 10.

2.13.5 X-factor

The X-factor (see section III.A of Reference 2) is used to account for all unusual observations that aren't already explained by one of the existing factors. The model parameters for the X-factor consist of the model for stability but with an inflated system noise covariance Q. The amount by which to inflate Q is the parameter ξ. Its value is learned by the MATLAB code using equation 10 of Reference 2.

2.13.6 Overwriting order of factors

When multiple factors are active at a given time, we use the notion of an ordering of the factors to determine which one affects each signal, as in Reference 2.

The ordering used here is

$$\text{X} - \text{factor} < \text{handling} < \text{suction} < \text{blood sample} < \text{damped trace} \tag{2.8}$$

where $f^{(a)} < f^{(b)}$ means that the parameters from $f^{(b)}$ can overwrite those set by $f^{(a)}$.

Acknowledgements

This work was funded by grant number CHZ/4/801 from the Chief Scientist Office (Scotland): Improving Decision Support for Treating Arterial Hypotension in Adult Patients during their Management in Intensive Care, May 2013–Apr 2015. The work of Konstantinos Georgatzis was supported by the Scottish Informatics and Computer Science Alliance (SICSA). Chris Hawthorne and Ian Piper received funding from AAGBI/Anaesthesia which allowed collection of pilot data for this project. We thank the Intensivists Prof Peter Andrews, Mr Laurence Dunn and Prof John Kinsella for their feedback in our review meetings, which helped to keep the project focused on the important questions.

References

[1] ixellence GmbH. ixTrend, Available from https://www.ixellence.com/index.php/en/products/ixtrend [Accessed 23 Sep 2015]; 2015.

[2] Quinn JA. *Bayesian condition monitoring in neonatal intensive care.* PhD thesis, University of Edinburgh, 2008.

[3] Shaw M. *A concise description of the clinical waveform pre-processing workflow*. Unpublished manuscript. 2013.

[4] Altman DG, Bland JM. Measurement in medicine: the analysis of method comparison studies. *J R Stat Soc Series D (The Statistician)* 1983;32(3):307–17.

[5] Murphy KP. Switching Kalman filters. Technical report. Available from https://www.cs.ubc.ca/~murphyk/Papers/skf.pdf [Accessed 23 Sep 2015]; 1998.

[6] Murphy KP. *Machine learning: a probabilistic perspective*. MIT Press; 2012.

[7] Lerner U, Parr R. Inference in hybrid networks: theoretical limits and practical algorithms. In: *Proceedings of the seventeenth annual conference on uncertainty in artificial intelligence*. 2001. p. 310–18.

[8] Georgatzis K, Williams CKI. Discriminative switching linear dynamical systems applied to physiological condition monitoring. In: Meila M, Heskes T, editors, In: *Proceedings of the thirty-first annual conference on uncertainty in artificial intelligence*. 2015, pp. 306–315.

[9] Särkkä S. *Bayesian filtering and smoothing*. Cambridge University Press; 2013.

[10] Breiman L. Random forests. *Mach Learn* 2001;45(1):5–32.
[11] Amari S-i. Integration of stochastic models by minimizing α-divergence. *Neural Comput* 2007;19(10):2780–96.
[12] Williams CKI, Stanculescu I. Automating the calibration of a neonatal condition monitoring system. In: Peleg M, Lavrac N, Combi C., editors, AIME, volume 6747 of *Lecture Notes in Computer Science*. Springer-Verlag Berlin Heidelberg; 2011, p. 240–9.
[13] Fawcett T, Provost F. Activity monitoring: noticing interesting changes in behavior. In: *Proceedings of the fifth ACM SIGKDD international conference on knowledge discovery and data mining (KDD'99)*. 1999. p. 53–62.
[14] Stanculescu IA, Williams CKI, Freer Y. Autoregressive hidden Markov Models for the early detection of neonatal sepsis. *IEEE J Biomed Health Inform* 2014;18(5):1560–70.
[15] Quinn JA, Williams CKI. Physiological monitoring with factorial switching linear dynamical systems. In: Barber D, Cemgil A and Chiappa S, editors, *Bayesian time series models*. Cambridge University Press; 2011, p. 182–204.
[16] Ghahramani Z, Hinton GE. Parameter estimation for linear dynamical systems. Technical report, University of Toronto, 1996.

Chapter 3

Signal processing and feature selection preprocessing for classification in noisy healthcare data

Qiao Li, Chengyu Liu, Julien Oster and Gari D. Clifford

3.1 Introduction

Although current healthcare practice is centered on human expert assessment of the correlations between parameter values and symptoms, there is a growing awareness within medical communities that the enormous quantity and variety of data available cannot be effectively assimilated and processed without automated or semi-automated assistance [1]. Automated systems have been in place in the intensive care unit (ICU), the operating room (OR) and clinical ward for several decades, including automated arrhythmia analysis of the bedside electrocardiogram (ECG) and low (or high) oxygen saturation warnings from the photoplethysmograph (PPG). However, each device acts in an isolated fashion with no reference to related signals or an individual's prior medical information, such as genetics or medical history. Since modern physiological monitoring devices are tuned to be highly sensitive, but prone to noise, a paradigm shift in monitoring technology is required, which allows for more intelligence in the device and less expert oversight [2]. Artifacts, noise and missing values are the main reasons for the high levels of false alarms [3]. Meanwhile, the explosion of mHealth in both abundant and resource-constrained countries is both a cause for concern and celebration [4–7]. While mHealth clearly has the potential to deliver information and diagnostic decision support to the poorly trained, it is not appropriate to simply translate the technologies which the trained clinician uses into the hands of nonexperts. In particular, it is important that the explosion of access does not lead to a flooding of the medical system with low-quality data and false negatives. Although telehealth has the potential to connect remote users with little training to trained experts, with the patient-to-doctor ratio being as low as 50,000:1 in parts of low-income countries, automated algorithms will be essential to cope with the number of recordings that are likely to be made available. Moreover, since the greatest (and often the only) chance for improving the quality of physiological data is at source, a rapid feedback to the recordist or user concerning the clinical viability of the data is needed. Therefore, data screening must occur at the front end using automated algorithms, prompting the user to retake recordings when quality is low.

In order to provide information for medical experts (or automated decision support systems) to make choices concerning patient care, the wealth of available data must be reduced to a set of distinct concepts and features. Although many parameters are derived from patient data "on the fly" and recorded for later review, trust metrics or signal quality measures associated with these parameters are rarely stored. Therefore, it is difficult to ascertain the credibility of a given parameter unless the original data from which the parameter was derived are available, either to visually verify the data or in order to derive independent quality metrics.

Noise reduction algorithms often introduce misleading distortions in medical time-series data and, therefore, they should be applied only when the data are determined to be too noisy for a feature extraction algorithm to be applied accurately. However, it is often necessary to extract features and compare them with a population norm, or a patient's history, in order to determine whether significant amounts of noise are present. A method for simultaneously (or recursively) extracting features and estimating noise levels is, therefore, appropriate.

Since robust methods for dealing with noisy data are not always available or sufficient, it is sometimes more appropriate to define a signal quality measure for a given data stream, and simply ignore the segments of data that have a signal quality below a given value. However, metrics for signal quality are both signal and application specific. Signal quality indices (SQIs) can generally be constructed by thresholding on known physiological limits such as the maximum field strength for the ECG, the maximum rate of change of the blood pressure or the distribution of energy in the frequency domain. However, it is the relationship between physiological parameters that provides the greatest opportunity to construct SQIs. For example, if heartbeats are detected in several ECGs and/or pulsatile waveforms within an expected period of time, all signals can be considered to be of reasonable quality. In Li *et al.* [8], we calibrated a set of ECG signal quality metrics (based on statistical, temporal, spectral and cross-spectral features of the ECG), so that a given value of an SQI metric was equated to known error in heart rate. A similar approach was also taken when processing the arterial blood pressure waveform and hence error bounds in derived estimates that rely on heart rate and blood pressure (such as the cardiac output) can easily be estimated from the standard compound error formula. Generally, data in the ICU are processed in isolation from other parameters and signal quality labels are therefore rarely constructed with reference to other signals. In our approach to SQI derivation, we have concentrated on the relationships between signals, such as the transit time between the R-peak in the ECG and the pulse onset in the arterial blood pressure waveform [9] as well as the inter-ECG lead relationships [8]. By comparing related signals and thresholding these relationships on known physiological limits, it is possible to determine whether the data are logically consistent. Since it is rare that a sequence of extracted features will randomly manifest in a physiologically plausible manner, internal consistency between signals can indicate high signal quality on the contributing leads.

Throughout this chapter, we illustrate our approach to signal processing and feature selection preprocessing for atrial fibrillation (AF) detection in noisy environments. AF is the most common cardiac arrhythmia, with a prevalence of 0.4–1% in the general population and increases with age [10]. AF is associated with a fivefold increased risk of stroke, and one in six strokes occurs in patients with AF. This pathology can be symptomatic, (e.g., palpitation and fatigue) but can also be asymptomatic, which makes AF currently under-diagnosed. ECG signals acquired during ambulatory recordings and more specifically with mHealth applications are prone to noise and artifacts. Such recordings are also performed in an uncontrolled environment and by nonexperts.

The goal of this study is therefore to assess the influence of preprocessing algorithms and noise on the estimation of RR intervals and how these noisy estimates of the RR time-series impact the detection of AF episodes by state-of-the-art automated algorithms.

3.2 Preprocessing and database

The preliminary task for AF detection in noisy environments is to identify a fiducial point in each heart beat, from which timing and sometimes morphology, parameters can be evaluated [1-3,11,12]. The easiest fiducial point to automatically identify in the ECG is the highest energy component; the R-peak or QRS complex, which represents ventricular depolarization. There are several standard, yet highly accurate techniques for performing QRS detection, which we now describe.

3.2.1 QRS detection

Three popular QRS detectors were used to detect the QRS complex of ECG.

1. jqrs: [11,12] consists of a window-based peak energy detector. The original band-pass filter was replaced with a QRS matched filter (Mexican hat) and an additional heuristic ensuring no detection was made during flat lines. A search-back procedure was added in case of suspected missed beats.
2. gqrs: (available on Physionet; https://www.physionet.org/physiotools/wag/gqrs-1.htm), which consists of a QRS matched filter with a custom built set of heuristics (such as search back). It was designed by George Moody, and is freely available on Physionet, but does not have an associated publication.
3. wqrs: [13] consists of a low-pass filter, a nonlinearly scaled curve length transformation and decision rules. It is also freely available on Physionet.

A majority voting of the results of the three detectors was evaluated to calculate the beat-by-beat RR intervals.

3.2.2 Signal quality assessment

The SQI of the ECG was calculated using a machine learning approach, which combines several simple quality metrics [14,15]. Of these, bSQI is the most important one and it consists of the comparison of two different peak detectors, jqrs and wqrs, one (wqrs) being more sensitive to noise than the other (jqrs). When both such detectors agree, the signal is generally therefore clean, and thus bSQI was used in this study. bSQI was computed on a 10-s sliding window with a 9-s overlap, resulting in a second-by-second evaluation of signal quality.

3.2.3 Datasets

Two databases were used in this study, the MIT-BIH atrial fibrillation database (AFDB) and the long-term AF database (LTAFDB), which are open access and available from www.physionet.org.

The AFDB includes 25 ECG recordings of human subjects with AF (mostly paroxysmal). Of these, 23 records include two ECG signals with rhythm and unaudited beat annotations. The rest two records are represented only by the rhythm and annotation files without ECG signals and are eliminated from this study. The individual ECG recordings are each 10 hours in duration, and contain two ECG signals each sampled at 250 samples per second with 12-bit resolution over a range of ± 10 millivolts. The rhythm annotation files were prepared manually; these contain rhythm annotations of types AFIB (atrial fibrillation), AFL (atrial flutter), J (AV junctional rhythm) and N (used to indicate all other rhythms). The LTAFDB includes 84 long-term ECG recordings of subjects with paroxysmal or sustained AF. Each record contains two simultaneously recorded ECG signals digitized at 128 Hz with 12-bit resolution over a 20 mV range; record durations vary but are typically 24–25 hours. The types of rhythm annotations include AFIB (atrial fibrillation), N (normal sinus rhythm), SVTA (supraventricular tachyarrhythmia), VT (ventricular tachycardia), B (ventricular bigeminy), T (ventricular trigeminy), IVR (idioventricular rhythm), AB (atrial bigeminy) and SBR (sinus bradycardia). In this study, we regard the AFIB annotation as AF (1) and all other rhythm annotations as Non-AF (0).

The design of machine learning algorithm for AF detection included a development phase and a validation phase. The AFDB was used in the development phase and the LTAFDB was used in the validation phase. We also recommend to validate the robustness of the algorithm on an unseen database which is different from the development phase.

In the development phase, the ECG in AFDB was analyzed by the three QRS detectors and a majority voting was performed to calculate beat-by-beat RR intervals. The first channel of ECG was analyzed except record 07162 which the voltage of QRS complex is low in the first channel and the second channel was used. The AF and Non-AF rhythms were marked segment-by-segment by a 30-s length analysis window. Here we selected a 30-s window due to fact that, to be considered clinically relevant, AF events usually must last 30 s or even longer [16]. Rhythms with lengths shorter than 30 s were discarded. The bSQI metric was computed on a second-by-second basis, and a unique score was derived for each window by the median of the bSQI value over the window. In order to avoid the influence of noise during the development phase, the low quality segments with a median bSQI lower than 0.85 were removed from the dataset. A resultant dataset with total 26,925 high quality segments was extracted from AFDB, including 10,541 AF segments and 16,384 Non-AF segments. The dataset was then split randomly into a training set and a test set, stratified by patients rather than by segments, as shown in Table 3.1. Stratification by patients ensures that the training

Table 3.1 *Datasets using in this study*

	Development phase (AFDB)						Validation phase (LTAFDB)	
	Training set (12 cases)		Test set (11 cases)		Total (23 cases)		Total (84 cases)	
	AF	Non-AF	AF	Non-AF	AF	Non-AF	AF	Non-AF
Segments	5,327	8,639	5,214	7,745	10,541	16,384	118,473	103,498
Total	13,966		12,959		26,925		221,971	

set and test set contain mutually exclusive patients and reduces the chances of over-training. A K-fold cross-validation, also stratified by patients, was also performed to avoid overfitting during the development phase.

In the validation phase, the first channel of ECG in LTAFDB was analyzed by three QRS detectors except records 00, 24, 56 and 62, in which the first channel was very noisy and so the second channel was used. Note we did not eliminate the noisy segments in the validation phase, so that the validation statistics reflect both a real-world scenario, with previously unseen patients containing noisy data. Importantly, an entirely separate database was used, ensuring differences in patient population and recording techniques. A validation dataset with total 221,971 segments was extracted from the LTAFDB, including 118,473 AF segments and 103,498 Non-AF segments.

3.2.4 Adding realistic noise to known data

To evaluate the influence of the noise to AF detection, we added the muscle artifact (MA) noise, simulated using the fecgsyn toolbox [17], to each of the ECG signals in the LTAFDB in the validation phase. Simulations with different signal-to-noise-ratio (SNR) levels (24, 21, 18, 15, 12, 9, 6, 3, 0, −3 dB) were performed.

3.3 Feature extraction

Feature extraction is the process of reducing a set of raw or preprocessed data into a smaller set of quantities (features) that represent the key qualities of the data. Features should be chosen (or found) such that they possess highly different values for each class of data that requires identification (or classification). Since there is an almost infinite number of statistics and metrics that can be extracted from a given set of data, prior knowledge of the system (e.g., physiology or noise profiles under certain conditions) is often used to guide feature extraction. For example, AF is characterized by a chaotic electrical conduction through the AV node and ventricular response, resulting in an unpredictable depolarization of the ventricles, and therefore the RR interval time-series. It is not completely unpredictable, and a probabilistic modeling of the

RR intervals during AF episodes has been recently suggested [18]. The use of the statistics of RR intervals for the detection of AF episodes has been proven to be possible, and several methods have been proposed [19–21]. In this study, we have chosen to use a superset of the 14 RR interval time-series features proposed in these earlier studies. Although this may not be exhaustive, it provides a tractable list from which we can then perform feature selection (to remove redundant or suboptimal features).

3.3.1 Time-domain features

The mean value (mRR), minimum value (minRR) and maximum value (maxRR) of RR intervals of the current RR segment, the median value of HR (medHR), the standard deviation of RR intervals (SDNN), the percentage of RR intervals larger than 50 ms (PNN50) and the square root of the mean squared differences of successive RR intervals (RMSSD) were used as time-domain features [22].

3.3.2 Frequency-domain features

Burg's autoregressive approach (with an order of 6) was used to produce the power spectrum for the RR segment. The power spectrum was integrated over two frequency ranges: the low-frequency power (0.04–0.15 Hz) and the high-frequency power (0.15 to 0.40 Hz). The normalized low-frequency power (LF_n), normalized high-frequency power (HF_n) and the ratio of low-frequency power to high-frequency power (LF/HF) were used as the frequency-domain features [22].

3.3.3 Nonlinear features

Coefficient of sample entropy (COSEn) and normalized fuzzy entropy (NFEn) were used as nonlinear features [23–25], with an embedding dimension $m = 1$. For a detailed discussion of COSEn and NFEn please refer to the Appendix 1.

The median of the variation in the absolute standard deviation from mean of heart rate in three adjacent RR segments with same length (denoted by the abbreviation MAD) [26], was used as another nonlinear feature. An AF evidence feature (AFEv), as a numeric representation of the Lorenz plot, a two-dimensional histogram, was also used [27, 28]. The MAD method requires that the length of RR segment should be perfectly divisible by 3. Therefore, each window was truncated so that the number of RR intervals was rounded to be as large as possible while being exactly divisible by three.

3.4 Feature selection

Feature selection is primarily performed to select relevant and informative features. It can have other motivations, including [29]:

- general data reduction, to limit storage requirements and increase algorithm speed;
- feature set reduction, to save resources in the next round of data collection or during utilization;

- performance improvement, to prevent over-training and improve predictive accuracy;
- data understanding, to gain knowledge about the process that generated the data or simply visualize the data.

There are three main categories of feature selection algorithms: filters, wrappers and embedded methods. Filter methods, or feature ranking methods, provide a complete order of the features using a relevance index, including correlation coefficients, classical test statistics (t-test, F-test, chi-squared, etc.), mutual information and information theory. Wrappers and embedded methods involve the predictor as part of the selection process. Wrappers utilize a learning machine as a "black box" to score subsets of features according to their predictive power. Embedded methods perform feature selection in the process of training and are usually specific to given learning machines.

In this study, we tested two feature selection methods corresponding to two machine learning algorithms, logistic regression and the support vector machine.

3.4.1 Forward likelihood ratio selection for logistic regression

Logistic regression (LR) is a statistical model for classification, which identifies the impact of multiple independent variables in classifying the membership of one of the multiple dependent categories. For binary logistic regression (BLR), the number of the dependent categories was limited to two. BLR can be considered an extension of linear regression, which struggles with dichotomous problems. This difficulty is overcome by applying a mathematical transformation of the output of the classifier, transforming it into a bounded value between 0 and 1 more appropriate for binary predictions.

In the current study, the output variable Y is a positive (1) or negative (0) diagnosis for AF: the posterior probability $P(y|X)$ for the input feature vector X is modeled by a logistic function, as follows:

$$P(Y=0|X) = \frac{1}{1+\exp(w^T X)} \tag{3.1}$$

$$P(Y=1|X) = \frac{\exp(w^T X)}{1+\exp(w^T X)} \tag{3.2}$$

where w is the vector of the regression coefficients.

The sigmoid function $S(t)$ is usually employed as the standard logistic function and is defined as:

$$S(t) = \frac{1}{1+\exp(-t)} \tag{3.3}$$

The likelihood ratio (also termed the "odds ratio") is defined as the natural logarithm of (3.1) and (3.2). Thus a linear dependence between conditional probabilities and predictive variables is established as:

$$\ln\frac{P(Y=1|X)}{P(Y=0|X)} = \ln\frac{\exp(w^T X)/(1+\exp(w^T X))}{1/(1+\exp(w^T X))} = w^T X \tag{3.4}$$

From (3.4), if $P(Y = 1|X) = P(Y = 0|X)$, i.e., the probabilities of belonging to the AF class and non-AF class are equal, the output of $w^T X$ will be 0. So we can use the training set to train the BLR model, determining the selected feature vector X and their regression coefficients vector w. Then we can set $z = w^T X$ and calculate the outputs for the RR segments of test set, identifying them as AF segments if $z > 0$ and as Non-AF segments if else.

The aforementioned BLR analysis was performed on SPSS version 19 to explore the potential predictable features for AF detection. All 14 features were tested. A forward likelihood ratio selection was used. Initially there are no features in the model. Then the feature with the largest likelihood was selected into the model. If the statistical difference was significant with the adding of this feature, the feature was reserved as a contributory feature. Then the feature with the largest likelihood in the remaining features was selected into the model and the comparison was also performed. The selection is ended if the newly added feature could not significantly improve the AF prediction results. The key weakness of this method is that it can be too greedy: features are fully added at each step, so correlated predictors are unlikely to be included in the model.

3.4.2 Recursive feature elimination for support vector machine

The fundamental idea of support vector machine (SVM) classifier is the construction of the optimal hyperplane $\mathbf{w}^T\mathbf{x} + b = 0$, which separates different classes with maximal margin [29,30].

The maximal margin can be defined as maximization of the minimum distance between vectors and the hyperplane:

$$\max_{\mathbf{w},b} \min \left\{ \|\mathbf{x} - \mathbf{x}_i\| : \mathbf{w}^T\mathbf{x} + b = 0, i = 1, \ldots, m \right\} \tag{3.5}$$

The $\mathbf{w}$ and b can be rescaled in a way that the point closest to the hyperplane lies on a hyperplane $\mathbf{w}^T\mathbf{x} + b = \pm 1$. Hence for every x_i we get: $\mathrm{y}_i[\mathbf{w}^T\mathbf{x}_i + b] \geq 1$, so the width of the margin is equal to $2/||\mathbf{w}||$. Equation (3.5) then can be restated as the optimization problem of objective function:

$$\min_{\mathbf{w},b} \tau(\mathbf{w}) = \frac{1}{2}\|\mathbf{w}\|^2 \tag{3.6}$$

With the following constraints:

$$\mathrm{y}_i[\mathbf{w}^T\mathbf{x}_i + b] \geq 1, i = 1, \ldots, m \tag{3.7}$$

To solve it, a Lagrangian is constructed:

$$L(\mathbf{w}, b, \alpha) = \frac{1}{2}\|\mathbf{w}\|^2 - \sum_{i=1}^{m} \alpha_i (y_i[\mathbf{x}_i^T\mathbf{w} + b] - 1) \tag{3.8}$$

where $\alpha_i > 0$ are Lagrange multipliers. Its minimization leads to:

$$\sum_{i=1}^{m} \alpha_i y_i = 0, \quad \mathbf{w} = \sum_{i=1}^{m} \alpha_i y_i \mathbf{x}_i \tag{3.9}$$

According to the Karush-Kuhn-Thucker conditions [31],

$$\alpha_i(y_i[\mathbf{x}_i^T\mathbf{w} + b] - 1) = 0, i = 1, \ldots, m \tag{3.10}$$

The non-zero α_i corresponds to $y_i[\mathbf{x}_i^T\mathbf{w} + b] = 1$. It means that the vectors which lie on the margin play the crucial role in the solution of the optimization problem. Such vectors are called support vectors.

After some substitutions the optimization problem can be transformed to the dual optimization problem:

$$\max_{\alpha} W(\alpha) = \sum_{i=1}^{m} \alpha_i - \frac{1}{2}\sum_{i,j=1}^{m} \alpha_i\alpha_j y_i y_j \mathbf{x}_i^T\mathbf{x}_j \tag{3.11}$$

with constraints:

$$\alpha_i > 0 \quad i = 1, \ldots, m, \quad \sum_{i=1}^{m} \alpha_i y_i = 0 \tag{3.12}$$

Using the solution of this problem the decision function can be written as:

$$f(\mathbf{x}) = \text{sgn}\left(\sum_{i=1}^{m} \alpha_i y_i \mathbf{x}^T\mathbf{x}_i + b\right) \tag{3.13}$$

By replacing the dot product $\mathbf{x}^T\mathbf{x}'$ by a kernel function $k(\mathbf{x}, \mathbf{x}')$, it extends the linear SVM to a nonlinear SVM. The new decision function is:

$$f(\mathbf{x}) = \text{sgn}\left(\sum_{i=1}^{m} \alpha_i y_i k(\mathbf{x}, \mathbf{x}_i) + b\right) \tag{3.14}$$

In this study, we used the Gaussian kernel:

$$k(\mathbf{x}, \mathbf{x}') = \exp[-\gamma \left\|\mathbf{x} - \mathbf{x}'\right\|^2] \tag{3.15}$$

A standardization of the features is necessary before SVM training. The following centering and scaling of the data is used: $x_i' = (x_i - \mu_i)/\sigma_i$, where μ_i and σ_i are the mean and the standard deviation of feature x_i over training set. Note that the same μ_i and σ_i over the training set are used over the test set too.

A recursive feature elimination (RFE) algorithm was used for feature selection which was proposed by Guyon *et al.* [32]. The RFE algorithm method attempts to find the best subset of size σ ($\sigma < N$) by a form of greedy backward selection. It operates by trying to choose the σ features which lead to the largest margin of class separation by an SVM classifier. This combinatorial problem is solved in a greedy fashion at each iteration of training by removing the input dimension that decreases the margin the least until only σ input dimensions remain.

For a nonlinear SVM, the margin is inversely proportional to the value $W^2(\alpha) := \sum \alpha_k\alpha_l y_k y_l k(\mathbf{x}_k, \mathbf{x}_l)$. The algorithm thus tries to remove features that lead to small values of this variable. An iterative procedure was performed as below.

Repeat

Train an SVM on training set

Given the solution α, calculate $W^2_{(-p)}(\alpha)$ for each feature p:

$$W^2_{(-p)}(\alpha) = \sum \alpha_k \alpha_l y_k y_l k(\mathbf{x}_k^{-p}, \mathbf{x}_l^{-p})$$

(where $\mathbf{x}_k^{-p}$ means training point k with feature p removed)
Remove the feature with smallest value of $W^2(\alpha) - W^2_{-p}(\alpha)$
Until σ feature remains.

3.5 Evaluation metrics

The accuracy of AF predictor can be evaluated by the following indices:

- Sensitivity: $Se = \text{TP}/(\text{TP} + \text{FN})$
- Specificity: $Sp = \text{TN}/(\text{TN} + \text{FP})$
- Accuracy: $Acc = (\text{TP} + \text{TN})/(\text{TP} + \text{FP} + \text{FN} + \text{TN})$
- AUROC: the area under the receiver operating characteristic (ROC) curve

where TP is the number of true positives, TN is the number of true negatives, FP is the number of false positives and FN is the number of false negatives.

3.6 Results

3.6.1 Feature results comparison between AF and Non-AF

Table 3.2 shows the average values of all features for the AF and Non-AF RR segments (with one standard deviation). A group t-test demonstrates that are significant

Table 3.2 Statistical group t-test results for comparison between the AF and Non-AF groups

Variable	AF	Non-AF
Number of RR segments	10,541	16,384
mRR (s)	0.68 ± 0.14*	0.83 ± 0.16
minRR (s)	0.44 ± 0.10*	0.70 ± 0.22
maxRR (s)	1.07 ± 0.33*	0.96 ± 0.34
medHR (beats/min)	96 ± 21*	75 ± 16
SDNN (s)	0.15 ± 0.06*	0.05 ± 0.08
PNN50 (%)	73 ± 13*	14 ± 21
RMSSD (s)	0.20 ± 0.09*	0.08 ± 0.12
LF_n	0.38 ± 0.14*	0.29 ± 0.21
HF_n	0.62 ± 0.14*	0.71 ± 0.21
LF/HF	0.70 ± 0.46	0.70 ± 1.26
COSEn	-0.93 ± 0.52*	-2.10 ± 0.87
NFEn	0.55 ± 1.00*	-3.03 ± 1.65
MAD ($\times 10^{-5}$)	21.2 ± 9.7*	2.5 ± 8.3
AFEv	32.5 ± 9.1*	-14.8 ± 14.3

Note: Data are presented by mean ± standard deviation (SD). "*" means significant differences compared with Non-AF group using a group t-test ($P < 0.01$).

Table 3.3 Feature selection results for the training set and the corresponding regression coefficients of binary logistic regression using forward likelihood ratio method. The results are given for each regression step

Regression step	Regression coefficients for the selected variables								
	Constant	PNN50	AFEv	MAD	NFEn	COSEn	mRR	HFn	LF/HF
1	−5.137	0.108	0	0	0	0	0	0	0
2	−5.184	0.030	0.235	0	0	0	0	0	0
3	−5.231	0.058	0.230	−9,481	0	0	0	0	0
4	−3.659	0.046	0.202	−10,365	0.797	0	0	0	0
5	−6.711	0.044	0.150	−12,518	3.210	−4.495	0	0	0
6	−10.193	0.019	0.180	−10,730	3.656	−5.419	4.187	0	0
7	−9.903	0.020	0.174	−10,617	3.764	−5.669	4.754	−1.396	0
8	−6.396	0.018	0.174	−10,231	3.688	−5.545	5.194	−5.632	−1.282

differences of all features ($P < 0.01$) between the two groups except for the LF/HF ratio.

3.6.2 Model development phase

3.6.2.1 Logistic regression result

Table 3.3 shows the feature selection results for the training set and the corresponding regression coefficients of BLR using the forward likelihood ratio method. The results are given for each regression step. After eight regression steps, eight features were identified as the most contributory features, including PNN50, AFEv, MAD, NFEn, COSEn, mRR, HFn and LF/HF in turn. As shown in Table 3.3, the final classification formula for a given AF segment is:

$$\begin{aligned} z = w^T X = & -6.396 + 0.018 \times \text{PNN50} + 0.174 \times \text{AFEv} - 10231 \\ & \times \text{MAD} + 3.688 \times \text{NFEn} - 5.545 \times \text{COSEn} + 5.194 \times \text{mRR} \\ & - 5.632 \times \text{HFn} - 1.282 \times \text{LF/HF} \end{aligned} \tag{3.16}$$

Table 3.4 provides statistics for the TP, FN, FP and TN as well as Se, Sp and Acc for both training and test sets with the evaluation for each regression step. Using (3.16), the final AF prediction results were 99.4% for Se, 98.8% for Sp and 99.0% for Acc for the training set, and were 97.1% for Se, 94.9% for Sp and 95.8% for Acc for the test set.

K-fold cross-validation

Table 3.5 shows the results for K-fold cross-validation (K = 9). For each of the nine subsets, the selected features and the corresponding regression coefficients of the BLR model using the forward likelihood ratio method are given, as well as the evaluation results for both training and test sets. Finally, the results for voting together the nine BLR models are given, with a final Se of 98.5%, Sp of 97.9% and Acc of 98.1% for all 26,925 RR segments.

Table 3.4 Results of the TP, FN, FP and TN numbers and the three indices (Se, Sp and Acc) for both training and test sets with the evaluation for each regression step

Regression step	Training data							Test data						
	TP	**FN**	**FP**	**TN**	**Se (%)**	**Sp (%)**	**Acc (%)**	**TP**	**FN**	**FP**	**TN**	**Se (%)**	**Sp (%)**	**Acc (%)**
1	5,136	191	356	8,283	96.4	95.9	96.1	4,990	224	1,171	6,574	95.7	84.9	89.2
2	5,299	28	157	8,482	99.5	98.2	98.7	5,071	143	384	7,361	97.3	95.0	95.9
3	5,288	39	126	8,513	99.3	98.5	98.8	5,068	146	424	7,321	97.2	94.5	95.6
4	5,292	35	128	8,511	99.3	98.5	98.8	5,069	145	387	7,358	97.2	95.0	95.9
5	5,299	28	116	8,523	99.5	98.7	99.0	5,067	147	421	7,324	97.2	94.6	95.6
6	5,297	30	101	8,538	99.4	98.8	99.1	5,042	172	406	7,339	96.7	94.8	95.5
7	5,298	29	105	8,534	99.5	98.8	99.0	5,054	160	395	7,350	96.9	94.9	95.7
8	5,294	33	100	8,539	99.4	98.8	99.0	5,063	151	397	7,348	97.1	94.9	95.8

Table 3.5 The results for the K-fold cross-validation

Variable	Subsets for K-fold cross-validation								
	1	**2**	**3**	**4**	**5**	**6**	**7**	**8**	**9**
Training									
TP	7,583	10,089	9,290	9,210	9,555	9,617	9,056	9,184	9,399
FN	143	169	131	143	132	174	170	134	149
FP	273	314	276	318	261	325	286	283	334
TN	15,401	12,894	14,835	14,894	13,388	13,301	14,981	14,884	13,824
Se (%)	98.1	98.4	98.6	98.5	98.6	98.2	98.2	98.6	98.4
Sp (%)	98.3	97.6	98.2	97.9	98.1	97.6	98.1	98.1	97.6
Acc (%)	98.2	97.9	98.3	98.1	98.3	97.9	98.1	98.3	98.0
Test									
TP	2,680	272	1,009	1,175	854	750	1,237	1,214	990
FN	135	11	111	13	0	0	78	9	3
FP	12	12	24	51	155	25	8	128	24
TN	698	3,164	1,249	1,121	2,580	2,733	1,109	1,089	2,202
Se (%)	95.2	96.1	90.1	98.9	100.0	100.0	94.1	99.3	99.7
Sp (%)	98.3	99.6	98.1	95.6	94.3	99.1	99.3	89.5	98.9
Acc (%)	95.8	99.3	94.4	97.3	95.7	99.3	96.5	94.4	99.2
Summary of all K models									
Total TP					10,181				
Total FN					360				
Total FP					439				
Total TN					15,945				
Mean Se (%)					97.0 ± 3.4				
Mean Sp (%)					97.0 ± 3.3				
Mean Acc (%)					96.9 ± 2.0				
Voting all K models									
TP					10,389				
FN					152				
FP					358				
TN					16,026				
Se (%)					98.6				
Sp (%)					97.8				
Acc (%)					98.1				

3.6.2.2 SVM result

RFE feature selection

The result of RFE feature selection for the SVM algorithm is shown in Table 3.6. In the beginning all features are included in the model. The order of feature removal was LFn, HFn, LF/HF, MAD, COSEn, mRR, medHR, NFEn, RMSSD, PNN50, maxRR, SDNN and then minRR during each iteration. AFEv is the last feature left in the model. After the sixth iteration, the AUROC reaches a maximum on the test set. There are then eight features remaining in the model; AFEv, minRR, SDNN, maxRR, PNN50, RMSSD, NFEn and medHR.

Table 3.6 Result of RFE feature selection. Bold type indicates the highest AUROC

Iterate step	Removed feature at each step	Training set				Test set			
		Se	Sp	Acc	AUROC	Se	Sp	Acc	AUROC
0	–	99.51	99.24	99.34	99.85	96.36	96.75	96.59	99.30
1	LFn	99.53	99.24	99.35	99.85	96.36	96.73	96.58	99.27
2	HFn	99.47	99.25	99.33	99.86	96.43	96.69	96.59	99.22
3	LF/HF	99.49	99.25	99.34	99.85	96.16	96.79	96.54	99.20
4	MAD	99.42	99.25	99.31	99.85	96.13	97.20	96.77	99.26
5	COSEn	99.42	99.18	99.27	99.86	96.28	97.24	96.85	99.29
6	mRR	99.38	99.18	99.26	99.85	96.36	97.17	96.84	**99.31**
7	medHR	99.40	99.20	99.28	99.81	96.24	96.53	96.41	99.11
8	NFEn	99.38	99.11	99.21	99.77	96.38	96.42	96.40	99.04
9	RMSSD	99.34	99.10	99.19	99.74	96.14	96.40	96.30	98.99
10	PNN50	99.32	99.05	99.16	99.72	96.99	96.41	96.64	99.16
11	maxRR	99.31	98.88	99.04	99.72	97.30	96.23	96.66	99.04
12	SDNN	99.27	98.72	98.93	99.62	97.62	95.20	96.17	98.47
13	minRR	99.32	98.33	98.71	99.31	98.12	94.40	95.89	98.05

Table 3.7 Result of K-fold cross-validation

K-fold iterate	Training set (8-fold)				Test set (1-fold)			
	Se	Sp	Acc	AUROC	Se	Sp	Acc	AUROC
1	98.46	98.87	98.74	99.79	93.57	98.87	94.64	99.04
2	98.71	98.45	98.56	99.75	94.70	99.28	98.90	99.45
3	98.93	99.05	99.00	99.75	85.27	98.51	92.31	98.37
4	98.59	98.53	98.55	99.75	98.99	97.10	98.05	99.78
5	98.70	98.83	98.77	99.76	99.88	96.67	97.44	99.74
6	98.53	98.38	98.44	99.70	99.73	99.93	99.89	100.00
7	98.53	98.76	98.67	99.74	93.38	99.28	96.09	99.68
8	98.84	98.83	98.84	99.80	99.35	90.06	94.71	99.56
9	98.60	98.50	98.54	99.76	99.70	98.92	99.16	99.77
Mean	98.65	98.69	98.68	99.76	96.06	97.62	96.80	99.49
Std	0.16	0.23	0.18	0.03	4.90	3.03	2.53	0.50

K-fold cross-validation

The result of K-fold cross-validation is shown in Table 3.7. Note that we used ninefold rather than 10-fold here is due to that the odd number is convenient for majority voting. After generating the nine SVM models, we classified the whole dataset again using the nine models and compared the result between the mean and the majority voting of the nine models. The results are shown in Table 3.8. It can be seen that the Acc of majority voting is only slightly superior to that of taking the mean (98.66% vs. 98.50%).

Table 3.8 *Comparison of mean and majority voting of nine models on the whole dataset*

	Se	**Sp**	**Acc**
Mean of K models	98.31 ± 0.64	98.62 ± 0.25	98.50 ± 0.14
Voting of K models	98.65	98.66	98.66

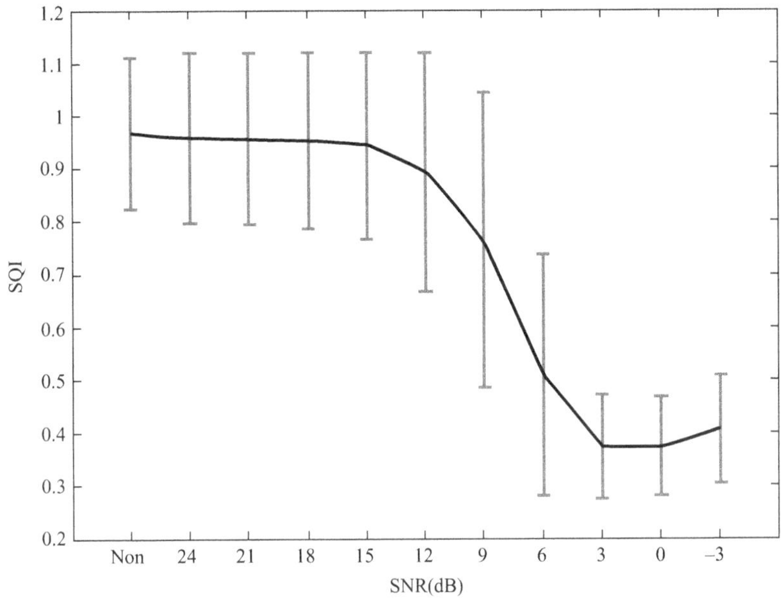

Figure 3.1 *SQI of the dataset along with the various SNR of adding noise*

3.6.3 Model validation phase

The models which were established in the development phase were validated on the unseen LTAFDB dataset with various additive noise (SNR) levels and with three different QRS detectors.

Figure 3.1 shows the mean and standard deviation of SQI of the dataset along with the various SNR levels. When the SNR ranges from 24 dB to 15 dB, the SQI remains at a high level (above 0.9), since these levels of adding noise have little influence on the QRS detection. When the SNR drops from 12 dB to 3 dB, the SQI drops by a large amount, from 0.89 to 0.37. Below 3 dB, the SQI plateaus, since both of the QRS detectors that were used for bSQI cannot correctly detect QRS complexes in extremely high noise situations.

Table 3.9 The result of Logistic regression models on LTAFDB dataset with and without adding noise (mean of K models)

Adding noise (dB)	jqrs			gqrs			wqrs			Voting (QRS)		
	Se	Sp	Acc	Se	Sp	Acc	Se	Sp	Acc	Se	Sp	Acc
Non	98.07	93.46	95.94	97.82	91.41	94.83	98.08	90.80	94.68	98.21	92.36	95.48
24	98.09	93.47	95.95	97.85	91.25	94.77	98.11	87.80	93.29	98.20	92.38	95.48
21	98.09	93.46	95.94	97.89	91.20	94.77	98.12	87.03	92.94	98.20	92.33	95.46
18	98.09	93.41	95.93	97.95	91.17	94.79	98.13	85.53	92.25	98.20	92.28	95.43
15	98.11	93.33	95.90	97.87	91.39	94.85	98.21	82.68	90.96	98.21	92.13	95.37
12	98.04	93.10	95.75	97.76	90.31	94.29	98.35	74.72	87.32	98.11	91.86	95.19
9	98.02	92.65	95.53	97.48	88.75	93.41	98.34	53.19	77.27	98.00	90.46	94.48
6	97.65	90.96	94.55	97.61	84.59	91.54	99.19	18.14	61.40	97.59	86.91	92.61
3	97.93	81.61	90.36	98.05	70.89	85.38	99.99	0.40	53.56	98.19	69.54	84.83
0	97.51	61.84	80.97	99.05	34.39	68.90	100.00	0.01	53.38	99.03	34.48	68.94
−3	98.35	31.50	67.38	99.99	0.57	53.63	100.00	0.00	53.37	99.96	0.60	53.63

Table 3.10 The result of Logistic regression models on LTAFDB dataset with and without adding noise (voting of K models)

Adding noise (dB)	jqrs			gqrs			wqrs			Voting (QRS)		
	Se	Sp	Acc	Se	Sp	Acc	Se	Sp	Acc	Se	Sp	Acc
Non	98.27	93.34	95.99	98.03	91.31	94.89	98.29	90.68	94.74	98.41	92.25	95.53
24	98.28	93.34	96.00	98.06	91.16	94.84	98.32	87.62	93.32	98.40	92.24	95.52
21	98.29	93.34	96.00	98.09	91.11	94.83	98.34	86.87	92.98	98.40	92.22	95.51
18	98.30	93.30	95.99	98.16	91.08	94.86	98.35	85.40	92.30	98.42	92.14	95.49
15	98.34	93.19	95.96	98.07	91.49	95.00	98.42	82.53	91.00	98.43	91.96	95.41
12	98.26	92.97	95.81	97.99	90.35	94.43	98.55	74.66	87.40	98.34	91.84	95.30
9	98.24	92.51	95.58	97.68	88.80	93.54	98.48	53.20	77.35	98.25	90.43	94.60
6	97.86	90.85	94.61	97.73	84.60	91.61	99.23	18.12	61.41	97.75	86.90	92.69
3	98.15	81.64	90.50	98.16	70.87	85.43	100.00	0.40	53.56	98.31	69.49	84.87
0	97.76	61.64	81.01	99.11	34.36	68.92	100.00	0.01	53.38	99.07	34.47	68.95
−3	98.55	31.21	67.35	99.99	0.57	53.63	100.00	0.00	53.37	99.97	0.59	53.63

Three QRS detectors and the majority voting of the three were used to analyze the LTAFDB dataset with and without adding noise. AF features were extracted from the RR intervals and were fed to the models which were established from the model development phase.

The results from the LR models are shown in Tables 3.9 and 3.10 and Figures 3.2–3.4.

The results from the SVM models are shown in Tables 3.11 and 3.12 and Figures 3.5–3.7.

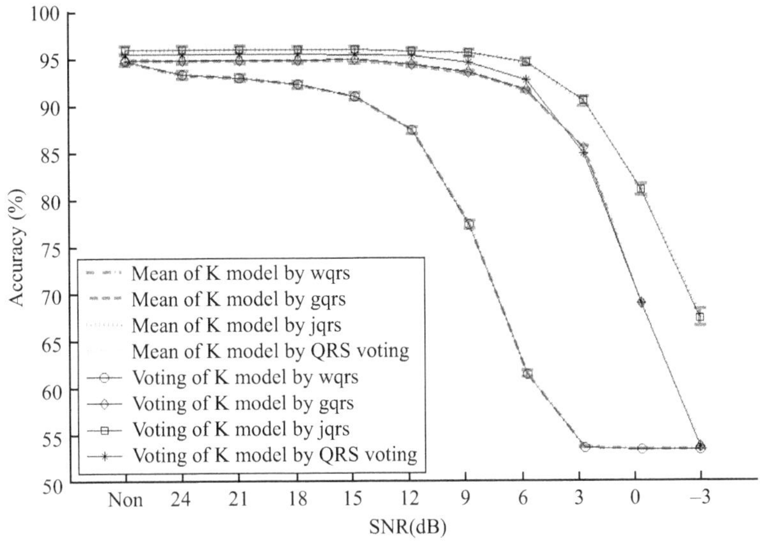

Figure 3.2 Accuracy of BLR models on LTAFDB dataset with added noise

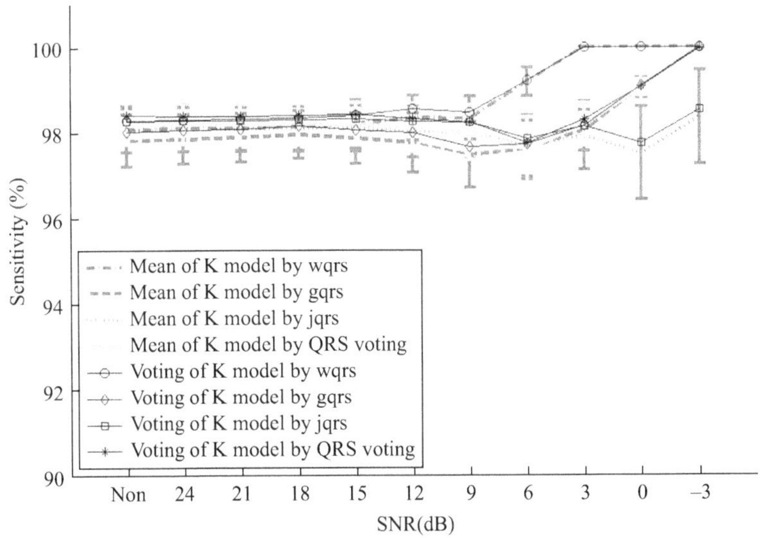

Figure 3.3 Sensitivity of BLR models on LTAFDB dataset with added noise

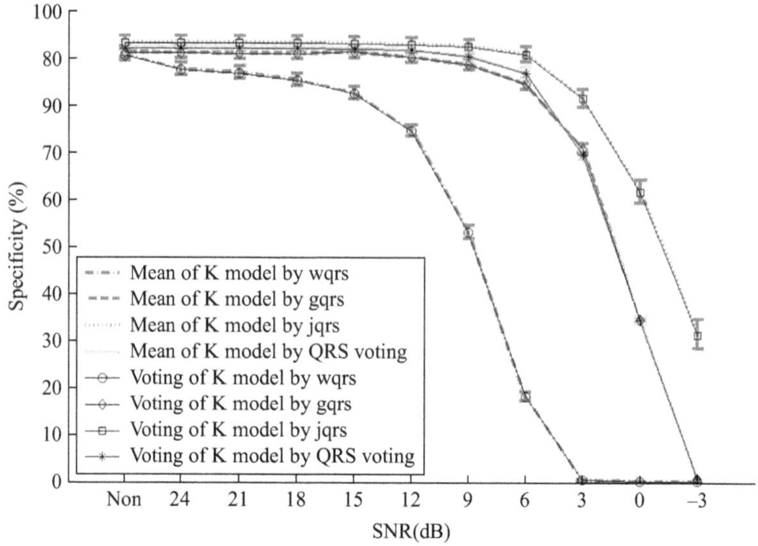

Figure 3.4 Specificity of BLR models on LTAFDB dataset with added noise

Table 3.11 The result of SVM models on LTAFDB dataset with and without adding noise (mean of K models)

Adding noise (dB)	jqrs			gqrs			wqrs			Voting (QRS)		
	Se	Sp	Acc	Se	Sp	Acc	Se	Sp	Acc	Se	Sp	Acc
Non	96.29	95.43	95.89	96.45	93.27	94.79	96.67	93.23	94.85	96.76	94.79	95.84
24	96.29	95.43	95.89	96.51	93.11	94.75	96.65	91.58	94.08	96.79	94.97	95.94
21	96.28	95.41	95.88	96.51	93.05	94.73	96.67	90.72	93.69	96.77	94.84	95.87
18	96.27	95.36	95.85	96.56	92.99	94.73	96.66	89.18	92.96	96.75	94.81	95.85
15	96.21	95.38	95.82	96.39	92.71	94.52	96.67	86.66	91.79	96.70	94.80	95.82
12	95.99	95.27	95.65	96.13	91.68	93.87	96.66	79.01	88.10	96.39	94.41	95.46
9	95.57	95.08	95.34	95.36	90.04	92.71	95.95	59.44	78.25	95.56	92.92	94.33
6	94.79	94.13	94.49	95.33	87.16	91.44	97.08	25.93	62.09	94.54	91.37	93.06
3	94.37	87.17	91.03	95.78	73.72	85.41	99.79	6.83	52.93	94.43	76.43	86.04
0	92.22	72.04	82.86	97.32	37.06	69.12	99.79	9.14	52.48	95.48	41.73	70.42
−3	91.11	46.00	70.21	99.86	0.91	53.64	99.59	11.23	52.46	98.95	2.34	53.90

Table 3.12 The result of SVM models on LTAFDB dataset with and without adding noise (voting of K models)

Adding noise (dB)	jqrs			gqrs			wqrs			Voting (QRS)		
	Se	**Sp**	**Acc**	**Se**	**Sp**	**Acc**	**Se**	**Sp**	**Acc**	**Se**	**Sp**	**Acc**
Non	96.69	95.36	96.07	96.45	93.20	94.93	96.67	93.14	95.02	97.13	94.71	96.00
24	96.68	95.32	96.05	96.51	93.02	94.88	96.65	91.52	94.25	97.16	94.88	96.09
21	96.68	95.31	96.04	96.51	92.95	94.85	96.67	90.53	93.81	97.15	94.75	96.02
18	96.66	95.24	96.00	96.56	92.89	94.85	96.66	88.82	93.00	97.12	94.71	96.00
15	96.61	95.26	95.99	96.39	92.63	94.63	96.67	86.17	91.77	97.07	94.70	95.96
12	96.42	95.16	95.84	96.13	91.56	93.99	96.66	78.31	88.10	96.77	94.34	95.64
9	96.08	94.98	95.57	95.36	89.96	92.84	95.95	57.75	78.12	96.00	92.83	94.52
6	95.27	94.07	94.71	95.33	87.07	91.48	97.08	22.55	62.33	94.83	91.37	93.22
3	94.93	87.00	91.25	95.78	73.69	85.48	99.79	1.03	53.74	94.74	76.23	86.11
0	93.08	71.71	83.17	97.32	37.01	69.20	99.79	0.22	53.36	95.89	41.30	70.44
−3	92.21	45.41	70.53	99.86	0.78	53.66	99.59	0.35	53.32	99.17	1.92	53.83

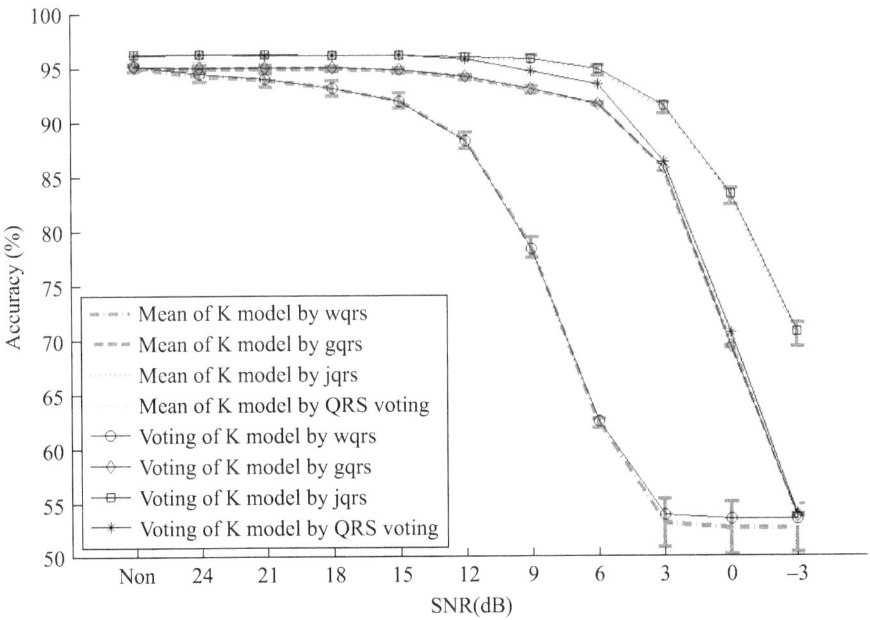

Figure 3.5 Accuracy of SVM models on LTAFDB dataset with added noise

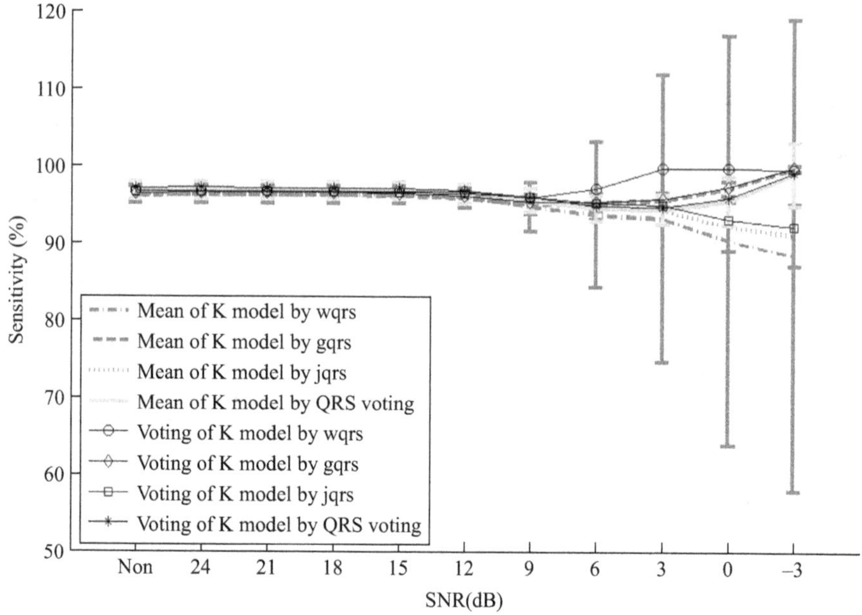

Figure 3.6 Sensitivity of SVM models on LTAFDB dataset with added noise

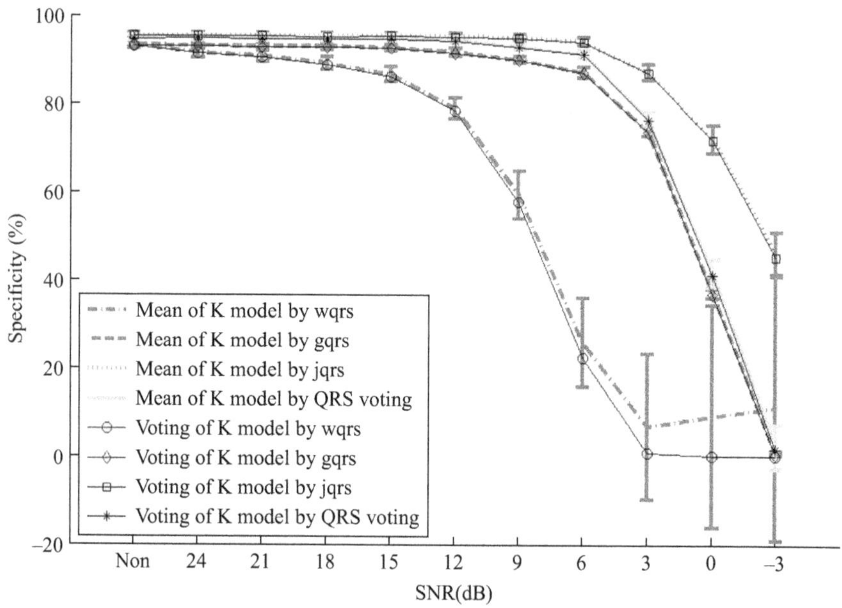

Figure 3.7 Specificity of SVM models on LTAFDB dataset with added noise

3.7 Discussion

Note that each of the K-folds gives similar results and therefore it is hard to select which K-fold is likely to give better results on the test set. (Although we report the performance on each test set, this information should not be used to select a model, because it now becomes an intermediate validation set, and more held out data are required to evaluate the actual out-of-sample performance.) There are several ways to deal with this, but essentially they boil down to a voting (and bagging) approach and using the out-of-bag error for estimating performance.

Unfortunately, in the absence of a new test sample, many researchers simply reapply the learning algorithm to the whole training set once the optimal cross-validated parameters have been found. However, overfitting is still possible since the data have already been used for model optimization. Alternatively, embedded methods, which allow feature ranking through a measure of variable importance, can be used. A typical example of this is Random Forests (RF), which is a form of bagging (although we have not explored RFs in this work).

In the examples we have presented here, we have taken the simplest approach and voted together each model developed on each fold together and cited results on the test set. In this case we find that we observe a modest rise in accuracy on the held out data from 96.9% to 98.1%. For more complex or nonlinear classifiers we may see larger improvements. However, there are also better ways to aggregate or vote together different classifiers, learning the physiological context in which each algorithm performs the best [33–35].

Finally we note that the use of real QRS detectors will result in errors in beat identification, even in low noise conditions. In reality, the noise can be extremely high from ambulatory activity, and so rejection of noisy segments needs to be considered very carefully. We refer the reader to Oster and Clifford [36] for more details on this subject. In this work, three popular QRS complex detection methods were evaluated on ECG signals with different SNRs. The "jqrs" method [11,12] consists of a window-based peak energy detector and essentially also a Pan and Tompkins (P&T)-like QRS detector [37]. Compared with the P&T method, it used a smaller window size (27 ms vs. 100 ms) thus inducing a better performance for rejecting false detections due to the high amplitude T waves. In the "jqrs" method, the original band-pass filter was replaced with a Mexican hat filter and an additional heuristic ensuring no detection was attempted during very low amplitude unvarying ECG (flat lines). A search-back procedure is also allowed in case of suspected missed beats. This combination provided the best performance among the three selected QRS complex detection methods. The "gqrs" method consists of a QRS matched filter with a custom built set of heuristics (such as search back). Unfortunately, despite the fact that open source code is available for inspection, this method does not have an associated publication, and is therefore difficult to comprehensively explain the implementation. The "wqrs" method [13] involves low-pass filtering of the ECG followed by a nonlinearly scaled curve length transformation and a series of decision rules. This method had the lowest performance of the three detectors on LTAFDB dataset, especially when the ECG signals were contaminated by realistic noise. From Figures 3.2–3.7, it can be easily seen that with the increase of SNR values, accuracy and specificity values of the "wqrs" method dropped rapidly. Although its sensitivity did not drop greatly, the standard deviations became much larger than the "jqrs" and "gqrs" methods. We also note that one may expect that the majority voting method would report better results than any of the independent QRS complex detection methods. From Tables 3.9–3.12, we can see that the voting method usually reported worse performances than "jqrs" method but better performance than other two independent methods. This may be because "wqrs" and "gqrs" respond to artifacts in a similar manner and are not truly independent. In fact, we have shown in earlier works that voting methods only provides substantial improvements over the best algorithm if each detection (or vote) is weighted based on the relative performance of the algorithm, particularly in the context of physiology and noise. For more details we refer the reader to Zhu *et al.* [33].

In conclusion we emphasize the following points:

1. Most literature reports over-trained data, and uses small numbers of patients drawn from a single database. Testing on completely unseen databases is required to provide some level of trust in the signal.
2. Most databases are handpicked to be clean. Testing on such data misrepresents the performance of an algorithm in the real world. Realistic noise should be titrated into the data and the performance of a classifier be tested as a function of such noise. (White and stationary noise is an unacceptable test.)
3. Signal quality metrics are important for identifying noisy periods of data and rejecting them from classification, or for allowing a classifier to learn the class output in the context of such noise. They also provide objective ways to assess the confidence intervals on the classifier's output.
4. Many databases contain expert annotations. Training and testing on these leads to an overly optimistic result. When automated algorithms are used to identify the features to present to a classifier during testing (mimicking the real world), significant drops in performance are observed.
5. Voting together classifiers or detectors improves the output, but generally only if you have large numbers of them, and/or can weight them using context (such as physiology and/or signal quality).

Appendix 1

Coefficient of sample entropy (COSEn)

COSEn was defined by Lake *et al.* [2,3] as an entropy measure derived from SampEn, designed specifically to detect AF in very short RR time series [2,3]. To avoid the lower confidence in entropy estimates due to low numbers of beats in shorter windows, and hence lower numbers of matches of length m and matches of length $m + 1$ due to the relatively small fixed r values, a measure called quadratic sample entropy (QSE), based on densities rather than probability estimates, was introduced in Reference 7. It normalized SampEn by the volume of each matching region, i.e., $(2r)^m$:

$$\begin{aligned} \text{QSE} &= -\ln\left(\frac{A^{m+1}(r)/(2r)^{m+1}}{B^m(r)/(2r)^m}\right) = -\ln\left(\frac{A^{m+1}(r)}{B^m(r)}\right) + \ln(2r) \\ &= \text{SampEn} + \ln(2r) \end{aligned} \tag{A1}$$

In addition, regression analyses showed that heart rate is independently associated with frequency of AF [21]. Hence, the COSEn measure uses the concept of density estimates of QSE but subtracts the natural logarithm of the mean RR interval from QSE as:

$$\text{COSEn} = \text{SampEn} + \ln(2r) - \ln(\text{mean(RR)}) \tag{A2}$$

where both r and mean(RR) use the unit of s.

Normalized fuzzy entropy (NFEn)

First, we generated quadratic fuzzy local measure entropy (QFLMEn) and quadratic fuzzy global measure entropy (QFGMEn) measures, based on the density estimates rather than probability estimates by normalizing FLMEn and FGMEn using the volume of each matching region, i.e., $(2r)^m$:

$$\begin{aligned} \text{QFLMEn} &= -\ln\left(\frac{AL^{m+1}(n_L, r_L)/(2r)^{m+1}}{BL^m(n_L, r_L)/(2r)^m}\right) = -\ln\left(\frac{AL^{m+1}(n_L, r_L)}{BL^m(n_L, r_L)}\right) + \ln(2r) \\ &= \text{FLMEn} + \ln(2r) \\ \text{QFGMEn} &= -\ln\left(\frac{AG^{m+1}(n_G, r_G)/(2r)^{m+1}}{BG^m(n_G, r_G)/(2r)^m}\right) = -\ln\left(\frac{AG^{m+1}(n_G, r_G)}{BG^m(n_G, r_G)}\right) + \ln(2r) \\ &= \text{FGMEn} + \ln(2r) \end{aligned} \tag{A3}$$

We also used the fact that heart rate is related to AF frequency and therefore subtracted the natural logarithm of the mean RR interval from QFLMEn and QFGMEn as:

$$\begin{aligned} \text{QFLMEn} &= \text{FLMEn} + \ln(2r) - \ln(\text{mean(RR)}) \\ \text{QFGMEn} &= \text{FGMEn} + \ln(2r) - \ln(\text{mean(RR)}) \end{aligned} \tag{A4}$$

And finally, NFEn is calculated as:

$$\begin{aligned} \text{NFEn} &= \text{QFLMEn} + \text{QFGMEn} \\ &= \text{FLMEn} + \text{FGMEn} + 2 \times \ln(2r) - 2 \times \ln(\text{mean(RR)}) \\ &= \text{FuzzyMEn} + 2 \times \ln(2r) - 2 \times \ln(\text{mean(RR)}) \end{aligned} \tag{A5}$$

References

[1] Clifford G.D., Long W.J., Moody G.B. and Szolovits P. Robust parameter extraction for decision support using multimodal intensive care data. *Philosophical Transactions of the Royal Society A*, 2009; 367(1887): 411–429.

[2] Clifford G.D., Behar J., Li Q. and Rezek I. Signal quality indices and data fusion for determining acceptability of electrocardiograms collected in noisy ambulatory environments. *Physiological Measurement,* 2012; 33: 1419–1433.

[3] Li Q. and Clifford G.D. Signal quality and data fusion for false alarm reduction in the intensive care unit. *Journal of Electrocardiology*, 2012; 45: 596–603.

[4] Fraser H.S. and Joaquin B. Implementing medical information systems in developing countries, what works and what doesn't. *AMIA Annual Symposium Proceedings*, 2010; 232–236.

[5] Gerber T., Olazabal V., Brown K. and Pablos-Mendez A. An agenda for action on global e-health. *Health Affairs*, 2010; 29: 233–236.

[6] Waegemann C.P. mHealth: the next generation of telemedicine? *Telemedicine Journal e-Health*, 2010; 16: 23–25.

[7] Tamrat T. and Kachnowski S. Special delivery: an analysis of mHealth in maternal and newborn health programs and their outcomes around the world. *Maternal and Child Health Journal*, 2012 Jul; 16(5): 1092–1101.

[8] Li Q., Mark R.G. and Clifford G.D. Robust heart rate estimation from multiple asynchronous noisy sources using signal quality indices and a Kalman filter. *Physiological Measurement,* 2008 Jan; 29(1): 15–32.

[9] Zong W., Moody G.B. and Mark R.G. Reduction of false arterial blood pressure alarms using signal quality assessment and relationships between the electrocardiogram and arterial blood pressure. *Medical and Biological Engineering & Computing,* 2004; 42: 698–706.

[10] Fuster V., Ryden L.E., Cannom D.S., *et al.* ACC/AHA/ESC 2006 guidelines for the management of patients with atrial fibrillation. *Circulation*, 2006; 8(9): 651–745.

[11] Behar J., Johnson A., Clifford G.D. and Oster J. A comparison of single channel fetal ECG extraction methods. *Annals of Biomedical Engineering*, 2014 Jun; 42(6): 1340–1353.

[12] Behar J., Oster J. and Clifford G.D. Combining and benchmarking methods of fetal ECG extraction without maternal or scalp electrode data. *Physiological Measurement*, 2014; 35: 1569.

[13] Zong W., Heldt T., Moody G.B. and Mark R.G. An open-source algorithm to detect onset of arterial blood pressure pulses. *Proceedings Computers in Cardiology*, 2003; 259–262.

[14] Behar J., Oster J., Li Q. and Clifford G.D. ECG signal quality during arrhythmia and its application to false alarm reduction. *IEEE Transactions on Biomedical Engineering*, 2013; 60(6): 1660–1666.

[15] Li Q., Rajagopalan C. and Clifford G.D. A machine learning approach to multi-level ECG signal quality classification. *Computer Methods and Programs in Biomedicine*, 2014 Dec; 117(3): 435–447.

[16] Carrara M., Carozzi L., Moss T.J., *et al.* Heart rate dynamics distinguish among atrial fibrillation, normal sinus rhythm and sinus rhythm with frequent ectopy. *Physiological Measurement*, 2015; 36(9): 1873–1888.

[17] Behar J., Andreotti F., Zaunseder S., Li Q., Oster J. and Clifford G.D. An ECG simulator for generating maternal-foetal activity mixtures on abdominal ECG recordings. *Physiological Measurement,* 2014; 35(8): 1537.

[18] Corino V.D., Sandberg F., Mainardi, L.T. and Sornmo, L. An atrioventricular node model for analysis of the ventricular response during atrial fibrillation. *Biomedical Engineering, IEEE Transactions* on, 2011; 58(12): 3386–3395.

[19] Lake D.E. and Moorman J.R. Accurate estimation of entropy in very short physiological time series: the problem of atrial fibrillation detection in implanted ventricular devices. *American Journal of Physiology-Heart and Circulatory Physiology*, 2011; 300(1): H319–H325.

[20] Sarkar S., Ritscher D. and Mehra R. A detector for a chronic implantable atrial tachyarrhythmia monitor. *IEEE Transactions on Biomedical Engineering*, 2008; 55(3): 1219–1224.

[21] Colloca R., Johnson A.E., Mainardi L. and Clifford G.D. A support vector machine approach for reliable detection of atrial fibrillation events. In *Computing in Cardiology Conference (CinC)*. New York: IEEE, 2013 (pp. 1047–1050).

[22] Task Force of the European Society of Cardiology. Heart rate variability standards of measurement, physiological interpretation, and clinical use, *European Heart Journal,* 1996; 17: 354–381.

[23] DeMazumder D., Lake D.E., Cheng A. *et al.* Dynamic analysis of cardiac rhythms for discriminating atrial fibrillation from lethal ventricular arrhythmias. *Circulation: Arrhythmia and Electrophysiology*, 2013; 6(3): 555–561.

[24] Lake D.E. and Moorman J.R. Accurate estimation of entropy in very short physiological time series: the problem of atrial fibrillation detection in implanted ventricular devices. *American Journal of Physiology Heart and Circulatory Physiology*, 2011; 300(1): H319–H325.

[25] Liu, C.Y., Oster J., Reinertsen E. *et al.*, Comparison of measures of entropy for atrial fibrillation detection (Under Review).

[26] D.T. Linker. Long-term monitoring for detection of atrial fibrillation. US Patent 7630756 B2, University of Washington, 2009.

[27] Sarkar S., Ritscher D. and Mehra R. A detector for a chronic implantable atrial tachyarrhythmia monitor. *IEEE Transactions on Biomedical Engineering*, 2008; 55(3): 1219–1224.

[28] Lake D.E. Renyi entropy measures of heart rate Gaussianity. *IEEE Transactions on Biomedical Engineering*, 2006; 53(1): 21–27.

[29] Guyon I., Gunn S., Nikravesh M. and Zadeh L.A. *Feature Extraction – Foundations and Applications*. Berlin Heidelberg: Springer, 2006.

[30] Boser B.E., Guyon I. and Vapnik V. A training algorithm for optimal margin classifiers. *Proceedings of Fifth Annual Workshop on Computational Learning Theory*, ACM, 1992: 144–152.

[31] Schölkopf B. and Smola A.J. *Learning with Kernels: Support Vector Machines, Regularization, Optimization, and Beyond*. Cambridge: MIT Press; 2001.

[32] Guyon I., Weston J., Barnhill S. and Vapnik V. Gene Selection for Cancer Classification using Support Vector Machines. *Machine Learning*, 2002; 46: 389–422.

[33] Zhu T., Johnson A.E., Behar J. and Clifford G.D. Crowd-sourced annotation of ECG signals using contextual information. *Annals of Biomedical Engineering*, 2014 Apr; 42(4): 871–884.

[34] Zhu T., Pimentel M.A.F., Clifford G.D. and Clifton, D.A. Bayesian fusion of algorithms for the robust estimation of respiratory rate from the photoplethysmogram. *37th Annual International Conference of the IEEE Engineering in Medicine and Biology Society (EMBC)*, IEEE, 2015: 6138–6141. doi:10.1109/EMBC.2015.7319793

[35] Zhu T., Dunkley N., Behar J. Clifton D.A. and Clifford, G.D. Fusing continuous-valued medical labels using a Bayesian model. *Annals of Biomedical Engineering*, 2015; 43(12): 2892–2902. doi:10.1007/s10439-015-1344-1.

[36] Oster J. and Clifford G.D. Impact of the presence of noise on RR interval-based atrial fibrillation detection. *Journal of Electrocardiology*, 2015; 48(6): 947–951.

[37] Pan J. and Tompkins W.J. A real-time QRS detection algorithm. *IEEE Transactions on Biomedical Engineering*, 1985; 32: 230–236.

Chapter 4
ECG model-based Bayesian filtering

Julien Oster

4.1 Background

The electrocardiogram (ECG) is a physiological signal representing the electrical activity of the heart. This signal is resulting from the depolarisation and repolarisation of the cardiac cells. Einthoven was the first to characterise the ECG signal, and its main constituting waves (P, Q, R, S and T waves) [1] and it earned him the Nobel Prize in Medicine in 1924.

With the digitisation of the ECG in the 1970s, and the current advent of eHealth technologies [2], the clinicians are faced with an explosion of data. This situation implies the need for the development of automatic or semi-automatic ECG interpretation, and explains why this field has been so prolific over the last decades [3].

The automatic analysis of ECG signal starts often with the detection of the most characteristic feature, the QRS complex [4]. This detection allows for the evaluation of the cardiac rhythm, by measuring the duration between two R peaks, which is called the RR interval, and the regularity of this cardiac rhythm. But it also offers the possibility for a deeper analysis of the cardiac cycle and the estimation of other biomarkers as depicted in Figure 4.1.

This field of research has been vastly explored during the last decades, and a wide range of methods has been applied. These techniques include adaptive filtering (AF) [5], wavelet transform [6], Principal Component Analysis [7], Independent Component Analysis [8], but also machine learning approaches such as neural networks [9], support vector machines [10], and graphical models like Hidden Markov Models [11].

In this chapter, a complete range of ECG signal analysis methods relying on the same theory, namely the Bayesian filtering theory, will be described. In a first section, this theory will be explained, along with the modelling of the ECG signal that is required for the application of Bayesian filtering. The following sections will focus on different applications of this theory, ranging from denoising to classification through delineation and source separation. This range of applications is already a demonstration of the versatility of the Bayesian filtering approaches.

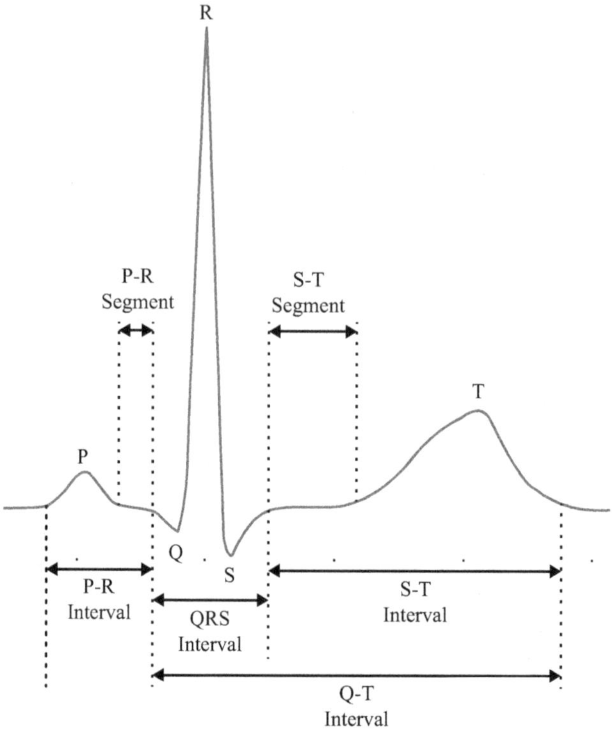

Figure 4.1 Representation of an ECG cycle, the five characteristics waves, and the main biomarkers

4.2 Theory

Bayesian filtering is a paradigm aiming at the estimation of hidden or latent variables that control a system. To apply such a technique, it is necessary to model the system, and derive what is called a state-space modelling. This state-space model informs on the evolution of the latent variables and also links these latent variables with the observations (or measurements) of the system. As will be seen later, Bayesian techniques are powerful tools, which offer more than only point estimates of the latent variables, but also provides information of the uncertainty of these estimations.

4.2.1 Bayesian filtering

Bayesian filtering is also often referred as state-space models, meaning that a system is completely controlled by an internal state $\mathbf{x}_k$. The model is given by its general form by a set of two equations:

$$\begin{cases} \mathbf{x}_k = f(\mathbf{x}_{k-1}, \mathbf{u}_{k-1}, \mathbf{w}_{k-1}, k-1) \\ \mathbf{y}_k = g(\mathbf{x}_k, \mathbf{v}_k, k) \end{cases}, \tag{4.1}$$

where $\mathbf{y}_k$ is the observation vector (or measurements), $\mathbf{w}_k$ is the state (or process) noise, $\mathbf{v}_k$ is the observation (or measurement) noise, $\mathbf{u}_k$ is a control (or input) vector and finally k is the current timestamp.

The upper equation is the evolution (or process) equation, and the lower the observation (or measurement) equation. It can be noted that both f and g functions are dependent of the time (hence the input k) and can also be noted f_k and g_k. A time-independent version of these equations can exist, and the model is then called stationary. Please note the control input $\mathbf{u}_k$ will not be considered further in this chapter.

Bayesian filtering aims at estimating the posterior probability $p(\mathbf{x_k}|\mathbf{y_{1:k}}, \theta_k)$, with θ_k being the parameters of the system $\{f_k, g_k, \mathbf{v}_k, \mathbf{w}_k\}$. This estimation is done recursively in two steps, a prediction step estimating the posterior probability $p(\mathbf{x_k}|\mathbf{y_{1:k-1}}, \theta_{k-1})$ by using the evolution equation, which is followed by correction step by using the observation equation and gives $p(\mathbf{x_k}|\mathbf{y_{1:k}}, \theta_k)$.

A special case of Bayesian filtering occurs when both f_k and g_k are linear and when the random variables are Gaussian. The problem is then called linear-Gaussian state-space model or a linear dynamical system, and the system can then be described by:

$$\begin{cases} \mathbf{x}_k = A_{k-1}\mathbf{x}_{k-1} + F_{k-1}\mathbf{w}_{k-1} \\ \mathbf{y}_k = C_k\mathbf{x}_k + G_k\mathbf{v}_k \end{cases}, \tag{4.2}$$

where both functions f and g are replaced by linear algebra operations (matrices).

The estimation of the posterior probability is then performed with the well-known Kalman filter equations (or algorithm) [12]:

$$\begin{aligned}
&\underline{\text{Prediction}} \\
\hat{\mathbf{x}}_{k|k-1} &= A_{k-1}\hat{\mathbf{x}}_{k-1|k-1}, \\
R_{k^-} &= A_{k-1}R_{k-1}A_{k-1}^T + F_{k-1}Q_{k-1}^w F_{k-1}^T, \\
&\underline{\text{Correction}} \\
K_k &= R_{k^-}C_k^T\left(C_kR_{k^-}C_k^T + G_kQ_{k-1}^v G_k^T\right)^{-1}, \\
\hat{\mathbf{x}}_{k|k} &= \hat{\mathbf{x}}_{k|k-1} + K_k\left(\mathbf{y}_k - C_k\hat{\mathbf{x}}_{k|k-1}\right), \\
R_k &= (I - K_kC_k)R_{k^-},
\end{aligned} \tag{4.3}$$

where Q_{k-1}^w is the covariance matrix of the process noise, $Q_{k-1}^w = cov(\mathbf{w}_{k-1}) = E[\mathbf{w}_{k-1}\mathbf{w}_{k-1}^T]$, $Q_{k-1}^v = cov(\mathbf{v}_{k-1})$, $R_{k^-} = cov(\hat{\mathbf{x}}_{k|k-1})$, $R_k = cov(\hat{\mathbf{x}}_{k|k})$, and K_k is called the Kalman gain.

4.2.2 Non-linear Bayesian filtering

The Kalman filter has been applied to a wide range of applications, and has been notoriously associated to the Apollo Space programme [13], therefore allowing men to land on the Moon. Nevertheless, the linear hypothesis is one of the biggest restrictions of its applications and several approaches have been proposed to overcome this limitation.

One of these solutions, called the Extended Kalman Filter (EKF), consists of the linearisation of both evolution and observation equations around the current estimates. The (4.1) is then linearised and rewritten as:

$$\begin{cases} \mathbf{x}_k = f(\hat{\mathbf{x}}_{k-1}, \hat{\mathbf{w}}_{k-1}, k-1) + A_{k-1}(\mathbf{x}_{k-1} - \hat{\mathbf{x}}_{k-1}) + F_{k-1}(\mathbf{w}_{k-1} - \hat{\mathbf{w}}_{k-1}) \\ \mathbf{y}_k = g(\hat{\mathbf{x}}_k, \hat{\mathbf{v}}_k, k) + C_k(\mathbf{x}_k - \hat{\mathbf{x}}_k) + G_k(\mathbf{v}_k - \hat{\mathbf{v}}_k) \end{cases}, \tag{4.4}$$

where

$$\begin{aligned} A_k &= \frac{\partial f(\mathbf{x}, \mathbf{w}, k)}{\partial \mathbf{x}}|_{\mathbf{x}=\hat{\mathbf{x}}_k} \\ F_k &= \frac{\partial f(\mathbf{x}, \mathbf{w}, k)}{\partial \mathbf{w}}|_{\mathbf{w}=\hat{\mathbf{w}}_k} \\ C_k &= \frac{\partial g(\mathbf{x}, \mathbf{v}, k)}{\partial \mathbf{x}}|_{\mathbf{x}=\hat{\mathbf{x}}_k} \\ G_k &= \frac{\partial g(\mathbf{x}, \mathbf{v}, k)}{\partial \mathbf{v}}|_{\mathbf{v}=\hat{\mathbf{v}}_k}. \end{aligned} \tag{4.5}$$

Using this linearised version, it is possible to get updates on the state by applying the Kalman filter algorithm or equations 4.3.

EKF, however, also has some limitations, mainly the fact that all functions are not differentiable, and as the derivatives cannot be computed, the different matrices can therefore not be estimated. A new range of Kalman filter has therefore been introduced and called Unscented Kalman Filter (UKF) [14]. UKF introduces σ-points ($\mathbf{x}^i$) and associated weights (ω_i), which represent a deterministic sampling of the state vector. The Kalman equations are then used to propagate the first and second order of the state, where the first order of the state $E[\mathbf{x}] = \sum_i \omega_i \mathbf{x}^i$, and the second order being $R_\mathbf{x} = \sum_i \omega_i (\mathbf{x}^i - E[\mathbf{x}])(\mathbf{x}^i - E[\mathbf{x}])^T$. The advantage of this approach is that first and second order of $\mathbf{y} = g(\mathbf{x})$ can be easily computed as $E[\mathbf{y}] = \sum_i \omega_i g(\mathbf{x}^i)$, and $R_\mathbf{y} = \sum_i \omega_i (g(\mathbf{x}^i) - E[\mathbf{y}])(g(\mathbf{x}^i) - E[\mathbf{y}])^T$.

Another class of non-linear Bayesian filtering has recently been introduced. It consists of a random sampling of the state vector, and let these samples evolve through the process equation and corrects them according the new observations made. This class of techniques is called particle filters, or Sequential Monte Carlo [15,16]. It offers the advantage of getting a more complete representation of the state vector distribution than only taking into account the first and second orders.

4.2.3 Switching Kalman filters

Bayesian filtering offers more than just a point estimate of the state vector. At each step, not only the latent variable estimate is updated, but also the uncertainty of this estimate (or the spread), which is given by the covariance matrix. Given the parameters of the state-space model, it is also possible to estimate the likelihood of a new observation having been generated by a given model, i.e. $p(\mathbf{y}_k | \mathbf{x}_k, \mathbf{y}_{1:k-1}, \boldsymbol{\theta}_k)$. It is therefore possible to estimate how likely a new observation has been generated by the given state-space modelling. In a system, where the state vector could jump between a finite number of modes (and be modelled with different state-space models), it would be possible to estimate the mode being the most likely to have generated a given observation. Such an approach is called Switching Kalman Filter (SKF).

SKF can be seen as an extension of Hidden Markov Models (HMM) [17]. As for HMM, there are (generally) finite number of latent states, called mode, and one aims at detecting the most likely latent mode from a set of observations. Nevertheless, SKF is more "advanced" than HMM, since each mode can be modelled by its own state-space formalism as a linear (or non-linear) dynamical system. In this section, we will briefly introduce the mechanism of SKF allowing for the selection of the most likely latent mode.

Let us call $C_k^{(i)}$ the observation matrix of the ith mode, such that $\mathbf{y}_k = C_k^{(i)}\mathbf{x}_k^{(i)} + G_k^{(i)}\mathbf{v}_k^{(i)}$ and let us denote $Q_k^{\mathbf{v}^{(\mathrm{i})}} = cov(\mathbf{v}_k^{(i)})$, the covariance matrix of the observation noise. The innovation at time k, is denoted $\tilde{\mathbf{y}}_k^{(i)} = \mathbf{y}_k^{(i)} - C_k^{(i)}\hat{\mathbf{x}}_k^{(i)}$ and $R_{\varepsilon,k}^{(i)}$ its covariance matrix, which can be computed with:

$$R_{\varepsilon,k}^{(i)} = G_k^{(i)} Q_k^{\mathbf{v}^{(i)}} G_k^{(i)^T} + C_k^{(i)} R_{k-}^{(i)} C_k^{(i)^T}, \tag{4.6}$$

with $R_{k-}^{(i)}$ being the *prior* state covariance matrix, which is computed step by step during the Kalman filter algorithm.

The residual likelihood for the ith mode, $l_k(i)$, can then be computed by:

$$l_k(i) = \frac{1}{\alpha} \frac{1}{\sqrt{2\pi \det(\mathbf{R}_{\varepsilon,k}^{(i)})}} \exp\left(-\frac{1}{2}\tilde{\mathbf{y}}_k^{(i)^T} \mathbf{R}_{\varepsilon,k}^{(i)^{-1}} \tilde{\mathbf{y}}_k^{(i)}\right), \tag{4.7}$$

with α being a normalisation factor, so that $\sum_i l_k(i) = 1$.

Monitoring this likelihood allows to select the most probable mode to have generated the new observations. Section 4.7 will show how this theory can be applied to ECG analysis for the detection of ventricular rhythms.

The next section will be devoted to the introduction of a dynamical modelling of the ECG signal. This model was the groundwork necessary for the development of effective Bayesian filtering applied to ECG analysis.

4.3 ECG model

McSharry *et al.* introduced a dynamical modelling of the ECG signal. This model was developed in order to simulate artificial signals [18], which could be used for the evaluation of different analysis techniques with a complete knowledge of the ground-truth of the underlying physiological signals. Not only precise measurements of Signal-to-Noise Ratio (SNR) were made possible but also accurate physiologically meaningful measurements such as QT, PR or QRS intervals, or ST levels for example.

The ECG has been modelled as a pseudo-periodic signal, with each heartbeat (or cycle) being modelled as a sum of Gaussian waves, and governed by a set of dynamical equations.

The first part of the modelling paper was dedicated to the creation of some realistic heart rhythm, and will not be explained further in this section, interested readers are referred to the original paper [18]. This part resulted in the creation of a variable ω, which represented the speed of the dynamical system.

The second part of the paper was devoted to the modelling of the ECG morphology. A typical heartbeat consists in a series of deflations, starting with a low amplitude P wave representing the depolarisation of the atria, followed by the high amplitude QRS complex representing the depolarisation of the ventricles, and finishing by a lower amplitude T wave representing the repolarisation of the ventricles.

Each of these three characteristic waves or components can be modelled as sum of multiple Gaussian waves, and it has been shown that two Gaussians can represent accurately each of the P and T waves, with three Gaussians being necessary for the modelling of the highest energy portion of the ECG, the QRS complex. A total of seven Gaussian waves have therefore been shown to be required for properly approximating the morphology of the ECG signals [19].

An ECG signal can therefore be represented by a set of equations, and modelled given a finite set of parameters:

$$\begin{cases} \dot{x} = \rho x - \omega y \\ \dot{y} = \rho y - \omega x \\ \dot{z} = -\sum_{i=1}^{7} \frac{\omega \Delta\theta_i}{b_i^2} g\left(\alpha_i, \Delta\theta_i, b_i\right) - (z - z_0) \end{cases}, \tag{4.8}$$

where $\rho = 1 - \sqrt{x^2 + y^2}$, ω is the angular speed or the speed of the dynamical system (given by the heart rhythm). z represents the ECG value in mV and α_i, b_i and ξ_i are the amplitude, width and angular position of the ith Gaussian, respectively, with $\Delta\theta_i = (\theta - \xi_i)(\mathrm{mod}\ 2\pi)$, where $\pi < \theta = a\tan 2(y, x) \leq \pi$ and with $g(a, b, c) = a\exp(-\frac{b^2}{2c^2})$ representing one Gaussian wave. z_0 was representing the baseline, and could serve for the modelling of the baseline wander by allowing it to evolve following a pseudo-periodical evolution at the respiratory frequency.

It is therefore possible to generate a synthetic ECG signal by selecting a small number of parameters, 21 (three per Gaussian wave), for the morphology of the heartbeat, and then use an omega function representing the heart rhythm to create a realistic ECG signal. An example of such simulation is depicted in Figure 4.2. These synthetic signals will then be used to assess the performance of existing ECG analysis techniques, and how noise can impact them, as these synthetic data can be distorted with different levels/types of noise, while knowing the ground-truth. But the model was later used also as the building block for new analysis techniques, parameters of this model were first estimated in an offline manner, using non-linear optimisation algorithms to estimate the parameters of the ECG model after having first localised the fiducial points [19,20]. This approach was applied to several problems, denoising, compression but also delineation or QT measurements [21].

In the following sections, we will present different applications for which the ECG-model based Bayesian filtering approach has been successfully applied, namely, denoising, delineation, source separation and ventricular beat detection.

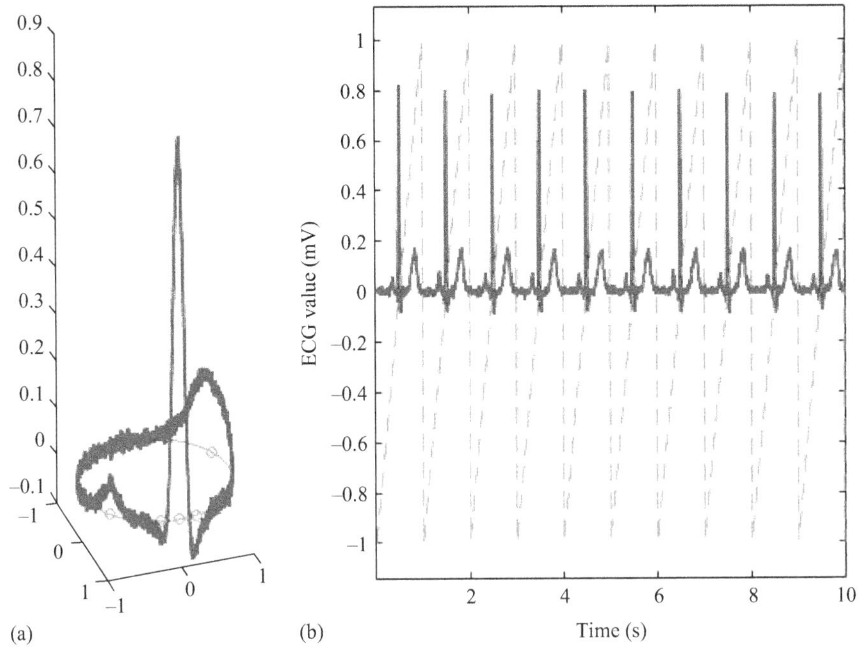

Figure 4.2 *Simulation of an ECG signal using the model. (a) 3D representation of ten simulated cycles. Circles represent the position of the five main waves. (b) Simulation of ten noisy ECG cycles, in dotted lines the representation of the scaled phase signal*

4.4 Denoising

4.4.1 Problem formulation

The dynamical equations are amazingly well suited for the state-space approach and a non-linear Bayesian approach was first proposed by Sameni *et al.* [22].

In order to apply the Bayesian filtering framework, it is necessary to define the state and observation vectors, and as will be seen later this design is preponderant and is offering the versatility of this approach. Let us define the state vector $\mathbf{x}_k = [\theta_k, z_k]$, where θ_k is the angular position in the cylindrical coordinates (or the phase in the cardiac cycle), and z_k represents the ECG value in mV at time k. The state-space formalism of this technique is defined by the following set of equations:

(i) the evolution equations are given by

$$\begin{cases} \theta_k = (\theta_{k-1} + \omega\delta) \mod 2\pi \\ z_k = -\sum_i \delta \dfrac{\omega \Delta\theta_{i,k-1}}{b_i^2} g\left(\alpha_i, \Delta\theta_{i,k-1}, b_i\right) + z_{k-1} + \eta \end{cases}, \tag{4.9}$$

where $\omega = 2\pi/RR$ the angular speed, δ the sampling period, and α_i, b_i and ξ_i are the amplitude, width and angular position of the ith Gaussian, respectively, with $\Delta\theta_{i,k-1} = (\theta_{k-1} - \xi_i)(\text{mod } 2\pi)$ and with $g(a, b, c) = a \exp(-\frac{b^2}{2c^2})$ a Gaussian wave.

(ii) the observation equations are defined by

$$\begin{cases} \varphi_k = \theta_k + v_{1,k} \\ s_k = z_k + v_{2,k} \end{cases}, \tag{4.10}$$

The observed signals, s_k is the ECG signal and φ_k is an artificial phase signal assigned linearly from 0 to 2π between two consecutive R waves and then rescaled between $-\pi$ and π.

There is therefore a need to create an artificial signal, which represents the cardiac phase. The R peaks are detected in a pre-processing step, and it is therefore assumed that this detection is possible and accurate even in noisy detections.

4.4.2 Parameter initialisation

The denoising technique, and the Bayesian filtering, depends heavily on a set of initial parameters. These parameters have a huge importance for the success of the technique, as they give us *prior* knowledge on the evolution of the signal. The main parameters to be determined are the three parameters associated to each of the Gaussian wave (α_i, b_i, ξ_i).

To be successfully applied, Bayesian filtering rely on a good parameter initialisation, which is usually performed on a small portion of the data at the beginning of the recording. A small number (usually 30) of ECG cycles represented as a function of the cardiac phase are stacked up. These stacks are used to determine a mean ECG template, and the standard deviation as function of the phase.

Once this mean ECG template has been estimated, it is possible to determine the Gaussian parameters by using a non-linear optimisation algorithm, as was suggested for the offline applications [19,20].

4.4.3 Benchmarking and results

Sameni *et al.* have created a small dataset of ECG signals in order to assess the denoising performance [22]. They extracted 190 30-s ECG segments from the MIT-BIH Normal Sinus Rhythm (NSR) database [23]. These segments were selected visually, by ensuring low noise level on the segments. The MIT-BIH NSR database contains long-term recordings from 18 subjects without significant arrhythmias.

Noise was added on top of these high quality segments, by using Muscle Artifact from the MIT-BIH Noise Stress Test (NST) database [23]. The noise amplitudes were adjusted in order to simulate different levels of noise with SNR ranging from 6 to 18 dB.

The Bayesian filtering approach results were compared to state-of-the-art techniques, such as simple Finite Impulse Response (FIR) filtering, AF, and wavelet decomposition (WD). Different Bayesian filter techniques were also compared, as the authors implemented Extended Kalman Filter (EKF), Extended Kalman Smoothing

Table 4.1 SNR results for the denoising with real muscle artefacts

SNR (dB) Input	**6.0**	**12.0**	**18.0**
FIR	5.9	9.7	11.7
AF	5.0	5.4	5.5
WD	6.9	12.9	18.9
EKF	10.0	14.1	18.8
EKS	12.0	15.5	19.5
UKF	9.5	13.8	18.7

(EKS) and Unscented Kalman Filter (UKF). The results obtained on this small dataset are assembled on Table 4.1.

The results demonstrated that the Bayesian filtering approaches outperform other techniques, especially in low SNR situations. It was also shown, that EKS gave best denoising results. Sameni *et al.* have also studied the effect of adaptive noise covariance parameters in order to cope with non-stationary noise levels, and interested readers are referred to their paper [22].

4.5 Delineation

The previous section has demonstrated the potential of ECG model-based Bayesian filtering for the estimation of the latent clean physiological signal. This cleaned version of the signal could then be used to apply "automatic" analysis techniques for the extraction of clinically valuable information, such as various intervals (QT, PR). Nevertheless, the Bayesian filtering approach offers the possibility to estimate such parameters more or less directly in the same time as the denoising takes place.

4.5.1 Problem formulation

The first approach for the delineation problem is to introduce a couple of extra state variables, which represent the independent waves characterising the ECG signal. That is dividing the previously introduced state vector z_k into three additive components $\{p_k, c_k, t_k\}$. The state-space model can then be modelled as follows.

The state equation is written as

$$\begin{cases} \theta_k = (\theta_{k-1} + \omega\delta) \mod 2\pi \\ p_k = -\sum_{i\in P} \delta \dfrac{\omega\Delta\theta_{i,k-1}}{b_i^2} g\left(\alpha_i, \Delta\theta_{i,k-1}, b_i\right) + p_{k-1} + \eta_p \\ c_k = -\sum_{i\in QRS} \delta \dfrac{\omega\Delta\theta_{i,k-1}}{b_i^2} g\left(\alpha_i, \Delta\theta_{i,k-1}, b_i\right) + c_{k-1} + \eta_c \\ t_k = -\sum_{i\in T} \delta \dfrac{\omega\Delta\theta_{i,k-1}}{b_i^2} g\left(\alpha_i, \Delta\theta_{i,k-1}, b_i\right) + c_{k-1} + \eta_t \end{cases}, \tag{4.11}$$

and the observation equation is

$$\begin{cases} \varphi_k = \theta_k + v_{1,k} \\ s_k = p_k + c_k + t_k + v_{2,k} \end{cases}. \tag{4.12}$$

The estimates of the three main waves are accessible to the user, and by processing them individually it is easy to estimate the starting and ending point of each of these already separated waves. But these clinical features could also be derived even more directly, by estimating the model parameters and their evolution with time. Bayesian filter is indeed a nice paradigm, which relies on a model description of the problem (and therefore a finite set of parameters) to estimate the posterior probability $p(\mathbf{x}_n|\mathbf{y}_{(1:n)}, \theta)$. But the estimation of the inherent parameters of the model could also be integrated in the filtering, by extending the state vector with these extra parameter variables, therefore estimating the posterior probability $p([\mathbf{x}_n, \theta_n]|\mathbf{y}_{(1:n)})$.

In the context of ECG signal processing, the main parameters of the model consist in the three parameters characterising each of the Gaussian waves. One of the main challenges when integrating a model parameter in the state vector, is how to model its evolution. The easiest solution is to assume that we have no insight in its evolution, and therefore assume a random walk evolution for this parameter. It is often wrongly assumed that a random walk implies that the parameter is not evolving or evolving slowly. But the evolution of a parameter following a random walk, can be seen as the diffusion of a gas particle, with a preferred direction (characterised by the mean of the Gaussian walk), and a given speed (characterised by the covariance).

$$\begin{cases} \theta_k = (\theta_{k-1} + \omega\delta) \mod 2\pi \\ z_k = -\sum_i \delta \dfrac{\omega \Delta\theta_{i,k-1}}{b_i^2} g\left(\alpha_i, \Delta\theta_{i,k-1}, b_i\right) + z_{k-1} + \eta \\ \alpha_{(i,k)} = \alpha_{(i,k-1)} + \chi_{\alpha_i} \\ b_{(i,k)} = b_{(i,k-1)} + \chi_{b_i} \\ \xi_{(i,k)} = \xi_{(i,k-1)} + \chi_{\xi_i} \end{cases}, \tag{4.13}$$

where $\{\chi_{\alpha_i}, \chi_{b_i}, \chi_{\xi_i}\}$ represent the noise for the random walks of the Gaussian wave parameters.

The estimation of the Gaussian parameters $\{\alpha_{(i,k)}, b_{(i,k)}, \xi_{(i,k)}\}$ can then be used to determine the starting and ending points of each of the three big waves (P, QRS and T). A probabilistic approach can be taken on this problem, by considering that each of the waves can be seen as a mixture of Gaussians, whose likelihood is given by:

$$p_W(x) = \sum_{i \in W} \pi_i \mathcal{N}(x|\xi_i, b_i), \tag{4.14}$$

where $\pi_i = \frac{|\alpha_i|}{\sum_i |\alpha_i|}$, and W represents the indices for the P wave, T wave and QRS complex. Given this representation, it is possible to calculate the start s_W and ending points e_W such that $p_W(x < s_W) = \varepsilon$ and $p_W(x > e_W) = \varepsilon$, with $\varepsilon = 0.01$, for example.

Table 4.2 Results for the ECG delineation. The distributions of the difference between the automatic and the manual annotations were approximated by normal distributions $\mathcal{N}(\mu, \sigma)$

Biomarker	μ (ms)	σ (ms)
QRS_{dur}	0	1.6
TP_{int}	0	1
QT_{int}	0	4

It has to be highlighted that the mixture of Gaussians has not to be confused with a sum of random variables following a Gaussian (normal) distribution, which also follows normal distribution as the authors have suggested when deriving the starting and ending points in [21].

Such an delineation method has been proposed by Sayadi and Shamsollahi [24], but for simplicity reasons they restricted the model to only five waves P, Q, R, S and T, the starting and ending points could therefore easily be computed analytically.

4.5.2 Benchmarking and results

In order to evaluate the performance of delineation, a subset of the MIT-BIH NSR database has been extracted [23]. Eighty 30-second ECG segments have been visually selected, by ensuring a low level of noise. A cardiologist expert annotated the data, by delineating the cycles, in order to extract some of the biomarkers. The automatic evaluation using the Bayesian filtering of some biomarkers (QRS duration QRS_{dur}, T-P interval TP_{int} and QT interval QT_{int}) were compared to the manual annotations. The distributions of the difference between the automatic and the manual annotations were approximated by normal distributions $\mathcal{N}(\mu, \sigma)$, and these variables are assembled in Table 4.2.

The results show that the delineation quality compares well with manual annotations, as most of the QT interval errors are lower than 12 ms, which compares well with manual annotation errors [25]. Sayadi *et al.* have also used this delineation approach for the extraction of fiducial points, in order to suppress baseline wander and have demonstrated the power of such an approach [26].

4.6 Source separation

In the previous sections, we have demonstrated the power of a model-based approach for the analysis of the ECG, for a better denoising and also for the estimation of some clinical parameters. In the previous applications, no *prior* knowledge on the noise has been added in the state-space equations, and the observation noise was a simple additive noise. However for some applications noise level could be higher, and could be more structured than simple white or coloured noise. In this section, we will describe the extension of the model-based approach for problems such as source separation. We will therefore assume that the "noise" has a pseudo-periodical structure as has the ECG. This pseudo-periodicity could be either identical or different from the ECG rhythm, that is the noise rhythm might be different from the cardiac rhythm.

4.6.1 Problem formulation

Some applications imply the simultaneous acquisition of multiple pseudo-periodical biosignals at once. These signals will therefore overlap, and for an accurate analysis of the signal of interest it will be necessary to separate all the sources. Different approaches have been suggested for source separation in biomedical applications, one of the most popular consists in applying ICA and relies on the assumption that each of the sources are statistically independent [27]. It is nevertheless possible to make stronger assumptions on the underlying sources, Sameni *et al.* have suggested a semi-blind approach using some *prior* knowledge on the rhythm of the biosignal to be analysed [28].

It is possible to make some stronger assumptions, and to imagine that the rhythm of both noise and signal are known, and that both their template can be estimated. Based on these assumptions, it is possible to apply the model-based filtering for an online estimation of the contribution of each of these sources. The state vectors have therefore to be extended, in order to integrate the parameters of the pseudo-periodical noise. The parameters for this state-space formalism are:

$$\begin{aligned}
\mathbf{x}_k &= [\theta_k^z, \theta_k^n, z_k, n_k, \{\alpha_{i,k}^z\}, \{b_{i,k}^z\}, \{\xi_{i,k}^z\}] \\
\mathbf{y}_k &= [\varphi_k^z, \varphi_k^n, s_k, s_k] \\
\mathbf{w}_k &= [\omega^z, \omega^z, \eta_k^z, \eta_k^n, \{\varepsilon_{\alpha,i}\}, \{\varepsilon_{b,i}\}, \{\varepsilon_{\xi,i}\}, \{\alpha_{i,k}^n\}, \{b_{i,k}^n\}, \{\xi_{i,k}^n\}] \\
\mathbf{v}_k &= [v_{1,k}, v_{2,k}, v_{3,k}, v_{4,k}],
\end{aligned} \tag{4.15}$$

which gives rise to the following process equations

$$\begin{cases}
\theta_k^z = (\theta_{k-1}^z + \omega^z \delta) \bmod 2\pi \\
\theta_k^n = (\theta_{k-1}^n + \omega^n \delta) \bmod 2\pi \\
z_k = z_{k-1} - \sum_i \delta \dfrac{\omega^z \Delta\Theta_{i,k-1}}{(b_{i,k-1}^z)^2} g\left(\alpha_{i,k-1}^z, \Delta\Theta_{i,k-1}, b_{i,k-1}^z\right) + \eta_k^z \\
n_k = n_{k-1} - \sum_i \delta \dfrac{\omega^n \Delta\theta_{i,k-1}}{(b_i^n)^2} g\left(\alpha_i^n, \Delta\theta_{i,k-1}, b_i^n\right) + \eta_k^n, \\
\alpha_{i,k}^z = \alpha_{i,k-1}^z + \varepsilon_{\alpha,i} \\
b_{i,k}^z = b_{i,k-1}^z + \varepsilon_{b,i} \\
\xi_{i,k}^z = \xi_{i,k-1}^z + \varepsilon_{\xi,i}
\end{cases} \tag{4.16}$$

and the observation equations

$$\begin{cases} \varphi_k^z = \theta_k^z + v_{1,k} \\ \varphi_k^n = \theta_k^n + v_{2,k} \\ s_k = z_k + n_k + v_{3,k}. \\ s_k = n_k + \sum_i g\left(\alpha_{i,k}^z, \Delta\Theta_{i,k}, b_{i,k}^z\right) + v_{4,k}, \end{cases} \tag{4.17}$$

It is interesting to note the observation equations have been extended as well. The presence of this fourth equation can be explained by a drifting phenomenon when this extra observation equation was missing, separation of the contribution of each source on a new observation. Some instabilities were leading to a drift on the signal and noise components. The idea behind the fourth equation is that the first "rough" approximation of the pseudo-periodical noise could be performed by suppressing the signal template from a new observation, that is $s_k - \sum_i g\left(\alpha_{i,k}^z, \Delta\Theta_{i,k}, b_{i,k}^z\right) = n_k + v_{4,k}$. This rough estimation could then be used in the second time to estimate the signal contribution z_k, by suppressing the first estimate of the noise from the new observation. The elegance of the Bayesian filtering approach allows to replace this iterative process by a single step, by adding this fourth equation. In order to account for the fact, that this extra-equation is a rough estimation of the noise component and less precise than equation two, one has only to increase the uncertainty of this equation, that is setting a higher noise covariance for v_4 than v_3.

4.6.2 Benchmarking and results

This approach has already been applied to two problems.

The first one consists in the acquisition of ECG during a Magnetic Resonance Imaging examination [29]. During such a procedure, the patient is located in a high static magnetic field. The movement of electrically charged particles, ions inside the blood flow, creates an electrical field which is picked up by the electrodes. This phenomenon, called MagnetoHydroDynamic (MHD) effect, superposes onto the ECG signal. The MHD effect is synchronised with the ECG, as the heart's electrical activity is triggering its contraction and therefore the blood flow. For this problem, there is no need to introduce φ_k^n, as the same phase variable could be used for both the signal (z_k) and the "noise" (n_k).

The performance of this approach was assessed on a very small subset of simulated pathological cases, using an in-house MHD generator [30]. The inversion of the T wave was simulated in one of these cases. It was assessed whether it is possible to automatically detect this inversion, the results are depicted in Figure 4.3. It can be seen that the T wave inversion has been automatically detected approximatively ten cycles after the inversion.

The second application consists in the extraction of the foetal ECG signal from abdominal signals [31]. These abdominal signals contain a mixture of both maternal ECG and foetal ECG, and it is therefore necessary to introduce the extra phase signal

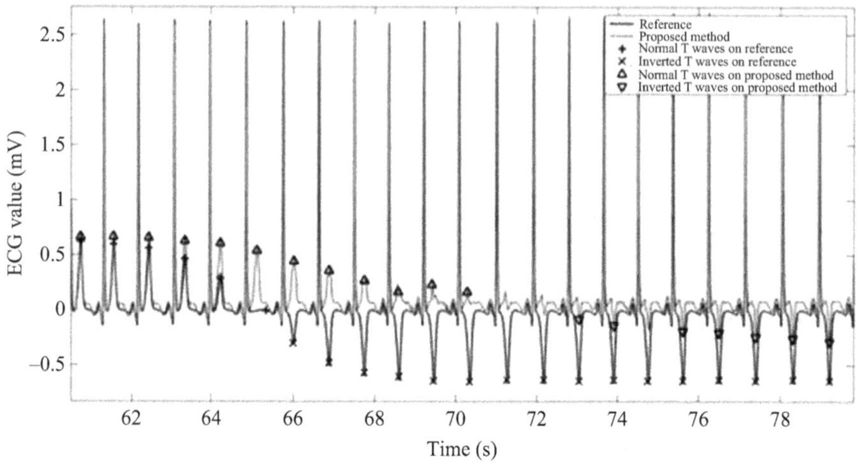

Figure 4.3 Results of ECG signal extraction, and automatic detection of a simulated T wave inversion. The annotations were obtained by using an automatic technique (ecgpuwave)

(φ_k^n), as the foetal cardiac rhythm is usually in the order of magnitude of twice the maternal ECG. The performance of this approach was assessed with SNR and QT interval measurements on a small dataset of simulated data, by using an in-house simulator [32], which is available on Physionet [23]. The Bayesian filtering approach outperformed other techniques, with a 14.1 dB SNR improvement and a median absolute error on QT measurements of 4.0 ms, well within the manual annotation error range.

4.7 Detection of pathological beats

As described in the previous sections, the ECG model-based filtering has been shown to be a powerful tool for the processing and analysis of ECG signals. Nevertheless, the performance of the different techniques relies on feeding the system with the correct *prior* knowledge, that is the morphology of the beats. However, the ECG can also be pathological, and therefore contains beats with a different morphology. The accuracy of the denoising and any other analysis would be greatly affected by such beats, and necessitate an improvement to the approach.

Bayesian filtering is a very versatile tool, in that it not only allows for estimating the hidden variables, but also informs on the level of confidence in these estimations. It offers the possibility to assess how a new observation is likely to have been generated by the ECG model and its given parameters. Bayesian filtering, relying on this property, have been proposed for novelty detection, that is detecting unexpected measurements in a time-series [33]. In our context, such an approach could therefore be used for the detection of noisy segments or episodes, but also pathological beats. This was the approach suggested by Sayadi *et al.* in order to detect Premature Ventricular Contraction, for whom the ECG morphology is different from the normal beats, which have been parameterised [34].

This technique is interesting, able to detect non-normal beats, but the processing or analysis of such beats is not possible, as no *prior* information is known for such beats. Some patients have very pathological rhythm, and the amount of pathological beats can be high (50% in case of bigeminy). An approach, which deals with such beats as being extremely unlikely and rare events, is therefore not optimal. It is thus necessary to extend this methodology to model pathological beats as well. SKF has already been described [17] and offers the possibility for such an extension, where the morphology of the normal and pathological beats can be modelled as different modes, and the mode with the highest likelihood over a given cardiac cycle can be selected. In this section, the heartbeat classification and filtering technique suggested in [35] will be described.

4.7.1 Problem formulation

Let us assume that a given number M of modes, which represent the morphology of each of the main type of heartbeats for one patient, is known. These morphologies being known, it is possible to estimate the state-space models for each of these modes. These M different Bayesian filtering can be run in parallel, and the likelihood can be computed for each new measurement as described in (4.7). Standard SKF allows to switch modes for every new samples, but physiologically such a switch only occurs at the start of a new heartbeat, that is the mode remains the same over a whole cardiac cycle. In order to simulate this behaviour, the mode cycle likelihood (l^C) computed over the cardiac cycle is given by:

$$l^C(i) = \int_{k_1}^{k_2} \exp\left(\left(\frac{\varphi_k - \pi/3}{\sigma_\theta}\right)^2\right) \times l_k(i)dk, \tag{4.18}$$

where φ is the artificial observed phase signal, k_1 is the sample such that $\varphi_{k_1} = -\pi$ and k_2 is defined such that $\varphi_{k_2} = \pi$, and σ_θ is a parameter defining the width of an exponential window.

The classification of the heartbeats is therefore achieved by selecting the mode with the highest cycle likelihood (l^C).

However, the ECG signals can be corrupted by noise or artefacts, or they might be some very unusual or rare events, which cannot be modelled easily. The SKF technique can be extended in order to allow some flexibility by including the possibility for novelty detection. Taking inspiration from Quinn *et al.* [36], an extra mode was introduced and called X-factor. The X-factor is a mode for which no *prior* information on the dynamics of the heartbeat is incorporated. The X-factor only relies on the smoothness of an ECG signal, and attacks the filtering problem with a target tracking angle. The ECG value is assumed to be the target, whose position (x_k) is evolving according to its speed (dx_k), which is modelled as following a random walk. The state-space formalism can be written as follows:

(i) evolution equations

$$\begin{cases} x_k = x_{k-1} + \dfrac{dx_{k-1}}{f_s} + \nu_{1,k} \\ dx_k = dx_{k-1} + \nu_{2,k} \end{cases}, \tag{4.19}$$

f_s being the sampling frequency, and $\nu_{\mathbf{k}}$ being the state noise.

(ii) observation equations

$$\{ s_k = x_k + v_{1,k}, \tag{4.20}$$

s_k being the observed signal (ECG) and $v_{1,k}$ the observation noise.

The SKF is finally run over $M + 1$ modes, and for each heartbeat the mode with the highest cycle likelihood is selected.

4.7.2 Parameter initialisation

In the previous section, we have assumed that the different modes were known, and that Gaussian parameters have been initialised properly. The procedure for this semi-automatic initialisation is described here.

First, the ECG signal has to be segmented around the R peaks, which are detected using standard detection algorithms. The segmentation is performed by mapping the RR intervals to a cyclic phase as described in [22], each cycle is then segmented from $-\pi$ to π radians.

Let us assume that a dominant class (heartbeat) and its typical morphology is known, if not this dominant class is supposed to be the first heartbeat of a given signal. Each new heartbeat is then compared to the dominant class morphology using a cross-correlation measure. If this value is over a given threshold, t_c, then the heartbeat is added to the dominant class. If not, a new class containing this new heartbeat is created. Subsequent cross-correlations are then performed on both classes. If the cross-correlation is not above t_c for either of the new groups, then the heartbeat is put in the third class. This process continues for all heartbeats.

At the end of this step, all the heartbeats have been assembled into different clusters. Only the relevant modes are kept for the estimation of the Gaussian parameters. The relevant modes are determined by counting the number of cycles in each cluster, and keeping only the clusters with a given number of cycles (t_r). The Gaussian parameters for each of the relevant modes are then estimated using the same process as described in the subsection 4.4.2.

The different classes have therefore been parameterised at this stage, and the only missing parameter is their label, that is whether the heartbeat is ventricular or normal. This labelling relies on the cardiologist or local expert to interpret the type

Table 4.3 Scores obtained on the DS2 (MIT-BIH arrhythmia database)

Technique	*Se*	*+P*	F_1
de Chazal [37]*	86.5	42.7	57.1
Llamedo *et al.* [38]*	95.3	28.6	44.0
automatic Llamedo *et al.* [39][a,*]	82.1	77.9	79.9
assisted Llamedo *et al.* [39]‡	91.4	96.9	94.1
SKF with X-factor[b,†]	90.5	99.96	95.2

[a]0.12% of the heartbeats were not classified.
[b]3.2% of the heartbeats were classified as X-factor, and therefore discarded for the computation of these statistics.
*These techniques are completely automatic.
‡12 cluster centroids were annotated by an expert.
†An average of 3 cluster centroids were annotated by an expert, with 5th percentile of 1 beat and 95th of 6 beats.

of each cluster, although automated approaches could also be possible. For instance, a heartbeat classifier based on features such as QRS width could be used [39,40], followed by a majority voting among all the heartbeats constituting a cluster.

4.7.3 Benchmarking and results

The method was assessed with respect to the performance of ventricular heartbeat classification. Confusion matrices were created for the SKF approach on a test sets (DS2 of the MIT-BIH arrhythmia database) separated from the train set. The proposed SKF approach was compared to state-of-the-art beat classification techniques described by Chazal *et al.* [37], Llamedo and Martínez [38], and the two techniques described by Llamedo and Martínez [39]. Although these techniques provide complete heartbeat classification, we have only considered their capability of ventricular beat classification, in order to compare with the SKF approach presented in this chapter.

The proposed technique detection of ventricular beats was assessed using the sensitivity (*Se*) and positive predictivity (*+P*) as suggested in [41], but also in terms of F_1 (which is the harmonic mean of *Se* and *+P*, and penalises False Positives and False Negatives equally).

The results are assembled in Table 4.3. It can be seen that the SKF results are higher than the other state-of-the-art techniques, the scores could even be improved if the Fusion beats were considered separately. Interested readers are referred to [35] for further results and analysis. Examples of the processing are depicted in Figure 4.4. A special emphasis on the interpretation of the X-factor and his role as signal quality index has been put in [42].

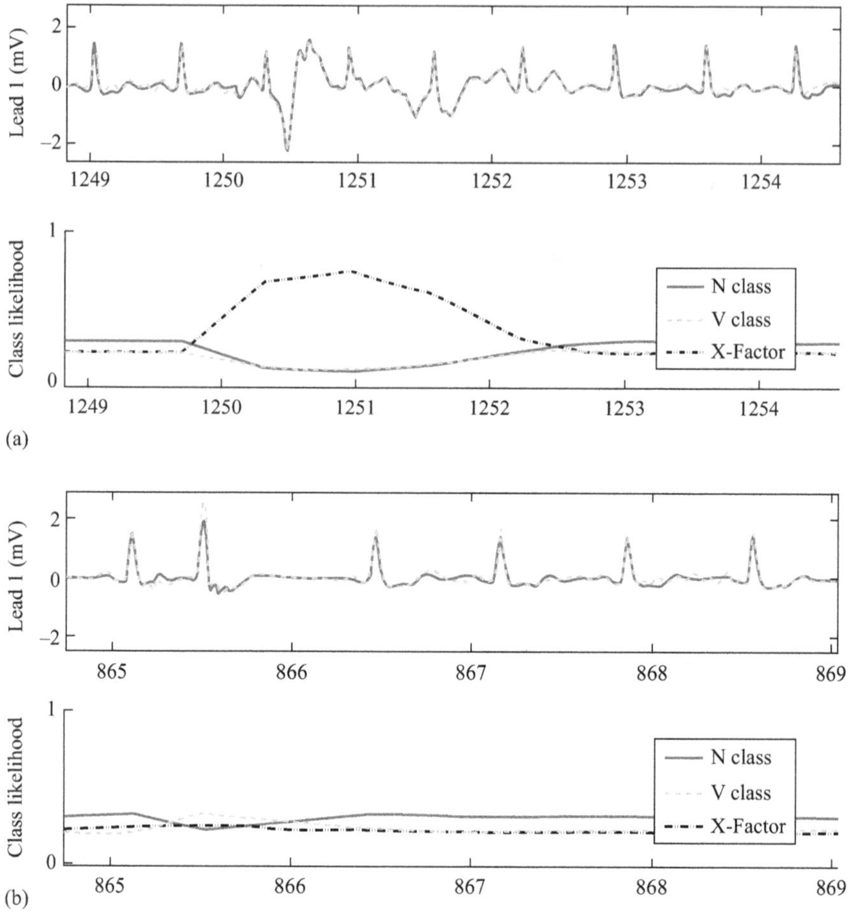

Figure 4.4 Example of the SKF filtering. The top row contains the ECG signal with both the raw signal (solid line) and the denoised signal (dashed line). The second row shows the class likelihood for each mode: normal beat (solid line), ventricular beat (dashed line) and X-factor (dash-dotted line). (a) An example of a noisy segment classified as X-factor. (b) An example of ventricular beat classification

4.8 Discussion

This chapter presented how the ECG model is well suited for Bayesian filtering, and how such an approach can be applied for several problems and analysis. As described in the Section 4.2.2, non-linear techniques need to be applied. Most of the papers only used the EKF for simplicity, and given that results obtained were satisfactory. However, the seminal paper by Sameni *et al.* has analysed the impact on the non-linear Bayesian filtering applied, and tested the effect of extended Kalman smoother, unscented Kalman filtering and particle filtering. It was shown that small improvements could be achieved using more complex techniques, but the significance of these improvements did not justify the increase of complexity. Interested readers are referred to the seminal paper by Sameni *et al.* on how to improve the filtering results, especially regarding the adjustment of the parameters to non-stationary situations, and varying level of noise.

The formalism of the methods presented in this chapter has been restricted to the analysis of a single ECG lead. However, the Bayesian filtering approach can easily be extended to multi-lead analysis. This extension can be done by adding a new observation per lead, that is measuring each new signal, and by adding new components in the state vector, for the representation of this new signal. The same phase signal and the angular position component will be used across all the leads. Bayesian filtering can therefore be used for the simultaneous processing of a whole 12 leads ECG signal. Moreover, this paradigm can be extended to any physiological signal, and is not restricted to ECG data. It has been shown that pulsatile signals can also be modelled by using Gaussian waves, and therefore be processed simultaneously with ECG signals [43,44]. Such an approach has been proposed for the analysis of physiological data acquired in Intensive Care Unit, in order to reduce false alarms [45].

The success of these Bayesian filtering techniques relies on a proper initialisation of the parameters. Bayesian filtering does indeed rely on *prior* knowledge of the system. In the given problem, the *prior* knowledge represents the dynamics of the signal, given by the parameters of the Gaussian waves. The initialisation has been the subject of some research, as the non-linear optimisation is highly dependent on the initial values. Clifford suggested the use of fiducial point detection for estimating the initial values [19,20], whereas Sameni *et al.* considered a semi-automatic approach by using manual initialisation of these values [22]. More recently, Andreotti *et al.* suggested wavelet delineation techniques for setting the initial values [46], whereas Behar *et al.* and Oster *et al.* considered a random search approach for the setting of the initial values [31,35,47]. Although the initialisation of the Gaussian wave parameters is one of the keys for the success of the technique, other parameters need to be set appropriately. The noise covariance matrices, both process and observation, are key parameters for an accurate filtering of the physiological signals. These matrices are adjusted so as to represent the level of confidence to have in each of the equations of the model. In noisy situations, it is effectively normal to have a higher level of trust in the process equation than in the noisy measurements and inversely in clean situations the measurements should be trusted more than the process equation. Sameni *et al.* discussed ways of dealing with the typical non-stationarities with physiological signals, and how the parameters can be adjusted with evolving levels of noise [22]. They discuss the possibility of using the innovation in order to adjust the measurement noise covariance. The use of external Signal Quality Index has also been suggested for optimally adjusting the noise parameters in state-space methods [42].

The ECG model-based filtering also relies on the observation of an artificial phase signal, which is created by detecting the position of the R peaks. It is often assumed that the detection of these peaks is an easy task. Although it is the most easily recognisable feature of an ECG signal, peak detection might still be a complicated task especially with high level of noise. Building an analysis technique on the knowledge of these R peaks positions is therefore a limitation for the Bayesian filtering approach. Moreover, the artificial phase is created as following a linear evolution between two R peaks, which is an overly simplistic assumption. Sameni *et al.* revealed that the filtering performance were affected during episodes of high rate variability, as in practice the ventricular diastolic phase is evolving more than the systolic phase. A solution has been suggested to this problem by incorporating the speed variable ω in the state vector [48]. By doing so, the technique is able to adjust the speed so as to simulate non-linear evolution of the phase. Nevertheless with such an approach, it was still recommended to observe the artificial phase signal. The use of Gaussian processes (GPs) has been recently suggested for solving the source separation problem, and extracting foetal ECG from abdominal recordings [49]. This approach is quite interesting, as it does not need the construction of the artificial phase signal, which is quite difficult in the case of fECG, where the foetal R peak amplitudes are low and therefore very difficult to detect without further processing.

A range of ECG analysis techniques have been described in this chapter. These techniques rely on the modelling of the dynamics of the ECG signal, and are based on Bayesian filtering. This approach has been shown to be highly versatile and offer an elegant solution for a wide range of ECG analysis applications, ranging from denoising [22,50,51], delineation [24], source separation [29,31] and classification [34,35,42].

References

[1] Einthoven W. The different forms of the human electrocardiogram and their signification. *Lancet* 1912; 179(4622):853–61.

[2] Clifford GD, Clifton D. Wireless technology in disease management and medicine, *Annu Rev Med* 2012;63:479–92.

[3] Clifford GD, Azuaje F, McSharry PE. (eds.). Advanced methods and tools for ECG Analysis. Artech House Publishing, Boston/London; 2006. 384pp. ISBN 1-58053-966-1.

[4] Kohler B-U, Hennig C, Orglmeister R. The principles of software QRS detection. *IEEE Eng Med Biol Mag* 2002;21(1):42–57.

[5] Thakor NV, Zhu Y-S. Applications of adaptive filtering to ECG analysis: noise cancellation and arrhythmia detection. *IEEE Trans Biomed Eng* 1991;38(8):785–94.

[6] Martínez JP, Almeida R, Olmos S, Rocha AP, Laguna P. A wavelet-based ECG delineator: evaluation on standard databases. *IEEE Trans Biomed Eng* 2004;51(4): 570–81.

[7] Moody GB, Mark RG. QRS morphology representation and noise estimation using the karhunen-loeve transform. In: Computers in cardiology 1989, proceedings, IEEE; 1989. p. 269–72.

[8] He T, Clifford G, Tarassenko L. Application of independent component analysis in removing artefacts from the electrocardiogram. *Neural Comput Appl* 2006;15(2):105–16.

[9] Clifford G, Tarassenko L, Townsend N. One-pass training of optimal architecture auto-associative neural network for detecting ectopic beats. *Electron Lett* 2001;37(18):1126–7.

[10] Mar T, Zaunseder S, Martínez JP, Llamedo M, Poll R. Optimization of ECG classification by means of feature selection. *IEEE Trans Biomed Eng* 2011;58(8):2168–77.

[11] Hughes NP, Tarassenko L, Roberts SJ. Markov models for automated ECG interval analysis. In: Advances in neural information processing systems. 2003.

[12] Kalman RE. A new approach to linear filtering and prediction problems. *J Fluids Eng* 1960;82(1):35–45.

[13] Grewal MS, Andrews AP. Applications of Kalman filtering in aerospace 1960 to the present [historical perspectives]. *IEEE Control Syst* 2010;30(3):69–78.

[14] Julier SJ, Uhlmann JK. Unscented filtering and nonlinear estimation. *Proc IEEE* 2004;92(3):401–22.

[15] Arulampalam MS, Maskell S, Gordon N, Clapp T. A tutorial on particle filters for online nonlinear/non-Gaussian Bayesian tracking. *IEEE Trans Signal Process* 2002;50(2):174–88.

[16] Doucet A, de Freitas N, Gordon N. Sequential Monte Carlo methods in practice. Springer, New York; 2001.

[17] Murphy K. Switching Kalman filters. Dept. of Computer Science, University of California, Berkeley, Technical Report; 1998.

[18] McSharry PE, Clifford GD, Tarassenko L, Smith LA. A dynamical model for generating synthetic electrocardiogram signals. *IEEE Trans Biomed Eng* 2003;50(3):289–94.

[19] Clifford G, Shoeb A, McSharry P, Janz B. Model-based filtering, compression and classification of the ECG. *Int J Bioelectromagn* 2005;7(1):158–61.

[20] Clifford GD. A novel framework for signal representation and source separation: applications to filtering and segmentation of biosignals. *J Biol Syst* 2006;14(2):169–83.

[21] Clifford G, Villarroel M. Model-based determination of QT intervals. In: Computers in cardiology, 2006, IEEE; 2006. p. 357–60.

[22] Sameni R, Shamsollahi MB, Jutten C, Clifford GD. A nonlinear Bayesian filtering framework for ECG denoising. *IEEE Trans Biomed Eng* 2007;54(12):2172–85.

[23] Goldberger AL, Amaral LA, Glass L, Hausdorff JM, Ivanov PC, Mark RG, *et al.* Physiobank, physiotoolkit, and physionet components of a new research resource for complex physiologic signals. *Circulation* 2000;101(23):e215–20.

[24] Sayadi O, Shamsollahi M. A model-based Bayesian framework for ECG beat segmentation. *Physiol Meas* 2009;30(3):335.

[25] Moody GB, Koch H, Steinhoff U. The physionet/computers in cardiology challenge 2006: Qt interval measurement. In: Computers in cardiology, 2006, IEEE; 2006. p. 313–16.

[26] Sayadi O, Shamsollahi MB. Model-based fiducial points extraction for baseline wandered electrocardiograms. *IEEE Trans Biomed Eng* 2008;55(1):347–51.

[27] James CJ, Hesse CW. Independent component analysis for biomedical signals. *Physiol Meas* 2005;26(1):R15.

[28] Sameni R, Jutten C, Shamsollahi MB. Multichannel electrocardiogram decomposition using periodic component analysis. *IEEE Trans Biomed Eng* 2008;55(8):1935–40.

[29] Oster J, Geist M, Pietquin O, Clifford GD. Filtering of pathological ventricular rhythms during MRI scanning. *Int J Bioelectromagn* 2013;15(1):54–9.

[30] Oster J, Llinares R, Payne S, Tse ZTH, Schmidt EJ, Clifford GD. Comparison of three artificial models of the magnetohydrodynamic effect on the electrocardiogram. *Comput Method Biomech Biomed Eng* 2015;18(13):1400–17.

[31] Behar J, Andreotti F, Oster J, Clifford GD. A Bayesian filtering framework for accurate extracting of the non-invasive fECG morphology. In: Computing in cardiology conference (CinC), 2014, IEEE; 2014. p. 53–6.

[32] Behar J, Andreotti F, Zaunseder S, Li Q, Oster J, Clifford GD. An ECG simulator for generating maternal-foetal activity mixtures on abdominal ECG recordings. *Physiol Meas* 2014;35(8):1537.

[33] Pimentel MA, Clifton DA, Clifton L, Tarassenko L. A review of novelty detection. *Signal Processing* 2014;99, 215–249.

[34] Sayadi O, Shamsollahi MB, Clifford GD. Robust detection of premature ventricular contractions using a wave-based Bayesian framework. *IEEE Trans Biomed Eng* 2010;57(2):353–62.

[35] Oster J, Behar J, Johnson AEW, Sayadi O, Nemati S, Clifford GD. Semi-supervised ECG beat classification and novelty detection based on switching Kalman filters. *IEEE Trans Biomed Eng* 2015;62:2125–34.

[36] Quinn J, Williams C, McIntosh N. Factorial switching linear dynamical systems applied to physiological condition monitoring. *IEEE Trans Pattern Anal Mach Intell*, IEEE Transactions on 2009;31(9):1537–51.

[37] de Chazal P, O'Dwyer M, Reilly RB. Automatic classification of heartbeats using ECG morphology and heartbeat interval features. *IEEE Trans Biomed Eng* 2004;51(7):1196–206.

[38] Llamedo M, Martínez JP. Heartbeat Classification using Feature Selection driven by Database generalization criteria. *IEEE Trans Biomed Eng* 2011;58(3):616–25.

[39] Llamedo M, Martínez JP. An automatic patient-adapted ecg heartbeat classifier allowing expert assistance. *IEEE Trans Biomed Eng* 2012;59(8):2312–20.

[40] Oster J., Tarassenko L. Automated ECG ventricular beat detection with switching Kalman Filters. In: Computing in Cardiology (Cinc). Vancouver, IEEE; 2016.

[41] ANSI/AAMI:EC57. Testing and reporting performance results of cardiac rhythm and ST-segment measurement algorithms; 1998.

[42] Oster J, Clifford G. Signal quality indices for state space electrophysiological signal processing and vice versa. *Adv State Space Meth Neural Clin Data* 2015;15:345–66.

[43] Clifford GD, cSharry PE. A realistic coupled nonlinear artificial ECG, BP, and respiratory signal generator for assessing noise performance of biomedical

signal processing algorithms. In: Second international symposium on fluctuations and noise, International Society for Optics and Photonics; 2004. p. 290–301.

[44] Sayadi O, Shamsollahi MB. Utility of a nonlinear joint dynamical framework to model a pair of coupled cardiovascular signals. *IEEE J Biomed Health Inform* 2013;17(4):881–90.

[45] Sayadi O, Shamsollahi MB. Life-threatening arrhythmia verification in ICU patients using the joint cardiovascular dynamical model and a Bayesian filter. *IEEE Trans Biomed Eng* 2011;58(10):2748–57.

[46] Andreotti F, Behar J, Oster J, Clifford GD, Malberg H, Zaunseder S. Optimized modelling of maternal ECG beats using the stationary wavelet transform. In: Computing in Cardiology Conference (CinC), 2014, IEEE; 2014. p. 325–8.

[47] Bergstra J, Bengio Y. Random search for hyper-parameter optimization. *J Mach Learn Res* 2012;13:281–305.

[48] Akhbari M, Shamsollahi MB, Jutten C, Coppa B. ECG denoising using angular velocity as a state and an observation in an extended Kalman filter framework, In: Engineering in Medicine and Biology Society (EMBC), 2012 Annual International Conference of the IEEE, IEEE; 2012. p. 2897–900.

[49] Noorzadeh S, Niknazar M, Rivet B, Fontecave-Jallon J, Guméry P-Y, Jutten C. Modeling quasi-periodic signals by a non-parametric model: application on fetal ECG extraction. In: Engineering in Medicine and Biology Society (EMBC), 36th Annual International Conference of the IEEE, IEEE; 2014. p. 1889–92.

[50] Oster J, Pietquin O, Kraemer M, Felblinger J. Nonlinear Bayesian filtering for denoising of electrocardiograms acquired in a magnetic resonance environment. *IEEE Trans Biomed Eng* 2010;57(7):1628–38.

[51] Sayadi O, Shamsollahi MB. ECG denoising and compression using a modified extended kalman filter structure. *IEEE Trans Biomed Eng* 2008;55(9):2240–8.

Chapter 5

The power of tensor decompositions in biomedical applications

Borbála Hunyadi, Sabine Van Huffel and Maarten De Vos

5.1 Introduction to tensors

Appropriately representing data is crucial for gaining insight and effectively approaching any given problem at hand. We will illustrate in this chapter the use of a particular representation, the tensor or higher order representation, for biomedical data analysis. Tensor algebraic concepts will be introduced by means of easily interpretable examples and visualizations of real-world biomedical problems. We also give a formal definition for the most important tensor notions and operations. For a wider number of examples outside biomedical applications, we refer the reader to References 1,2.

A single observation is represented by a scalar value s. For example, the brain potential of a given subject observed at a particular electroencephalogram (EEG) electrode 300 ms after a visual stimulus onset can be 1.7 μV. However, a single potential value cannot tell much about the overall brain response. We may want to make a series of observations or measure a signal over time, in which case our data is represented by a vector $v \in R^{I_1}$. To continue the previous example, the brain activity at this electrode observed within 0.5 s after the stimulus, sampled at 250 Hz, results in a vector of length 125. Further, we may want to observe the brain activity at different locations over the scalp. The multichannel EEG signal is now represented in a matrix $B \in \mathbb{R}^{I_1 \times I_2}$ where I_1 is the number of recording electrodes. Repeated experiments can provide information about an even bigger picture, such as the adaptation of the brain to consecutive stimuli. Such data is represented in a third-order array or tensor $T \in \mathbb{R}^{I_1 \times I_2 \times I_3}$, where I_3 is the number of consecutive experiments. The concept can be generalized to even higher order tensors $T \in \mathbb{R}^{I_1 \times I_2 \times \cdots \times I_n}$ by explicitly including more *modes*, for example when performing EEG measurements in different subjects, under different recording conditions, etc.

It is clear that in many situations the observed data naturally takes the form of a tensor. One may be tempted to store and handle such data as a series of matrices. *Matrix unfolding* (see Figure 5.1) may allow easier visualization on a 2D screen, and can be manipulated by means of well-established linear algebra tools. However, persisting

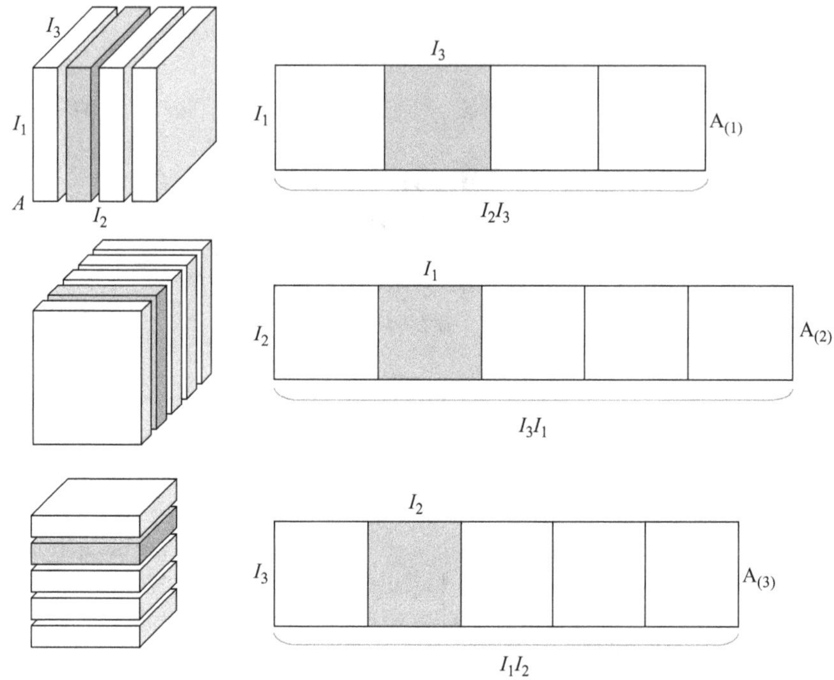

Figure 5.1 The three possible unfoldings of a 3D tensor into matrices along the three different modes

with the original tensor representations can be very beneficial for the following two reasons.

First, a tensor representation allows to preserve some crucial information residing in the multiway structure. For example, the brain response in a certain cognitive task may be modulated by different levels of difficulty, and may show differences in various pathological conditions. These two effects can be studied separately using different matrix representations, i.e. with a matrix which stores the brain response of each patient in each row, and another matrix with the brain responses at each difficulty level in each row, respectively. However, one should realize that the brain responses may be modulated differently in the different pathological groups. The interaction of these two effects will be hidden in a traditional matrix decomposition while it will become clear when studying the data in the inherent tensor representation, where the brain responses are stored along the *rows*, the patients are organized along the *columns* and the different difficulty levels are organized along the *tubes* (Figure 5.2).

The second motivation for holding on to tensor representation is related to some interesting mathematical properties of tensor manipulation techniques. We are going to demonstrate these in the following section.

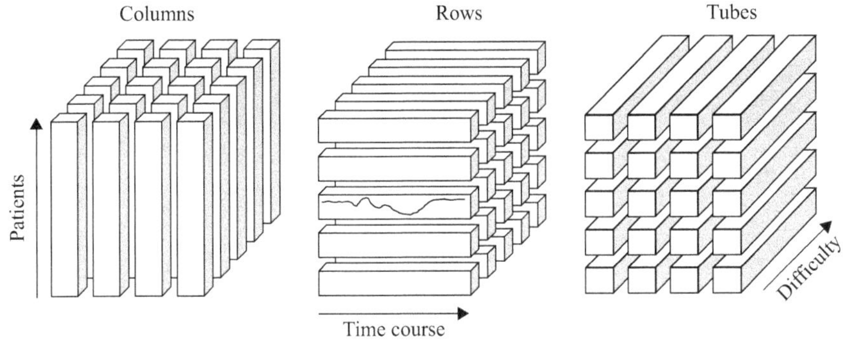

Figure 5.2 The data in a 3D tensor are arranged along the different modes in so-called rows, columns and tubes. In biomedical applications, the variation in different physical quantities is represented in each mode. For example, in a cognitive EEG experiment the time course of the EEG response is stored along the direction of the rows, data from different patients are organized along the columns and the different difficulty levels are organized along the tubes

5.2 Tensor decomposition techniques

5.2.1 Decomposition of matrices

Some of very common challenges in biomedical data processing include the high dimensionality of the data and low signal-to-noise ratios, due to the presence of measurement and physiological noise, superimposed on the signals under study. A basic concept in linear algebra is the singular value decomposition (SVD), which might offer some benefit when tackling these problems. Formally, the SVD of a matrix $M \in \mathbb{R}^{I_1 \times I_2}$ is the following factorization:

$$M = USV^T \tag{5.1}$$

where $U \in \mathbb{R}^{I_1 \times I_1}$ and $V \in \mathbb{R}^{I_2 \times I_2}$ are orthogonal matrices, V^T is the transpose of V and S is a non-negative diagonal matrix. The columns of U and V, denoted by $\mathbf{u}_i$ and $\mathbf{u}_i$, are called the left and right singular vectors of M, respectively. The diagonal elements of S, denoted as s_i, appear in decreasing order and are called the singular values of M. Given that the singular values are distinct, the decomposition is unique up to the joint reflection of u_i and v_i. The number of non-zero singular values is equal to the rank of the matrix, i.e. to the number of linearly independent columns/rows of the matrix. M can also be written as the weighted sum of the outer products of the singular vectors:

$$M = \sum \sigma_r \mathbf{u}_r \circ \mathbf{v}_r \tag{5.2}$$

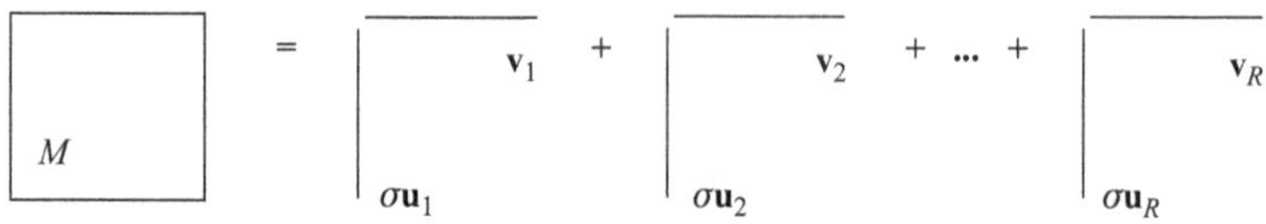

Figure 5.3 SVD of a matrix M in R rank-1 terms

Notice that each term in the summation is rank-1. In fact, the rank R of a matrix M can also be defined as the minimal number of rank-1 terms whose sum equals M. This decomposition is visualized in Figure 5.3.

Truncating the SVD to the first $\rho < R$ terms gives rise to a matrix Y which is the best *rank-ρ* approximation of the matrix M in the least squares sense, i.e. $\|X - Y\|^2$ is minimal. As such, SVD is an interesting tool for data compression: a considerable amount of variance in the data can be preserved by storing only the first ρ singular vectors and values. This amounts to the storage of $\rho(1 + I_1 + I_2)$ elements instead of $I_1 I_2$ elements. Moreover, small singular values typically correspond to noise, therefore, truncation at a well-chosen rank has denoising effects.

Now let us consider the problem of processing multidimensional observations which arise as a linear mixture of a number of underlying source signals. Formally, let $x(t) = [x_1(t), \ldots, x_p(t))] \in \mathbb{R}^P$ be the observed signal at time instant t and $s(t) = [s_1(t), \ldots, s_N(t)] \in \mathbb{R}^N$ the underlying sources. Then $x(t)$ can be written as

$$x(t) = As(t) \tag{5.3}$$

where A is an unknown mapping from R^N to R^P. In *blind source separation* the goal is to find the sources $s(t)$ and the mapping or mixing matrix A. The above equation can also be written in a matrix form, in which case we talk about the *factorization of the matrix X*:

$$X = AS \tag{5.4}$$

Note that there are in general an infinite number of solutions for the matrix factorization problem. That is, if AS is a valid solution, then for any invertible matrix M:

$$X = (AM)(M^{-1}S) = \widetilde{A}\widetilde{S} \tag{5.5}$$

However, in blind source separation (BSS), the uniqueness of the obtained solution is crucial. We aim to be able to interpret the results, i.e. match $\mathbf{s}(t)$ (the rows of S) with the true underlying sources, and perhaps remove sources of no interest and reconstruct the clean signal.

In order to find a unique solution for the BSS problem, various decomposition techniques impose different constraints. For example, the so-called principal component analysis (PCA) assumes that the sources underlying the observed signals are mutually uncorrelated. Therefore, it projects the data onto a new, orthonormal basis. Note, still, that there is no unique solution to this problem, as any rotation of the obtained basis is a valid solution as well. This phenomenon is called the rotational invariance property of PCA. One possible solution is to take the right singular vectors, i.e. the columns of V from the SVD of X.

Another popular class of methods, independent component analysis (ICA), imposes a statistical diversity among the underlying sources. In case the observations are non-negative, as well as the sources and the mixing system are presumably non-negative, non-negative matrix factorization (NMF) may provide a solution. However, the success of these approaches strongly depends on the validity of these assumptions, which, unfortunately, are often violated in reality.

5.2.2 Decomposition of tensors

In this section, we will generalize the above matrix concepts to tensors. Focusing on different properties of the SVD, we will obtain two different generalizations for it. The new higher order decompositions will share some powerful properties with SVD. In fact, a possible generalization of the SVD even resolves the ambiguity issue of matrix factorization, as tensor factorizations are unique under mild conditions.

5.2.2.1 Higher order SVD

First, we will give a generalization of SVD considering (5.1). That is, we are looking for a series of orthogonal projections which will transform the tensor $\mathcal{X}$ into an all-orthogonal and ordered tensor $\mathcal{S}$. Every $\mathcal{X} \in \mathbb{R}^{I_1 \times I_2 \times \cdots \times I_N}$ can be approximated by the product

$$\mathcal{X} = \mathcal{S} \times_1 U_1^{(1)} \times_2 U_1^{(2)} \cdots \times_N U_1^{(N)} \tag{5.6}$$

where the operator $\times_n$ denotes the mode-n product between a tensor $\mathcal{T} \in \mathbb{R}^{I_1 \times I_2 \times \cdots \times I_N}$ and a matrix $U \in \mathbb{R}^{J_n \times I_n}$, defined as

$$(\mathcal{T} \times_n U)_{i_1 i_2 \ldots j_n \ldots i_N} = \sum_{i_n} t_{i_1 i_2 \ldots i_n \ldots i_N} u_{j_n i_n} \tag{5.7}$$

Analogously to the product of two matrices, U makes linear combinations of the columns of $\mathcal{T}$. The product in (5.6), termed higher order singular value decomposition (HOSVD), has the following properties:

- $U^{(n)} = \left[\mathbf{u}_1^{(n)} \mathbf{u}_2^{(n)} \cdots \mathbf{u}_{I_n}^{(2)}\right]$
- $\mathcal{S} \in \mathbb{R}^{I_1 \times I_2 \times \cdots \times I_N}$ is a tensor with subtensors $\mathcal{S}_{i_n=\alpha}$, obtained by fixing the nth index to α, show the following properties:
  - all-orthogonality:
    $\langle \mathcal{S}_{i_n=\alpha}, \mathcal{S}_{i_n=\beta} \rangle = 0$ when $\alpha \neq \beta$
  - ordering:
    $\|\mathcal{S}_{i_n=1}\| \geq \|\mathcal{S}_{i_n=}2\| \geq \cdots \geq \|\mathcal{S}_{i_n=I_n}\| \geq 0$
    for all n.

The Frobenius-norms of $\|\mathcal{S}_{i_n=i}\|$ are called the n-mode singular values of $\mathcal{X}$ and the vectors $\mathbf{u}_i^n$ are the n-mode singular vectors. The values $I_1, I_2, \ldots, I_N$ correspond to the ranks of the different matrix unfoldings of $\mathcal{X}$ along the different modes. The n-tuple I_n is called the multilinear rank of the tensor $\mathcal{X}$. A graphical representation of the decomposition in case of a third-order tensor is given in Figure 5.4.

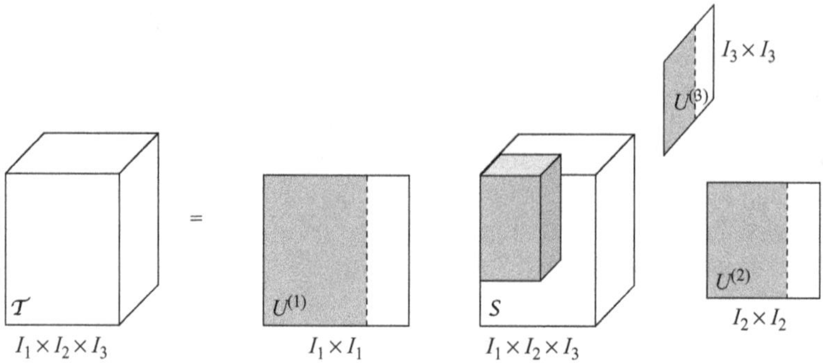

Figure 5.4 Visualization of the higher order singular value decomposition of a third-order tensor $\mathcal{T}$

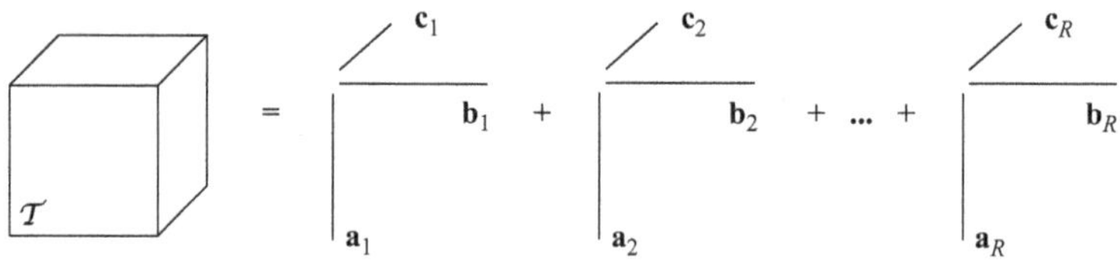

Figure 5.5 CPD of a tensor $\mathcal{T}$ in R rank-1 terms

By dropping the orthogonality constraints, we arrive to the so-called Tucker3 model:

$$\mathcal{X} = \mathcal{G} \times_1 V_1^{(1)} \times_2 V_1^{(2)} \cdots \times_N V_1^{(N)} + \mathcal{E} \tag{5.8}$$

Choosing a core tensor $\mathcal{G}$ with smaller dimensions than $\mathcal{X}$, but keeping the error $\mathcal{E}$ sufficiently small, one obtains a good compressed estimate of the original dataset. Therefore, HOSVD is often used for dimensionality reduction and feature extraction.

5.2.2.2 Canonical polyadic decomposition

Another possible generalization of matrix SVD for tensors is considering (5.2), i.e. expansion as a sum of rank-1 terms.

As we have seen in the previous sections, the problem of matrix decomposition is ill posed and additional constraints are needed in order to obtain a unique solution. Interestingly, tensors admit unique decompositions under mild conditions.

Canonical polyadic decomposition (CPD) approximates a third-order tensor $\mathcal{T} \in \mathbb{R}^{I_1 \times I_2 \times I_3}$ with a sum of R rank-1 tensors:

$$\mathcal{T} \approx \sum_{r=1}^{R} \mathbf{a}_r \circ \mathbf{b}_r \circ \mathbf{c}_r \tag{5.9}$$

CPD is visualized in Figure 5.5. Note that the definition is formulated for third-order tensors; however, the model can be extended to higher order tensors in a

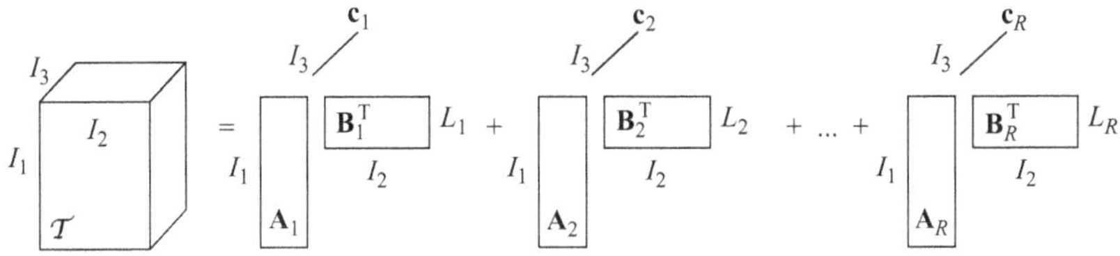

Figure 5.6 BTD-($L_r, L_r, 1$) of a tensor $\mathcal{T}$

straightforward manner. The rank of the tensor is defined as the smallest R for which (5.9) is exact.

The advantage of the CPD model is its uniqueness up to permutation and scaling under the usually fulfilled conditions [3]. A more general framework for uniqueness has been recently presented in References 4, 5.

5.2.2.3 Block term decomposition

The block term decomposition (BTD), introduced in References 6–8, generalizes CPD, as it allows components of low multilinear rank, as opposed to the rank-1 model of CPD. In this chapter, we consider one particular case, decomposition into rank-($L_r, L_r, 1$) terms.

The rank-($L_r, L_r, 1$) BTD of a third-order tensor $\mathcal{T} \in \mathbb{R}^{I_1 \times I_2 \times I_3}$ into a sum of rank-($L_r, L_r, 1$) terms ($1 \leq r \leq R$) is given as

$$\mathcal{T} \approx \sum_{r=1}^{R} \left(\mathbf{A}_r \cdot \mathbf{B}_r^T\right) \circ \mathbf{c}_r \tag{5.10}$$

in which the matrix $\mathbf{D}_r = \mathbf{A}_r \cdot \mathbf{B}_r^T \in \mathbb{R}^{I_1 \times I_2}$ has rank L_r and the vector $\mathbf{c}_r$ is non-zero. In addition to permutation and scaling, inherited from the CPD, the factors $\mathbf{A}_r$ may be post-multiplied by any non-singular matrix $\mathbf{F}_r \in \mathbb{R}^{L_r \times L_r}$, provided that $\mathbf{B}_r^T$ is pre-multiplied by the inverse of $\mathbf{F}_r$. When the matrices $[\mathbf{A}_1 \cdots \mathbf{A}_R]$ and $[\mathbf{B}_1 \cdots \mathbf{B}_R]$ are full column rank and the matrix $[\mathbf{c}_1 \cdots \mathbf{c}_R]$ does not contain collinear columns, the decomposition is guaranteed to be unique up to the above indeterminacies.

Figure 5.6 visualizes the decomposition of a tensor in rank-($L_r, L_r, 1$) terms.

The uniqueness of the decomposition is paramount for BSS, as it allows to give physical interpretation to the results and match the resulting components to true underlying processes. In the matrix case, uniqueness is ensured by various constrains such as orthogonality or independence, which often has no physical meaning or is a too strong assumptions. However, the weaker uniqueness conditions of CPD and BTD are met for a wide range of parameters. This makes these tensor decompositions very interesting tools for various BSS applications in biomedical analysis problems.

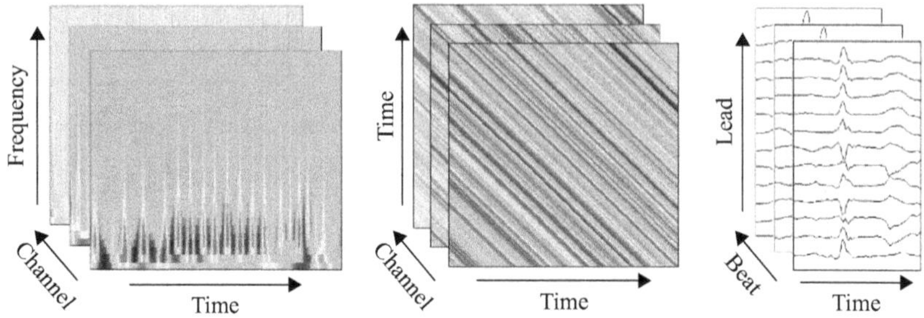

Figure 5.7 Biomedical data are often represented in a tensor. A multichannel EEG measurement may be expanded into the frequency dimension using wavelet transform, resulting in a channel × time × frequency tensor (left). A channel × Hankel matrix representation may be used to model the multichannel EEG as a sum of exponentially damped sinusoids (middle). Epoched multichannel measurements naturally take the form of a tensor. For example, a 12 lead ECG recording segmented around each heartbeat forms a lead × time × beat tensor (right)

5.3 Construction of tensors in biomedical applications

There are several ways to organize biomedical data in a tensor. Often this organization comes naturally from the way the data was collected. At other times a specific tensorization method is applied in order to convey additional information about the data, which is thought to be of interest in the given problem. We will provide several examples of both approaches, some of which are also visualized in Figure 5.7.

5.4 Naturally occurring tensors

5.4.1 Genomic data

Genome-scale signals, such as mRNA expression levels, protein's DNA-binding occupancy levels or copy number variations can be recorded using DNA microarrays. These signals provide information about cellular processes, which may characterize normal or pathological regulatory mechanisms. A single sample of DNA microarray probes the signal of a certain number of genes. Samples may be analysed from multiple patients. Repeated probing under different experimental conditions can give additional insight, such as collecting samples at different time points during different oxidative stress conditions [9]. A tensorial framework allows to integrate these experimental conditions and analyse them simultaneously. Depending on the number of different experimental conditions we wish to vary, we might represent the data as a higher order tensor with dimensions *patients* × *genes* × *experimental condition* 1 × ⋯ × *experimental condition* N.

5.4.2 Repeated multichannel measurements

As already mentioned, biomedical data comes naturally in a multiway form in case of repeated multichannel measurements. For example, the brain activity in response to the task paradigm can be studied using functional magnetic resonance imaging (fMRI). The fMRI signals are measured in a large number of voxels (points on a high-resolution 3D grid defined over the volume of the brain). In order to study the modulation of brain responses to a particular stimulation sequence, Beckmann and Smith [10] organized continuous multisession and multi-subject fMRI data in a *voxel* × *time* × *session* and *voxel* × *time* × *subject* tensor. One can assume that the same task elicits a similar response in the same brain regions across subjects and with similar timing in repeated experiments. However, the strength of the activation may vary in different subjects, or in consecutive sessions performed by the same subjects. In other words, we expect that each source in the brain has the same temporal and spatial signature, and these signatures are scaled over the different subjects or sessions, giving rise to a *rank*-1 structure. As such, the CPD model in (5.9) is appropriate to analyse data. Choosing the appropriate number of components R, each term in the CPD decomposition corresponds to a distinct brain source. Their spatial and temporal characteristics, as well as the modulation over the repetitions can be studied using the signatures $\mathbf{a}_r$, $\mathbf{b}_r$ and $\mathbf{c}_r$.

5.4.3 Epoched multichannel measurements

Relevant information sometimes resides in well-defined epochs within the continuous data, rather than throughout the whole measurement. This is the case for example in event-related potential (ERP) data, where the brain response in each trial, observed on EEG (or MEG), follows a specific waveform within a few hundred milliseconds time-locked to the stimulus onset. During a typical experiment, a few hundred stimuli are presented to a subject. In order to analyse the EEG, the continuous data is broken down in epochs with a predefined window length around the stimuli. Such data is naturally organized in a *channel* × *time* × *trial* tensor. The decomposition of such a tensor can help to find patterns which are representative for one type of stimulus, but not for the other. This information can be utilized in order to recognize users' intention based on their brain responses to different stimuli in a brain–computer interface (BCI) setting [11,12] or extract the localization of repeated spikes during a neonatal seizure [13,14]. Similarly, in case of ECG measurements, it may be important to study the variations in the ECG waveform of the consecutive heartbeats. For example, an alternating pattern in the amplitude of consecutive T waves, called T wave alternans, is a possible indicator for risk of sudden cardiac death. A convenient way to do so is segmenting the ECG into single beats. After appropriate alignment of the T waves, the multi-lead ECG data is represented in a *lead* × *time* × *beats* tensor. In case the patient has T wave alternans, this will be indicated by the presence of an ABABAB pattern in the trial mode signature of an $R = 1$ CPD model [15].

5.5 Tensor expansion of matrix data

We have seen that multichannel time series naturally take the form of a *channel* × *time* matrix. There are several different approaches to extend this to a tensorial representation by expanding the time course into an extra dimension, with the aim of conveying additional information about the signal.

5.5.1 Frequency transformation

The frequency content of biomedical signals often carries crucial information. This information can be conveyed by expanding the time series by means of a time–frequency transformation. This has been exploited in various ways. In a study aiming at classifying different pathological heartbeats, the ECG signal was analysed using a short-time Fourier transformation to construct a *channel* × *time* × *frequency* tensor [16]. Alternatively, wavelet transformation [17,18] or Wigner–Ville distribution [19] is often used to expand the EEG matrix into a tensor. A particularly elegant example is the extraction of stereotypical oscillatory brain sources in the alpha and theta bands, related to resting and mental arithmetic, as revealed by the CPD of wavelet transformed EEG [20]. Studying wavelet transformed ERP data in various subjects and sessions, represented in a five-way tensor, helped to reveal a quantitative difference in occipital gamma-band response between different conditions of a visual paradigm [21]. It could also facilitate the classification of different ERPs in a BCI [22].

A frequency transformation can also be applied over space. Local spatial Fourier transform computed on the EEG matrix gives rise to a *space* × *time* × *wave* × *vector* tensor. This formulation will allow to separate sources with correlated but shortly delayed activities, which is the case when interictal epileptic activity spreads between two regions [23].

5.5.2 Hankel structure

A less intuitive but also powerful way of deriving a tensor representation is by means of the Hankel decomposition. Biomedical signals may be modelled as the sum of exponentially damped sinusoids [24–26]. Such signal model allows unique BSS in rank-$(L_r, L_r, 1)$ terms [27]. To exploit the desired structure, each channel signal, $\mathbf{a}_{ch} = [a_{ch}(1)\ a_{ch}(2)\ \cdots\ a_{ch}(S)]$, $ch = 1, \ldots, I_1$, is mapped to a Hankel matrix as follows:

$$\begin{bmatrix} a_{ch}(1) & a_{ch}(2) & a_{ch}(3) & \cdots & a_{ch}(I_3) \\ a_{ch}(2) & a_{ch}(3) & \cdots & a_{ch}(I_3) & a_{ch}(I_3+1) \\ a_{ch}(3) & \cdots & a_{ch}(I_3) & a_{ch}(I_3+1) & a_{ch}(I_3+2) \\ \vdots & \ddots & \ddots & \ddots & \ddots \\ a_{ch}(I_2) & a_{ch}(I_2+1) & \cdots & a_{ch}(S-1) & a_{ch}(S) \end{bmatrix}$$

One can show that the Hankel matrix associated with a signal generated by L_r distinct poles is *rank-*L_r. For example, the Hankel matrix of a pure exponential is rank-1, while the one of a pure sinusoid or an exponentially damped sinusoid is rank-2. Noisy or non-stationary signals such as chirps give rise to Hankel matrices of higher rank. Since the Hankel mapping is linear, and assuming that the channel signals are linear combinations of the underlying sources, the above matrix is the linear combination of the Hankel matrices associated with the sources. It follows that the multichannel EEG data, represented by a tensor in the form of *Hankel matrix* × *channels*, can be decomposed in block terms of $(L_r, L_r, 1)$ (equation (5.10)) in order to retrieve the original sources. Indeed, it was shown that BTD combined with Hankel tensor representation of EEG successfully extracts and localizes epileptic seizure sources [28], and can also reliably estimate arterial activity from surface ECG for the purpose of analysing arterial fibrillation in cardiology patients [29].

5.5.3 Representation by means of a feature set

Sometimes very specific knowledge is available about which properties of the signal are interesting for a given problem. For example, it has been shown that multiscale entropy (MSE), which can characterize the complexity of a signal at different time scales, shows differences between the electrical brain activity of patients with Alzheimer's disease and healthy controls. Therefore, multichannel MEG measurements of various patients and controls can be analysed where the MSE values are organized in a *subject* × *channel* × *temporal scale* tensor. Subsequent tensor decomposition reveals a characteristic filter, defined by the combination of the spatial and temporal factors. By projecting the data from a new subject onto this subspace, the resulting weight value can give an indication about the class membership of the subject [30]. In different problems, various different signal characteristics or features may be of interest. For example, various time and frequency domain features may be extracted from consecutive EEG windows in order to characterize normal versus epileptic seizure patterns [31]. This way, the multichannel EEG matrix is expanded to a *channel* × *epoch* × *feature* tensor.

5.6 Successful decompositions of biomedical data tensors

Once we have an appropriate tensor representation, a suitable tensor decomposition method must be chosen. The optimal choice depends on three main considerations: the purpose of the data analysis, the a priori information available, and the structure of the data. In case of exploratory data analysis, aiming at understanding hidden factors in the data, or extracting the sources underlying an observed signal, fully unsupervised tensor decompositions would be the method of choice. If some a priori knowledge is available, such as non-negativity of the sources, constraints on the factor matrices can be imposed. For example, non-negative CPD and additional l_1-regularization successfully differentiates tumour tissue types using magnetic resonance spectroscopic imaging [32]. Sometimes complementary observations, e.g. recordings of different signal modalities are available. Knowledge may be transferred between these modalities using coupled tensors decompositions. Labelled data represents even stronger a priori knowledge, which will allow us to use supervised tensor decomposition when the goal is to differentiate classes in grouped data. Finally, the parameters of the tensor decomposition must be set carefully. We will dedicate a separate section to this topic in Section 5.10. In the following sections, we illustrate the use of these different decompositions with several examples.

5.7 Unsupervised tensor decompositions

5.7.1 Blind source separation

Electroencephalography (EEG) measures the changes in brain's electrical activity over time using electrodes placed over the scalp. The electrical potentials, propagating in all directions from their sources, travel through different tissues before reaching the scalp. Therefore, the signals measured at the electrodes are a mixture of the attenuated electrical activity of various brain sources. Besides, EEG also picks up other physiological sources such as muscle (electromyography – EMG) or eye (electrooculography – EOG) activity. It is also very sensitive to non-physiological artefacts, such as power line noise or electrode movement. Therefore, the interpretation of the EEG is often difficult and requires careful preprocessing.

One of the most important applications of EEG is recording and studying epileptic seizure activity. The voltage distribution over the electrodes can give an indication about the location of the seizure source. However, due to involuntary movements and discomfort of the patient, these recordings are often contaminated by artefacts. Below we illustrate how unsupervised tensor decompositions can help to separate the distinct sources underlying the noisy EEG and characterize the seizure source.

The epileptic seizure activity is known as an oscillatory phenomenon, consisting of rhythmical waves in a frequency band below 30 Hz which evolve in amplitude, frequency, and location [33]. Consider for example the seizure segment depicted in Figure 5.8a. The seizure pattern, most prominent on the T1 channel, begins with a few distinct sharp waves. Between 2 and 4 s after the start of the segment, the waves occur more rhythmically four times every second. Later on, from 7 s, the waves become sharper and shorter, repeating more rapidly, at a rate of 8 Hz. Despite of the clear frequency evolution, a short seizure segment, such as the pattern between 2 and 3 s, can be considered stationary. The continuous wavelet transform (CWT) of this stationary seizure segment, visualized in Figure 5.8b, results in an approximately rank-1 $time \times frequency$ matrix where large coefficients are present only at certain frequency scales, corresponding to the rhythm of the seizure pattern. These large coefficients are distributed along the whole length of the segment, following the actual phase of the oscillation. Moreover, we can assume that within this short segment the seizure does not spread yet from its source to other brain regions. Therefore, the seizure pattern will be the most prominent on the channel which is nearby the true source, and will also be visible on adjacent channels, although with moderate amplitude. The voltage distribution of the seizure pattern over the channels thus gives an indication of the location of the seizure source. Notice that if these assumptions are correct, then the seizure pattern can be represented by a rank-1 third-order tensor, which is the outer product of a frequency signature, a temporal signature and a spatial signature.

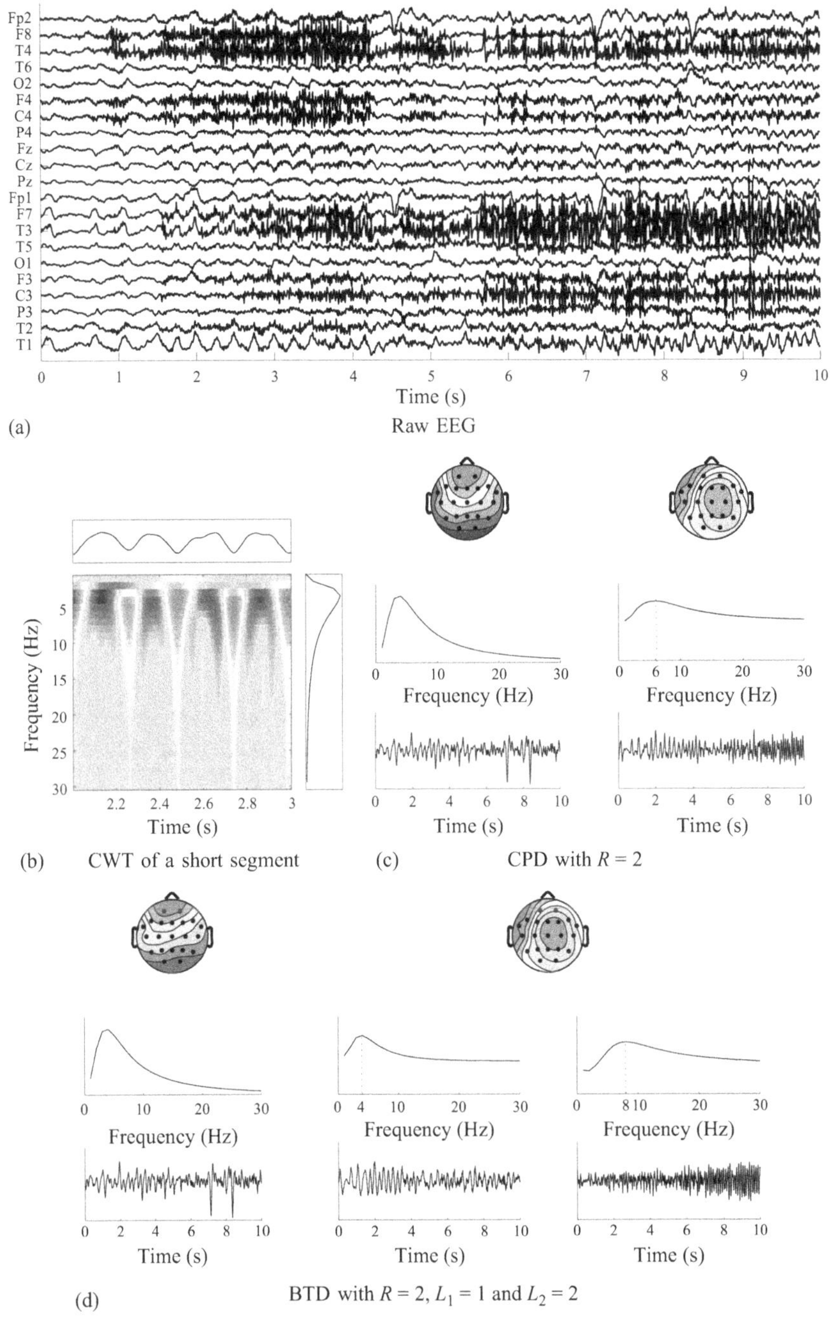

Figure 5.8 *(a) An EEG segment showing epileptic seizure activity. (b) Continuous wavelet transform of a stationary segment is an essentially rank-1 matrix. (c) CPD extracts eye and seizure activity with two components. (d) BTD extracts very similar eye activity, but captures more detailed features of the frequency content of the seizure pattern*

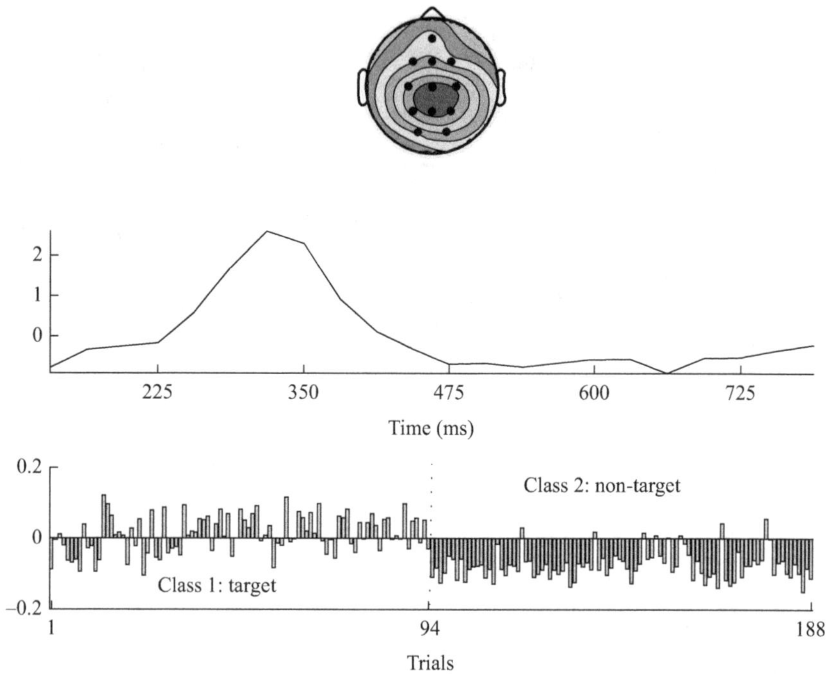

Figure 5.9 Rank-1 CPD of a auditory ERP dataset. The spatial mode and temporal mode factors show a stereotypical P300 scalp topography and time course. Target (attended) and non-target (non-attended) trials are classified with 73.4% accuracy based on the trial mode factor

Based on these considerations, epileptic seizures were successfully localized using the spatial signature of the CPD of the wavelet transformed multichannel EEG segment at seizure onset [17,18]. The CPD of the seizure in the previous example is shown in Figure 5.8c. Observing the time course in comparison with the raw EEG segment and the spatial signature with frontal dominance, it is clear that the first component captures eye blinks. The second component represents the seizure source. An oscillatory pattern is observed on the temporal signature, which is similar to the T1 channel of the raw EEG. Moreover, the spatial signature shows an anterior temporal onset, which is in agreement with the pathology of the patient. However, note that the frequency signature, showing a wide peak around 6 Hz, is not very informative about the spectral content of the seizure. This is because the rank-1 components of a CPD model cannot capture the evolving nature of the pattern. A BTD offers more flexibility, as it allows components of higher rank. In Figure 5.8d, we show the decomposition of the same EEG segment into block terms. The first rank-1 term captures the eye blinks, as in CPD. However, choosing the second term as rank-(2, 2, 1), a more detailed characterization of the seizure pattern is possible. The temporal signature on the left contains early slow activity, while the one on the right captures the late fast oscillatory pattern of the seizure. The frequency characteristics can be directly seen from the frequency signatures, namely, the 4 Hz peak on the left and the 8 Hz peak in the right frequency signature.

5.7.2 Unsupervised classification

Tensor decompositions can be used for unsupervised classification as well. Let us consider a classification problem, where the data points to be classified are represented as an N-dimensional feature set. Then, the entire dataset can be organized in an $(N + 1)$-dimensional tensor, where the indices of the data points are along the last mode. After applying an appropriate tensor decomposition method, the signature of the last mode can give an indication about the class membership. This approach has been successful to classify attended and non-attended trials in an auditory BCI dataset [34]. Different data representations were explored, including a *channel* $\times$ *time* $\times$ *trial*, and a *channel* $\times$ *frequency* $\times$ *trial* tensor, obtained by applying fast Fourier transform on each ERP time course. In Figure 5.9, we illustrate the ERP classification, achieved by a rank-1 CPD on the former representation. The spatial mode and temporal mode factors show a stereotypical P300 scalp topography and time course. Target (attended) and non-target (non-attended) trials are classified with over 70% accuracy based on the trial mode factor.

5.8 Supervised tensor decompositions

The tensor decompositions discussed before are extremely powerful as they provide a concise view on the underlying, intrinsic structure of the data. This is particularly useful for exploratory data analysis, independent of the type of data, as it will reveal the underlying natural low-dimensional representation by means of a Tucker, CPD or BTD decomposition in a fully unsupervised way. When considering supervised learning methods, one thinks of a traditional classification problem where the goal is to learn the boundary between classes based on given labels in the dataset. Such a boundary is characterized by the decision function, derived from the labelled datasets. Hence, traditional classifiers learn from labelled data to classify new data points into the corresponding classes. However, the properties of higher order models might also be exploited in a supervised way, and might in certain cases outperform traditional supervised methods. The goal is to fuse known class labels and the intrinsic structure of the data in order to provide class labels of unseen data in a more robust way than when machine learning techniques that do not exploit structure would have been used. Different groups have proposed some individual approaches to combine tensorial frameworks within learning problems, e.g. References 35, 36. Certain types of structured learning can also be formalized in a general framework. When the assumed underlying structure relates to a CPD model, higher dimensional learning tasks on multidimensional arrays might be reformulated to problems where the classification solution is a solution of an optimization problem constrained by the structure

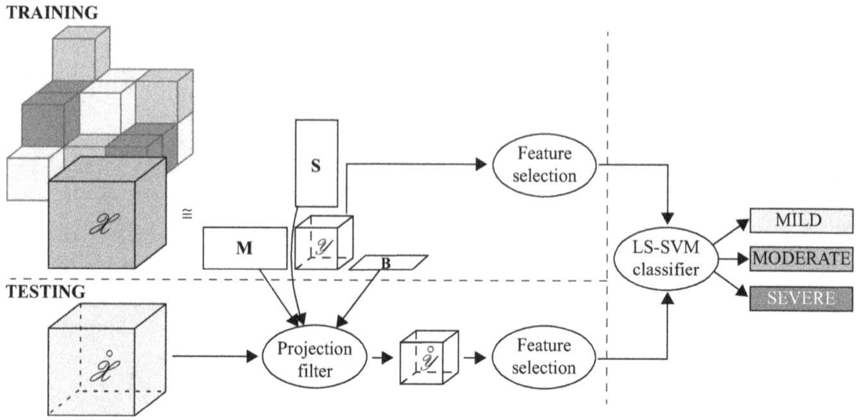

Figure 5.10 An example of how tensor decompositions can be used for a classification problem. Three types of tensors, represented in three shades of gray are used as training examples to discriminate between three classes. These training examples can be decomposed in a tensor decomposition that reduces the dimensionality and in the same time aims to maximize class differences. This leads to projection matrices that can be used to evaluate the class of an unseen example

[24,37]. Alternatively, the Tucker decomposition can also incorporate discriminative constraints in its generalization known as the higher order discriminant analysis (HODA). Rather than only aiming to model the underlying variance as good as possible, HODA estimates a multidimensional decomposition where the subspaces in the different modes encode for optimal separability of the different classes. This can be seen as a generalization of classical linear discriminant analysis (LDA) where every data sample is represented in a higher dimensional way. Such a method has been successfully used to discriminate between different neonatal EEG states [38]. A flow chart of the classification is visualized in Figure 5.10, where a Tucker decomposition is computed on the tensor constructed by concatenating different higher dimensional training samples. After decomposition, an additional classifier can be used on the most discriminative features from the core tensor. Reducing the dimensionality and preserving class-discriminative features can lead to a particularly robust method for classification in high-dimensional spaces.

5.9 Coupled tensor decompositions

In order to understand a complex biomedical system, multimodal measurements might be beneficial, which are able to capture complementary aspects of the same system. For instance, simultaneous EEG and fMRI measurements are highly beneficial for studying brain function, as the former has good temporal resolution, and the latter good spatial resolution. In addition, brain anatomy or structure may be studied using MRI or DTI images. Several strategies exist to fuse the different modalities. For diverse datasets, a parallel processing of the individual modalities takes place, followed by a decision making step. Alternatively, in an integrative approach knowledge from one modality is used as a constraint in the analysis of the other. Finally, a data fusion approach allows a symmetrical interaction between the modalities [39]. Integration and fusion may be achieved through the coupled decomposition of the different modalities. This approach requires that the datasets are linked through a common dimension. In the following sections, we discuss a few examples, illustrating the benefit of this common link in time, in space, or variability among multiple subjects.

5.9.1 Coupling of multi-subject data

Coupling in a multi-subject database may be achieved by exploiting the subject-by-subject variability. More specifically, it is plausible that the different mental tasks involve more intense neural processing in one subject than in another. Moreover, one can assume that the relative level of involvement appears both in the strength of the EEG as well as in the strength of the fMRI response. Therefore, in case one arranges the measurements in a *subject* × *EEG response* and a *subject* × *fMRI response* matrix, each matrix is generated as a mixture of the same underlying neural sources by the same mixing matrix. This is the principle behind the jointICA approach, which fuses fMRI and ERP data into spatiotemporal snapshots to describe the dynamic relationship between hemodynamic and electromagnetic brain sources [40].

A limitation of the jointICA technique is the fact that it uses a single EEG channel, overlooking spatial information from the EEG. Multichannel EEG information can be incorporated via horizontal or vertical channel concatenation [41], or, formulating the problem as a coupled matrix-tensor factorization (CMTF) [42,43].

Below we illustrate how the CMTF scheme can characterize various spatiotemporal brain sources during interictal epileptic discharges (IEDs) measured by EEG-fMRI. Traditionally, epileptic EEG-fMRI is analysed within the general linear model (GLM) framework, where a regressor is defined based on the timing of the interictal spikes observed in the EEG. This regressor is then used to find voxels showing similar blood oxygen level dependent (BOLD) fMRI signal fluctuations. The GLM results often show widespread activations in the brain, which is partly explained by the mismatch between the temporal dynamics of EEG and fMRI. As the BOLD signal in response to a transient neural event peaks after several seconds, fMRI cannot differentiate the nuances of all underlying neural processes which are reflected in the millisecond resolution EEG. In fact, an IED often starts with a sharp spike followed by a slow wave. Source localization studies have shown that the spike propagates within a few tens of milliseconds. Moreover, slow waves are considered to be related to inhibitory activity. Therefore, we argue that both the IED and the GLM maps capture a mixture of underlying neural activity. In order to disentangle these sources, similar consideration are made as in jointICA, explained above. That is, we work with a group of

10 temporal lobe epilepsy cases, assuming that the same neural processes are reflected in the EEG and fMRI, and the strength of the neural processes vary in each patient. Average IEDs from each patient are organized in a *channel* × *time* × *patients* tensor. The GLM-based activations maps of each patient are masked using a thresholded average GLM-based map, the images are vectorized and stored in a *voxels* × *patients* matrix. A CMTF is performed, where the two modalities share the same factor in the *patient* mode. A rank of $R = 2$ was chosen based on the core consistency diagnostic [44] of the EEG. The patient mode factors were fixed according to the patient-by-patient amplitudes of the spike and the slow wave.

The results of the decomposition are shown in Figure 5.11. Comparing the EEG sources with the grand average IED, one can observe that the first source captures the spike, while the second source captures the slow wave activity. Note the close resemblance of the spatial signatures (top left) and the scalp distributions of the spike and the slow wave in the grand average IED (top right). The average GLM-based activation maps is shown in the bottom left. Widespread activations are present in the right temporal lobe and in the occipital lobe. The first fMRI source, corresponding to the spike, shows predominantly temporal lobe activation. Interestingly, the second fMRI source, corresponding to the slow wave, captures the activation in the occipital lobe. Previous tractography studies have shown strong structural connection between the temporal lobe and the occipital lobe, as well as occipital activations in temporal lobe epilepsy (TLE). However, to our knowledge, a relationship between slow waves and occipital lobe activations has not been established. Further analysis is needed to confirm and interpret our results. Nevertheless, we believe that the joint factorization of EEG and fMRI can lead to new insights in the characterization of epileptic network activity.

5.9.2 Temporal coupling

Continuous EEG and fMRI data may be integrated based on the assumption that they capture the same changes in brain activity over time. As the sampling rate and the dynamics of the EEG and fMRI signals are different, some preprocessing is necessary. The following procedure was proposed in Reference 45, one of the first studies to fuse multimodal neuroimaging data. The EEG signal recorded during a single fMRI image was defined as a segment. Then, a time-varying EEG spectrum was computed over the consecutive EEG segments, forming a *channel* × *frequency* × *time* EEG tensor. The fMRI images were vectorized and the consecutive images were organized in a *voxel* × *time* matrix. As such, the time mode of the two datasets is aligned. Finally, the coupled decomposition was formulated mathematically as a multiway partial least squares (N-PLS) problem, i.e. the simultaneous factorization of the fMRI matrix and a CPD of the EEG tensor, with a constraint that maximizes the covariance between the temporal signatures of the EEG (independent variable) and the fMRI (dependent variable). The study identified possible brain regions which participate in generating or controlling spontaneous brain rhythms such as alpha activity.

Ocular artefacts often obscure the EEG data. There are many approaches to remove such artefacts, among which one of the most robust ways is estimating the eye movements based on simultaneously recorded EOG. The estimation can be formulated

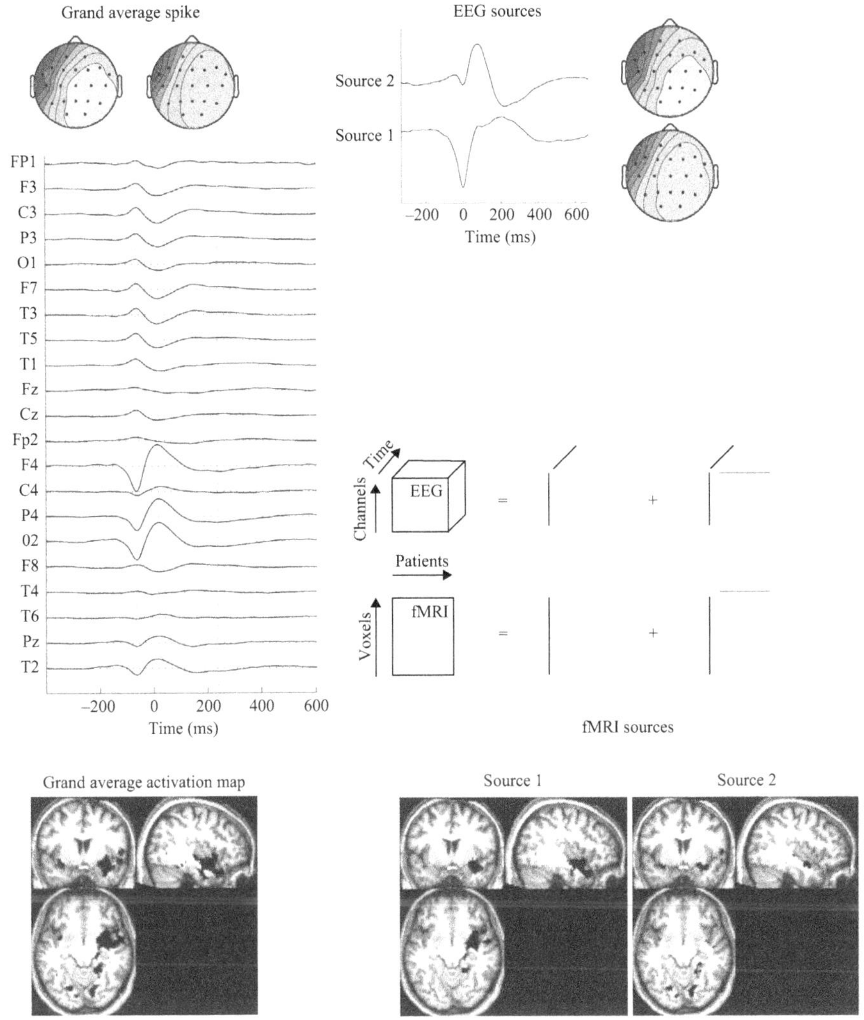

Figure 5.11 *Coupled tensor-matrix factorization (CMTF) was performed on an EEG-fMRI dataset recorded in temporal lobe epilepsy patients. The schematic representation of the factorization into two components, where the modalities share the same factors in patient mode, is shown in the middle. The multichannel average IEDs and GLM-based fMRI activation maps of each patient form the input tensor and matrix, respectively. The grand average IED and grand average activation map are shown in the left. The resulting EEG and fMRI sources are shown in the top and bottom right, respectively*

as a CMTF problem. As the effect of eye movement is not exactly the same on the EEG and EOG signals, Rivet *et al.* [46] proposed a relaxed CMTF solution, which estimates correlated shared factors, instead of equivalent ones. Additionally, their formulation also allows that the first or second derivatives of the factors are correlated rather than the original factors themselves. It was shown in both synthetic and real signals that refining coupling based on such similarities rather than equivalence have improved the estimation of the factors.

5.9.3 Spatial coupling

In the previous example, the EEG-fMRI integration was carried out using the common temporal dimension as a link between the two datasets. Alternatively, the decomposition may be coupled along the common spatial dimension, as proposed in Reference 47. In order to account for the different spatial resolution of the EEG and fMRI, fMRI data at voxels on the cortical grid of the EEG source space were extracted. Then, the integration is solved as a CMTF problem. The authors have applied a special formulation, which takes into account not only coincidence but also diversity among the modalities, by allowing one common component, one individual EEG and one individual fMRI component.

5.10 Practical considerations

The previous sections clearly illustrated the power of using tensor decompositions in a variety of cases. In all examples, the final result for the optimal models was shown. However, it is important to highlight a few practical issues that are crucial for obtaining these results, and that might not be clear when one is not familiar with this class of methods.

5.11 Parameter selection

The appropriate choice of model parameters is crucial for obtaining an interpretable and useful result. Whereas in supervised classification the optimal parameters may be determined using cross-validation, choosing the model parameters is a more difficult question in unsupervised problems.

Different representations of the same dataset have different algebraic properties, therefore, the chosen tensorization will influence the optimal number of components and ranks. For example, oscillatory sources represented in a Hankel matrix will certainly be different from rank-1, therefore, a BTD must be chosen. Besides mathematical considerations, background knowledge from the application field may help to estimate the number of terms as the expected number of underlying sources. For instance, in case of a seizure localization problem, one may expect that only a few distinct sources exist, including a seizure, an artefact and a background activity source. Apart from utilizing such heuristics, several automated techniques exist to estimate the tensor ranks. For a brief overview of different techniques, we refer the

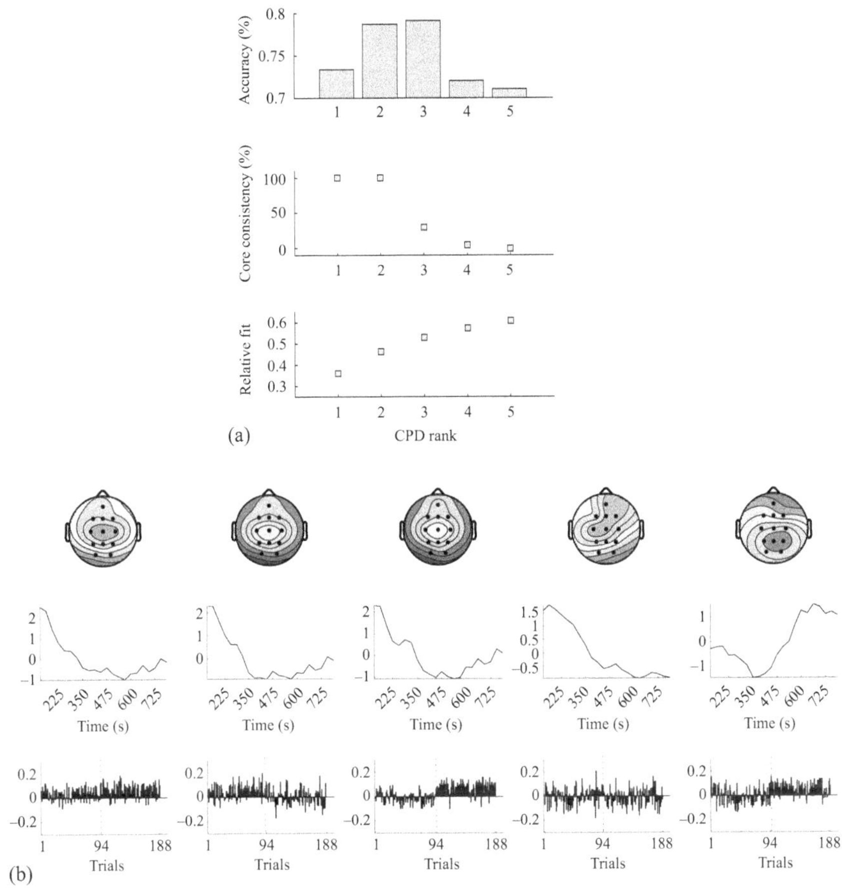

Figure 5.12 The same P300 classification problem is considered as in Section 5.7.2. (a) Classification accuracy, core consistency and fit of CPD models with increasing rank. (b) Rank-5 CPD of the same auditory ERP dataset as shown in Figure 5.9. Trials were sorted based on their true class membership: trials 1–94 are targets, while trials 95–188 are non-targets. The trial mode weights represent predictions.

reader to Reference 28 and references therein. Below we will illustrate the effect of different model parameter selection in a practical example.

Let us consider the P300 classification problem discussed previously in Section 5.7.2. A CPD was performed for different ranks between 1 and 5. The relative fit of the model and the core consistency [44] was computed for each model. We assume that one component captures the P300 source while other components model noise and other brain sources. It is not known a priori which component captures the P300, therefore, the classification of the trials was attempted using each trial signature separately. We report the best classification for each model, i.e. we assume that in a real application we will find a way to automatically select the relevant component. The results are shown in Figure 5.12a.

Recall that a classification accuracy of 73.4% was achieved already using a rank-1 CPD. When fitting a rank-2 CPD model on the data, the relative fit increases from 0.36 to 0.46 and the accuracy reaches 79%. It seems that the second component models some significant effects in the data, and this leaves more room for the first component to capture additional P300-specific variability in the data compared to the rank-1 model. The very high-core consistency values indicate that both the rank-1 and rank-2 solutions follow a CPD model, i.e. a trilinear interaction between the signatures sufficiently describes the data. However, the core consistency drops to 30% for a rank-3 model, suggesting that a considerable amount of non-trilinear variability is present in the data. Nevertheless, the P300 characteristics are still captured reliably, yielding a 79% accuracy. Finally, although model fit increases slightly, core consistency values around zero indicate invalid models. Indeed, classification accuracy drops as well. Figure 5.12b depicts the components obtained with a rank-5 model. It is easily observed that the spatial and the temporal signatures of the first three components are highly correlated. When correlations in multiple factors are observed, one should check whether two or more terms nearly cancel each other. This phenomenon is called degeneracy and may indicate that the CPD rank is set too high.

5.12 Initialization

Tensor decompositions are computed using optimization algorithms: an initial guess is updated iteratively in a well-chosen direction, in order to minimize the objective function value, given as the fit of the model. The iterative procedure stops when the step size or the relative change of the objective function value is smaller than a predefined value. A tensor decomposition is a non-linear and non-convex problem. As such, even though theoretically unique, there is no guarantee that the optimization algorithm will find the unique solution. In fact, the algorithm may converge to a local minimum. A good initialization is important to make sure that the algorithm converges fast to a good optimum. In general, it is recommended to run the decomposition algorithm multiple times from different initializations. Then, the best solution can be selected as the one with the smallest objective function value. Good initializations include generating pseudo-random factor matrices drawn for uniform or standard normal distributions, orthogonalizing such factors using QR factorization [48], or computing the initial factors based on HOSVD or using generalized eigenvalue decomposition. For more details and references, we refer the reader to Reference 49.

5.13 Tools and algorithms

Below we list a few useful MATLAB® toolboxes, which implement the tensor decomposition methods mentioned in this chapter. The Tensorlab toolbox for MATLAB [50] offers various different optimization algorithms to compute a CPD or a BTD, including the popular alternating least squares method, or the non-linear least squares algorithm [48]. Furthermore, its structured data fusion module allows to implement coupled matrix and tensor decompositions, as well as to incorporate various constraints. Besides the built-in options, such as non-negativity, orthogonal, polynomial, Hankel, etc., its domain-specific language allows the users to implement their own desired factor structures.

The MATLAB Tensor Toolbox [51] extends MATLAB built-in capabilities to manipulate multidimensional arrays. Different classes are implemented in order to efficiently handle dense, sparse and factored tensors either as a Tucker-type or CPD-type approach.

Finally, the Tensor Toolbox for Feature Extraction and Applications [52] implements efficient tensor decompositions for multilinear discriminative feature extraction based on constrained Tucker/CP models.

Acknowledgements

The research leading to these results has received funding from the European Research Council under the European Union's Seventh Framework Programme (FP7/2007-2013)/ERC Advanced Grant: BIOTENSORS (no. 339804). This paper reflects only the authors' views and the Union is not liable for any use that may be made of the contained information. Figures 5.5, 5.6 and parts of 5.9. were originally published in [28] by SpringerOpen, Spinger-Verlag, GmbH.

References

[1] Andrzej Cichocki, Danilo Mandic, Huy Anh Phan, Cesar Caiafa, Guoxu Zhou, Qibin Zhao and Lieven De Lathauwer. Tensor decompositions for signal processing applications: From two-way to multiway component analysis. *IEEE Signal Processing Magazine*, 32(2): 145–163, 2015.

[2] Tamara G. Kolda and Brett W. Bader. Tensor decompositions and applications. *SIAM Review*, 51(3):455–500, 2009.

[3] Joseph B. Kruskal. Three-way arrays: Rank and uniqueness of trilinear decompositions, with application to arithmetic complexity and statistics. *Linear Algebra and Its Applications*, 18(2):95–138, 1977.

[4] Ignat Domanov and Lieven De Lathauwer. On the uniqueness of the canonical polyadic decomposition – Part II: Overall uniqueness. *SIAM Journal on Matrix Analysis and Applications*, 34(3):876–903, 2013.

[5] Ignat Domanov and Lieven De Lathauwer. On the uniqueness of the canonical polyadic decomposition – Part I: Basic results and uniqueness of one factor matrix. *SIAM Journal on Matrix Analysis and Applications*, 34(3):855–875, 2013.

[6] Lieven De Lathauwer. Decompositions of a higher-order tensor in block terms – Part I: Lemmas for partitioned matrices. *SIAM Journal on Matrix Analysis and Applications*, 30(3):1022–1033, 2008.

[7] Lieven De Lathauwer. Decompositions of a higher-order tensor in block terms – Part II: Definitions and uniqueness. *SIAM Journal on Matrix Analysis and Applications*, 30(3):1033–1066, 2008.

[8] Lieven De Lathauwer and Dimitri Nion. Decompositions of a higher-order tensor in block terms – Part III: Alternating least squares algorithms. *SIAM Journal on Matrix Analysis and Applications*, 30(3):1067–1083, 2008.

[9] Larsson Omberg, Gene H. Golub, and Orly Alter. A tensor higher-order singular value decomposition for integrative analysis of DNA microarray data from different studies. *Proceedings of the National Academy of Sciences*, 104(47):18371–18376, 2007.

[10] Christian F. Beckmann and Stephen M. Smith. Tensorial extensions of independent component analysis for multisubject {FMRI} analysis. *NeuroImage*, 25(1):294–311, 2005.

[11] Rob Zink, Borbála Hunyadi, Sabine Van Huffel and Maarten De Vos. Tensor-based classification of an auditory mobile BCI without a subject-specific calibration. *Journal of Neural Engineering*, 13(2): 026005, 2016.

[12] Katrien Vanderperren, Bogdan Mijović, Nikolai Novitskiy, *et al.* Single trial ERP reading based on parallel factor analysis. *Psychophysiology*, 50(1): 97–110, 2013.

[13] Wouter Deburchgraeve, Perumpillichira J. Cherian, Maarten De Vos, *et al.* Neonatal seizure localization using PARAFAC decomposition. *Clinical Neurophysiology*, 120(10):1787–1796, 2009.

[14] Ivana Despotovic, Perumpillichira J. Cherian, Maarten Vos, *et al.* Relationship of EEG sources of neonatal seizures to acute perinatal brain lesions seen on MRI: A pilot study. *Human Brain Mapping*, 34(10):2402–2417, 2013.

[15] Griet Goovaerts, Carolina Varon, Bert Vandenberk, Rik Willems, and Sabine Van Huffel. Tensor-based detection of T wave alternans in multilead ECG signals. In *Computing in Cardiology Conference (CinC), 2014*, pages 185–188. Piscataway, NJ: IEEE, 2014.

[16] Kai Huang and Liqing Zhang. Cardiology knowledge free ECG feature extraction using generalized tensor rank one discriminant analysis. *EURASIP Journal on Advances in Signal Processing*, 2014(1):1–15, 2014.

[17] Evrim Acar, Canan Aykut-Bingol, Haluk Bingol, Rasmus Bro, and Bülent Yener. Multiway analysis of epilepsy tensors. *Bioinformatics*, 23(13):i10–i18, 2007.

[18] Maarten De Vos, Anneleen Vergult, Lieven De Lathauwer, *et al.* Canonical decomposition of ictal scalp EEG reliably detects the seizure onset zone. *NeuroImage*, 37:844–854, 2007.

[19] Martin Weis, Florian Römer, Martin Haardt, Dunja Jannek, and Peter Husar. Multi-dimensional space–time–frequency component analysis of event related EEG data using closed-form PARAFAC. In *Acoustics, Speech and Signal Processing, 2009. ICASSP 2009, Taipei, Taiwan. IEEE International Conference on*, pages 349–352, Apr. 2009.

[20] Fumikazu Miwakeichi, Eduardo Martinez-Montes, Pedro A. Valdes-Sosa, Nobuaki Nishiyama, Hiroaki Mizuhara, and Yoko Yamaguchi. Decomposing

EEG data into space–time–frequency components using parallel factor analysis. *NeuroImage*, 22(3):1035–1045, 2004.

[21] Morten Mørup, Lars K. Hansen, Christoph S. Hermann, Josef Parnas, and Sidse M. Arnfred. Parallel factor analysis as an exploratory tool for wavelet transformed event-related EEG. *NeuroImage*, 29(3):938–947, 2006.

[22] Hyekyoung Lee, Young-Deok Kim, Andrzej Cichocki, and Seungjin Choi. Nonnegative tensor factorization for continuous EEG classification. *International Journal of Neural Systems*, 17(4):305–317, 2007. PMID: 17696294.

[23] Hanna Becker, Laurent Albera, Pierre Comon, *et al.* EEG extended source localization: Tensor-based vs. conventional methods. *NeuroImage*, 96:143–157, 2014.

[24] Borbála Hunyadi, Marco Signoretto, Stefan Debener, Sabine Van Huffel, and Maarten De Vos. Classification of structured EEG tensors using nuclear norm regularization: Improving P300 classification. In *2013 International Workshop on Pattern Recognition in Neuroimaging (PRNI)*, Philadelphia, PA, pages 98–101, 2013.

[25] Wim De Clercq, Bart Vanrumste, Jean-Marie Papy, Wim Van Paesschen, and Sabine Van Huffel. Modeling common dynamics in multichannel signals with applications to artifact and background removal in EEG recordings. *Biomedical Engineering, IEEE Transactions on*, 52(12):2006–2015, 2005.

[26] Piotr J. Franaszczuk and Katarzyna J. Blinowska. Linear model of brain electrical activity – EEG as a superposition of damped oscillatory modes. *Biological Cybernetics*, 53(1):19–25, 1985.

[27] Lieven De Lathauwer. Blind separation of exponential polynomials and the decomposition of a tensor in rank-$(L_r, L_r, 1)$ terms. *SIAM Journal on Matrix Analysis and Applications*, 32(4):1451–1474, 2011.

[28] Borbála Hunyadi, Daan Camps, Laurent Sorber, *et al.* Block term decomposition for modelling epileptic seizures. *EURASIP Journal on Advances in Signal Processing*, 2014(1):1–19, 2014.

[29] Lucas N. Ribeiro, Antonio R. Hidalgo-Munoz, and Vicente Zarzoso. Atrial signal extraction in atrial fibrillation electrocardiograms using a tensor decomposition approach. In *37th Annual International Conference of the IEEE Engineering in Medicine and Biology Society (EMBC)*, Milan, Italy, pages 6987–6990, Aug. 2015.

[30] Javier Escudero, Evrim Acar, Alberto Fernandez, and Rasmus Bro. Multiscale entropy analysis of resting-state magnetoencephalogram with tensor factorisations in Alzheimer's disease. *Brain Research Bulletin*, Vol. 119, Part B, pages 136–144, 2015.

[31] Evrim Acar, Canan Aykut-Bingol, Haluk Bingol, Rasmus Bro, and Bülent Yener. Seizure recognition on epilepsy feature tensor. In *Engineering in Medicine and Biology Society, 2007. EMBS 2007. 29th Annual International Conference of the IEEE*, pages 4273–4276, Aug. 2007.

[32] H.N. Bharath, Diana M. Sima., Nicolas Sauwen, Uwe Himmelreich, Lieven De Lathauwer, Sabine Van Huffel. Tensor based tumor tissue type differentiation using magnetic resonance spectroscopic imaging. In *37th Annual International*

Conference of the IEEE Engineering in Medicine and Biology Society (EMBC), Milan, Italy, Aug. 2015, pages 7003–7006, 2015.

[33] John M. Stern and Jerome Engel. *An Atlas of EEG Patterns*. Philadelphia, PA: Lippincott Williams & Wilkins, 2005.

[34] Rob Zink, Borbála Hunyadi, Sabine Van Huffel, and Maarten De Vos. Exploring CPD based unsupervised classification for auditory BCI with mobile EEG. In *Neural Engineering (NER), 2015 Seventh International IEEE/EMBS Conference on*, pages 53–56, Montpellier, France, Apr. 2015.

[35] Dacheng Tao, Xuelong Li, Xindong Wu, Weiming Hu, and Stephen J. Maybank. Supervised tensor learning. *Knowledge and Information Systems*, 13:1–42, 2007.

[36] David R. Hardoon and John Shawe-Taylor. Decomposing the tensor kernel support vector machine for neuroscience data with structured labels. *Machine Learning*, 79(1–2):29–46, 2010.

[37] Marco Signoretto, Quoc Tran Dinh, Lieven De Lathauwer, and Johan A.K. Suykens. Learning with tensors: A framework based on convex optimization and spectral regularization. *Machine Learning*, 94(3):303–351.

[38] Vladimir Matic, Perumpillichira J. Cherian, Ninah Koolen, *et al.* Holistic approach for automated background EEG assessment in asphyxiated full-term infants. *Journal of Neural Engineering*, 11(6):066007, 2014.

[39] Dana Lahat, Tülay Adali, and Christian Jutten. Multimodal data fusion: An overview of methods, challenges, and prospects. *Proceedings of the IEEE*, 103(9):1449–1477, Sep. 2015.

[40] Vince D. Calhoun, Tulay Adali, G. D. Pearlson, and K. A. Kiehl. Neuronal chronometry of target detection: Fusion of hemodynamic and event–related potential data. *NeuroImage*, 30(2):544–553, 2006.

[41] Wout Swinnen, Borbála Hunyadi, Esra Acar, Sabine Van Huffe, and Maarten De Vos. Incorporating higher dimensionality in joint decomposition of EEG and fMRI. In *22nd European Signal Processing Conference (EUSIPCO)*, Lisbon, 2014, pp. 121–125. IEEE, 2014.

[42] Evrim Acar, Tamara G. Kolda, and Daniel M. Dunlavy. All-at-once optimization for coupled matrix and tensor factorizations. *arXiv preprint arXiv:1105.3422*, 2011.

[43] Borbála Hunyadi, Wim Van Paesschen, Maarten De Vos, and Sabine Van Huffel. Fusion of electroencephalography and functional magnetic resonance imaging to explore epileptic network activity. In *24th European Signal Processing Conference (EUSIPCO)*, Budapest, 2016.

[44] Rasmus Bro and Henk A. L. Kiers. A new efficient method for determining the number of components in PARAFAC models. *Journal of Chemometrics*, 17(5):274–286, 2003.

[45] Eduardo Martínez-Montes, Pedro A. Valdás-Sosa, Fumikazu Miwakeichi, Robin I. Goldman, and Mark S. Cohen. Concurrent EEG/fMRI analysis by multiway partial least squares. *NeuroImage*, 22(3):1023–1034, 2004.

[46] Bertrand Rivet, Marc Duda, Anne Guerin-Dugue, Christian Jutten, and Pierre Comon. Multimodal approach to estimate the ocular movements during

EEG recordings: A coupled tensor factorization method. In *37th Annual International Conference of the IEEE Engineering in Medicine and Biology Society (EMBC)*, Milan, Italy, pages 6983–6986, Aug. 2015.

[47] Esin Karahan, Pedro A. Rojas-Lopez, Maria L. Bringas-Vega, Pedro A. Valdes-Hernandez, and Pedro A. Valdes-Sosa. Tensor analysis and fusion of multimodal brain images. *Proceedings of the IEEE*, 103(9):1531–1559, Sep. 2015.

[48] Laurent Sorber, Marc Van Barel, and Lieven De Lathauwer. Optimization-based algorithms for tensor decompositions: Canonical polyadic decomposition, decomposition in rank-$(L_r, L_r, 1)$ terms and a new generalization. *SIAM Journal on Optimization*, 23(2):695–720, 2013.

[49] Stefan Kindermann and Carmeliza Navasca. New algorithms for tensor decomposition based on a reduced functional. *Numerical Linear Algebra with Applications*, 21(3):340–374, 2014.

[50] Nico Vervliet, Otto Debals, Laurent Sorber, Marc Van Barel and Lieven De Lathauwer. Tensorlab 3.0, Available online, Mar. 2016. URL: http://www.tensorlab.net/ (accessed August 1, 2016).

[51] Brett W. Bader, Tamara G. Kolda, *et al.* MATLAB tensor toolbox version 2.6. http://www.sandia.gov/~tgkolda/TensorToolbox (accessed August 1, 2016), Feb. 2015.

[52] Anh Huy Phan. NFEA: Tensor toolbox for feature extraction and applications. http://www.bsp.brain.riken.jp/~phan/nfea/nfea.html (accessed August 1, 2016), Feb. 2011.

Chapter 6
Patient physiological monitoring with machine learning

Marco A. F. Pimentel and David A. Clifton

The task of discovering novel medical knowledge from complex, large-scale and high-dimensional patient data, collected during care episodes, is central to innovation in medicine. The recognition of complex trajectories in multivariate time-series data requires effective models and representations for the analysis and matching of functional data. In this chapter, we describe a method based on Gaussian processes for exploratory data analysis using the observational physiological time-series data.

The method focuses on a representation of unevenly sampled *trajectories* that allows for revealing physiological recovery patterns in a database of vital signs acquired from post-operative patients. While our primary motivation comes from clinical data, this approach may be applicable to other time-series domains. We first describe methods that have been proposed in the literature for the same purpose. We then provide a brief summary of Gaussian processes, and describe our proposed approach for performing "clustering" of patients' trajectories.

6.1 Introduction

The task of knowledge discovery from time-series data is important for "tracking" the health status of post-operative patients. An enormous amount of work has been devoted to the task of modelling time-series data.

The autoregressive model is a basic means of analysing time-series data, which specifies that the output variable depends linearly on its previous values. Other examples include state-space models, which are based on the notion that there is an unobserved state of the system, or latent state, that evolves through time and which may only be observed indirectly. For example, the health status of a patient can only be observed through "noisy" observations of the patient's physiology and mental status.

The most basic state-space model with a continuous-valued latent state is the linear dynamical system (LDS), which is the discrete-time analogue of a linear differential equation. The hidden Markov model (HMM) [1] is the discrete-state space analogue of an LDS. Quinn *et al.* [2] applied an extension of an LDS model to the problem of monitoring the condition of premature infants receiving intensive care.

A factorial-switching LDS model (equivalent to a switching Kalman filter) was described and tested with continuous time-series data collected from bedside monitors. This model was developed into a hierarchical factorial-switching LDS [3] by adding a set of higher-level variables to model correlations in the physiological factors in order to detect sepsis in ICU patients. Lehman *et al.* [4] used a switching vector autoregressive framework to systematically learn and identify continuously acquired arterial blood pressure data dynamics. These can possibly be recurrent within the same patient and shared across an entire cohort of ICU patients.

Work by Willsky *et al.* [5,6] uses Bayesian nonparametric models for capturing the generation of continuous-valued time-series. This method uses an HMM for segmenting time-series data, where the latter are characterised by autoregressive models. Beta processes, which provide prior distributions in the unit interval, are then used to share observation models across several series. Thus, this *BP-AR-HMM* model is used to capture variability between series by sampling subsets of low-level features that are specific to individual series. Lehman *et al.* [7] used this model to discover shared dynamics in ICU patients' continuously acquired blood pressure time-series data. A different Bayesian nonparametric method for exploratory data analysis and feature construction in continuous time-series has been proposed in Reference 8. This method builds on the framework of latent Dirichlet allocation and its extension to hierarchical Dirichlet processes, which allows the characterisation of each series as switching between latent "modes," where each mode is characterised as a distribution over features that specify the series dynamics. The model was applied to heart-rate data collected from premature infants admitted to a neonatal ICU. A different probabilistic model, the *continuous shape template model*, has also been applied for discovering time-series' segments that can repeat within and across different series of continuous heart-rate data [9].

Although conceptually sound, it is unclear how such approaches cope with irregularly sampled data and missing data. As opposed to equally spaced time-series, on which the methods described above have been applied, irregularly sampled time-series data are characterised by variable intervals between successive measurements; i.e., the spacing of observation times is not constant. Different time-series typically contain different numbers of observations and the times at which observations were recorded may not be aligned. Furthermore, periods of missing data are common in clinical scenarios. The properties of these data mean that most common machine learning algorithms and models for supervised and unsupervised learning cannot be directly applied.

One solution to these problems is offered by Gaussian processes. Gaussian processes are a Bayesian modelling technique that has been widely used for various machine learning tasks, such as dimensionality reduction, non-linear classification, and regression [10,11]. It is a nonparametric method, informally suggesting that the number of parameters in the model can grow with the number of observed data. Compared to other related techniques, Gaussian process models have the advantage that prior knowledge of the functional behaviour (e.g., periodicity or smoothness) may be easily expressed. The Bayesian nature of its formulation also means that inference is performed within a probabilistic framework, allowing us to reason in the presence of noise, incompleteness, and artefacts, all of which are characteristic of the data recorded in hospital settings.

Gaussian processes have been used for modelling physiological time-series data. Clifton *et al.* [12,13] used Gaussian process regression to cope with artefactual and missing vital-sign data, and incorporated the Gaussian process posterior in their novelty detection schemes. Stegle *et al.* [14] proposed a robust regression model for noisy heart-rate data based on Gaussian processes and a preliminary clustering procedure that learns the structure of outliers and noise bursts. In the work described in chapter 6 of Reference 15, trend analysis was performed using dependent Gaussian processes, in which the correlation between two or more physiological variables is used to obtain improved regression results. Clifton *et al.* [16] extended extreme value theory such that a function-wise approach to novelty detection was taken, as opposed to point-wise approaches that are most commonly described in the literature. The method was illustrated using Gaussian process regression, which offers a probabilistic framework in which distributions over a function space are defined. Gaussian process regression has also been used for the ranking of gene expressions [17].

In this work, we propose a representation of vital-sign trajectories using Gaussian process regression, which may be used for the recognition of "normal" and "abnormal" patterns of physiological trends. Figure 6.1 illustrates the components of our proposed approach. We model the evolution of the unevenly sampled physiological trajectories using Gaussian process regression, and we introduce a kernel similarity measurement for the comparison of the latent functions based on the likelihoods of the data points in each trajectory. This *patient-to-patient* similarity measurement can be used for the functional characterisation of vital-sign trajectories, which may then be used for recognising known trajectories and identifying unknown trajectories as would be required for identifying "abnormal" vital-sign time-series.

6.2 Methodology

In the following sections we describe our proposed approach and analysis conducted.

6.2.1 Dataset

For this analysis we selected a cohort of post-operative patients who stayed for a minimum of 24 hours on the post-operative ward (after upper-gastrointestinal surgery for removal of cancer), and for a period no longer than 20 days (which corresponds approximately to the 95th quantile for the length of stay on the ward of the entire cohort of patients considered, $N = 407$). The rationale for this was to exclude both very short or very long stayers from our analysis and focus on a more "homogeneous" cohort of patients with regard to length of stay. For the analysis considered in this work, we also excluded patients who died on the ward, had an emergency admission to the Intensive Care Unit (ICU), or cardiac arrest. This resulted in a total of 326 patients that were included in this analysis. For all patients, the first day of their vital-sign trajectories corresponds to the day on which surgery took place.

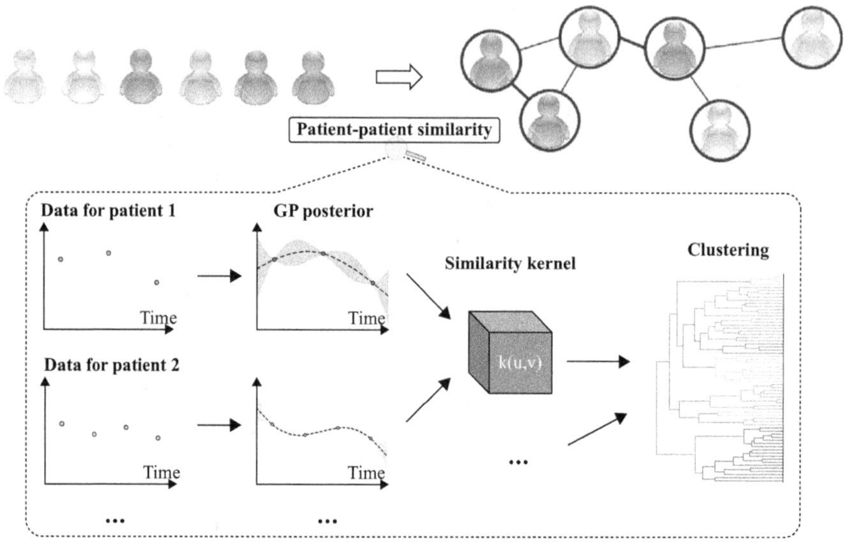

Figure 6.1 Overview of our approach for the functional characterisation of vital-sign trajectories with Gaussian processes

Although the proposed approach can be applied to multivariate time-series data, given the small size of the dataset we demonstrate the proposed approach using univariate observational data from our cohort of post-operative patients. We can, however, take into account the contribution of all five vital signs (and not focus only on a single vital sign). For this, we consider the output of a model constructed using our proposed approach described in Reference 18, which provides a parsimonious representation of the overall physiological trajectories for each patient. In short, a multivariate model of normality based on pre-discharge vital-sign data from patients (who were discharged alive), $\mathbf{U}$, is constructed using kernel density estimates [19,20]; then, for each patient, the likelihood $p(\mathbf{u}_i|\mathbf{U},\sigma)$ of each observation set $\mathbf{u}_i$ (with $i = 0, ..., N$) with respect to this model is computed, and the correspondent novelty score $z(\mathbf{u}_i)$ is finally obtained: $z(\mathbf{u}_i) = -\log p(\mathbf{u}_i|\mathbf{U},\theta)$.

Thus, for each patient, we obtain a "univariate", unevenly sampled time-series of novelty score values; i.e., a collection n pairs of $(t, z(\mathbf{u}))$, where t corresponds to the time of the observation set $\mathbf{u}$, and n is the number of observation sets for that patient. The details of how the model is constructed have previously been described (see Reference 18).

6.2.2 Gaussian processes

We provide a brief summary of Gaussian processes in this section. It therefore makes a rather compressed introduction to the topic. A more thorough introduction is available in Reference 11.

When performing a regression task we assume there exists some optimal prediction function $f \in \mathscr{X} \to \mathscr{Y}$, possibly with a noise distribution. In linear regression, we assume that the outputs $\mathbf{y}$ are a linear function of the inputs $\mathbf{X}$, with some parameters $\boldsymbol{\theta}$, usually fewer than the number of training examples $N : |\boldsymbol{\theta}| \ll N$. However, for many real-world datasets a simple parametric form, such as a linear form, is an unrealistic assumption. Therefore, we would like to have models that can learn general functions f. Since the functions may not be summarised by a small (fixed) number of parameters $\boldsymbol{\theta}$, maximum likelihood estimation of the parameters may cause overfitting. In fact, in a Gaussian process, the effective number of parameters is often infinite. Therefore, in order to perform inference we need to place a prior probability distribution on functions. We make predictions using our posterior on an underlying predictive function f given a set of training examples in the form of input-output pairs: $\mathscr{D} = \{(\mathbf{x}_i \in \mathbb{R}^D, y_i \in \mathbb{R})\}_{i=1}^N$.

Gaussian processes provide a distribution over real-valued functions which is widely used for non-linear regression and classification tasks [11]. By definition, a function $f : \mathscr{X} \to \mathbb{R}$ is distributed according to a Gaussian process if and only if $p(f(\mathbf{x}_1), \ldots, f(\mathbf{x}_N))$, the density of that function's values at any N points $\mathbf{x}_i \in \mathscr{X}$, is multivariate Gaussian. This allows Gaussian processes to be parameterised tractably by a mean function $m(\mathbf{x})$ and a covariance kernel function $\mathbf{K}(\mathbf{x}_i, \mathbf{x}_j)$ specifying the correlations within any finite point set, such that

$$\mathbf{y} = f(\mathbf{x}) \sim \mathscr{GP}\big(m(\mathbf{x}), \mathbf{K}(\mathbf{x}_i, \mathbf{x}_j)\big), \tag{6.1}$$

with possibly some Gaussian observation noise. Note that the covariance matrix $\mathbf{K}$, or Gram matrix, whose entries $\mathbf{K}_{ij}$ are often thought of as the "similarity" between inputs $\mathbf{x}_i$ and $\mathbf{x}_j$, encodes our prior knowledge concerning the functional behaviour we wish to model. Without loss of generality, the prior mean function is typically set to zero: $m(\mathbf{x}) = 0$. The most commonly used covariance function is the squared-exponential,[1]

$$k_{SE}(\mathbf{x}_i, \mathbf{x}_j) = \sigma_0^2 \exp\left(-\frac{\| \mathbf{x}_i - \mathbf{x}_j \|^2}{2\ell^2}\right), \tag{6.2}$$

where $\boldsymbol{\theta} = \{\sigma_0, \ell\}$ are hyperparameters modelling the y-scaling and x-scaling (or time-scale if the data are time-series), respectively, and where $\| \cdot \|$ denotes the Euclidean norm. The squared-exponential covariance function is said to be *stationary* because it only depends on the difference between points $\mathbf{x}_i - \mathbf{x}_j$, rather than on their absolute value. In general, covariance functions have to fulfil Mercer's theorem, meaning that $\mathbf{K}(\mathbf{x}_i, \mathbf{x}_j)$ has to be symmetric and positive semidefinite, and therefore $k_{SE}(\cdot, \cdot)$ is a valid kernel. Many mathematical operations, such as summation or taking a product, preserve positive definiteness and can therefore be used for combining basic kernels to make more complex kernels. A survey of covariance functions can be found in chapter 4 of Reference 11.

[1] It is also known as the exponentiated-quadratic, or the Gaussian kernel function.

Given a training set $\mathscr{D}$, using the standard conditioning rules for a Gaussian distribution, we can obtain the predictive distribution on a new observation y_* at test input $\mathbf{x}_*$:

$$\begin{bmatrix} \mathbf{y} \\ y_* \end{bmatrix} = \mathcal{N}\left(\begin{bmatrix} 0 \\ 0 \end{bmatrix}, \begin{bmatrix} \mathbf{K} & \mathbf{K}_* \\ \mathbf{K}_*^\top & \mathbf{K}_{**} \end{bmatrix} \right) \tag{6.3}$$

implying

$$p(y_*|\mathbf{x}_*, \mathbf{X}, \mathbf{y}) \sim \mathcal{N}(\mu_*, \sigma_*^2), \text{ with} \tag{6.4}$$

$$\mu_* = \mathbf{K}_*^\top \mathbf{K}^{-1} \mathbf{y} \in \mathbb{R}, \tag{6.5}$$

$$\sigma_*^2 = \mathbf{K}_{**} - \mathbf{K}_*^\top \mathbf{K}^{-1} \mathbf{K}_* \in \mathbb{R}^+. \tag{6.6}$$

Here, $\mathbf{K}_* = k(\mathbf{X}, \mathbf{x}_*) \in \mathbb{R}^{N+1}$ is the cross-covariance between the test input $\mathbf{x}_*$ and the training inputs $\mathbf{X}$; $\mathbf{K}_{**} = k(\mathbf{x}_*, \mathbf{x}_*) \in \mathbb{R}^+$ is the prior variance of $\mathbf{x}_*$.

The values of the hyperparameters $\boldsymbol{\theta}$ may be optimised by, for example, minimising the negative log marginal likelihood (NLML) which is defined as

$$\text{NLML} = -\log p(\mathbf{y}|\mathbf{x}, \boldsymbol{\theta}) \tag{6.7}$$

$$= \frac{1}{2}\log|\mathbf{K}| + \frac{1}{2}\mathbf{y}^\top \mathbf{K}^{-1}\mathbf{y} + \frac{N}{2}\log(2\pi) \tag{6.8}$$

This is sometimes called the type-II maximum likelihood (if we remove the negative logarithm). Interpreting the NLML as a cost function reveals that the first term penalises model complexity and the second term penalises low data likelihood (i.e., low data fitness). Bias-variance trade-off is therefore performed by minimising the NLML, which is commonly achieved using gradient descent. In a full Bayesian treatment, we should integrate out the hyperparameters. Unfortunately, this cannot be performed analytically in general, e.g., for the input scale. Sampling methods, or other approximations, are usually used to estimate these integrals [11].

In our experiments, we used a single squared-exponential covariance function and a zero-mean function to capture the overall physiological recovery of post-operative patients. During training, each time-series was centred by removing the mean of the time-series data to achieve a zero-mean function. The hyperparameters $\{\sigma_0^2, \ell\}$ were selected using a grid-search optimiser for minimising the NLML: $\sigma_o^2 \in [3, 4, 5, ..., 15]$ (in units of $z(\mathbf{x})$) and $\ell \in [2.0, 2.5, 3.0, ..., 5.0]$ (in units of days). We then evaluated the resulting function over a uniform grid of test points $\mathbf{x}_*$ sampled every hour within the range $\mathbf{x}_*^n \in [t_1, t_f]$, where t_1 and t_f correspond to the time of the first and last observations for patient n. Figure 6.2 shows a few examples of the regression results obtained with our dataset using this procedure.

We observe that small (daily) variations of the novelty scores are smoothed by use of this approach. Nevertheless, the model is able to capture the overall trajectory of recovery of the patients. For example, patient 31 exhibits a high initial physiological derangement following major surgery, and a clear return to normality (decrease in the physiological novelty score), as a result of recovery on the ward. Patient 105, on the other hand, appears to be within the normal range of novelty score values throughout their stay on the ward.

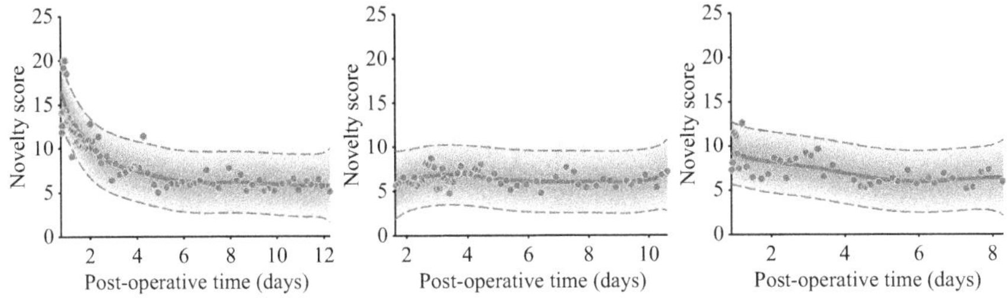

Figure 6.2 Examples of the Gaussian process posteriors obtained for the novelty scores of three post-operative patients. Circles correspond to the raw data. Thick lines correspond to the posterior means, and dashed lines mark the 95% confidence area for the computed posterior mean. Shaded areas denote the uncertainty level of the mean (darker areas, uncertainty is lower). (a) Patient 31; (b) Patient 105; (c) Patient 373

6.2.3 Time-series clustering

In this section we describe our proposed approach for performing clustering of the Gaussian process posteriors over the uniform grid of test points (sampled every hour).

To quantify the similarity of time-series we make use of kernels. Kernel-based classifiers, like any other classification scheme, should be robust against invariances and distortions. Dynamic time warping (DTW), a method based on dynamic programming [21], has been previously combined with kernel methods [22,23].

Let $\mathscr{X}^{\mathbb{N}}$ be the set of discrete-time time-series taking values in an arbitrary space $\mathscr{X}$. One can try to align two time-series $\mathbf{u} = (u_1, ..., u_n)$ and $\mathbf{v} = (v_1, ..., v_m)$ of lengths n and m, respectively, in various ways by distorting them. An alignment π of length $|\pi| = p$ between two sequences $\mathbf{u}$ and $\mathbf{v}$ (with $p \leq n + m - 1$ since the two series have $n + m$ points and they are matched at least at one point in time) is a pair of increasing integer vectors (π_1, π_2) such that $1 \leq \pi_1(1) \leq ... \leq \pi_1(p) = n$ and $1 \leq \pi_2(1) \leq ... \leq \pi_2(p) = m$, with unitary increments and no simultaneous repetitions (we use the notation of Reference 24). We write $\mathscr{A}(\mathbf{u}, \mathbf{v})$ for the set of all possible alignments between $\mathbf{u}$ and $\mathbf{v}$, which can be conveniently represented by paths in an $n \times m$ matrix. Following the well-known DTW metric, the *cost* of the alignment can be defined by means of a distance ϕ that measures the discrepancy between any two points u_i and v_j, such that

$$D_{\mathbf{u},\mathbf{v}}(\boldsymbol{\pi}) = \sum_{i=1}^{|\pi|} \phi(u_{\pi_1(i)}, v_{\pi_2(i)}) \tag{6.9}$$

Dynamic programming algorithms provide an efficient way to compute the optimal path $\boldsymbol{\pi}^*$ which gives the minimum cost among all possible alignments,

$$\boldsymbol{\pi}^* = \arg\min_{\pi \in \mathscr{A}(\mathbf{u},\mathbf{v})} \frac{1}{|\boldsymbol{\pi}|} D_{\mathbf{u},\mathbf{v}}(\boldsymbol{\pi}) \tag{6.10}$$

Different kernel distances (or scores) ϕ have been proposed in the literature to compute the similarity between time-series based on DTW, such as the negative squared Euclidean distance $\phi(u, v) = -||u - v||^2$ [22],

$$k_{DTW_1}(\mathbf{u}, \mathbf{v}) = \exp\left(-\underset{\pi \in \mathscr{A}(\mathbf{u},\mathbf{v})}{\arg\min} \frac{1}{|\pi|} \sum_{i=1}^{|\pi|} ||u_{\pi_1(i)} - v_{\pi_2(i)}||^2\right), \tag{6.11}$$

or a Gaussian kernel [23],

$$k_{DTW_2}(\mathbf{u}, \mathbf{v}) = \underset{\pi \in \mathscr{A}(\mathbf{u},\mathbf{v})}{\arg\max} \frac{1}{|\pi|} \sum_{i=1}^{|\pi|} \exp\left(-\frac{1}{\sigma^2} ||u_{\pi_1(i)} - v_{\pi_2(i)}||^2\right). \tag{6.12}$$

The global alignment (GA) kernel, proposed by Cuturi *et al.* [25], assumes that the alignment that gives the minimum cost may be sensitive to peculiarities of the time-series and intends to take advantage of all possible alignments weighted exponentially. Hence, it is defined as the sum of exponentiated costs of the individual alignments, such that

$$k_{GA}(\mathbf{u}, \mathbf{v}) = \sum_{\pi \in \mathscr{A}(\mathbf{u},\mathbf{v})} \exp\left(-D_{\mathbf{u},\mathbf{v}}(\pi)\right) \tag{6.13}$$

$$= \sum_{\pi \in \mathscr{A}(\mathbf{u},\mathbf{v})} \exp\left(-\sum_{i=1}^{|\pi|} \phi(u_{\pi_1(i)}, v_{\pi_2(i)})\right) \tag{6.14}$$

$$= \sum_{\pi \in \mathscr{A}(\mathbf{u},\mathbf{v})} \prod_{i=1}^{|\pi|} k(u_{\pi_1(i)}, v_{\pi_2(i)}) \tag{6.15}$$

where $k = \exp -\phi$. It has been argued that k_{GA} runs over the whole spectrum of the costs and leads to a smoother measure than the minimum of the costs, i.e., the DTW distance [25].

In our implementation, we use the kernel suggested in Reference 24,

$$k(u, v) = \exp(-\phi_\sigma(u, v)), \tag{6.16}$$

$$\phi_\sigma(u, v) = \frac{1}{2\sigma^2} d(u, v) + \log\left(2 - e^{-\frac{1}{2\sigma^2} d(u,v)}\right) \tag{6.17}$$

where the bandwidth σ of the kernel can be set as a multiple of a simple estimate of the median (Euclidean) distance of different points observed in different time-series of the training set, scaled by the square root of the median length of time-series in the training set,[2] as suggested in Reference 24; $d(u, v)$ corresponds to the distance between any two points of the time-series $\mathbf{u}$ and $\mathbf{v}$. Cuturi *et al.* [25] used $d(u, v) = ||u - v||^2$. In our case, as previously described, the time-series or trajectories obtained with the Gaussian process framework are characterised by a mean function and a measure of the uncertainty in the trajectory estimation, which handles the incompleteness, noise and artefacts underlying the observational data considered. That is, because we used

[2]That is, $\hat{\sigma} = \text{median}(||u - v||)\sqrt{L}$, where L corresponds to the median length of the time-series in $\mathscr{X}$.

a Gaussian likelihood function, each point u_i in a given trajectory $\mathbf{u}$, is defined by $u_i \sim \mathcal{N}(m_{u_i}, \Sigma_{u_i})$. In order to take this into account, we use the 2-Wasserstein distance between two Gaussian distributions [26], which is given by

$$d(u,v) = d(\mathcal{N}(m_u, \Sigma_u), \mathcal{N}(m_v, \Sigma_v)) = ||m_u - m_v||^2 + ||\Sigma_u^{1/2} - \Sigma_v^{1/2}||_F^2 \quad (6.18)$$

where $||\cdot||_F$ is the *Frobenius* (also called *Hilbert-Schmidt*) norm.

Using the measure of discrepancy (or similarity) described above, classification or clustering of the trajectories may be performed. There are a large number of clustering methods proposed in the literature. In this work, we use an *agglomerative hierarchical clustering* method. Other partitioning techniques, such as k-means or model-based clustering, share the property that objects in a dataset are partitioned into a specific number of clusters at a single step. In contrast, hierarchical clustering methods produce a cluster tree; i.e., a series of nested clusters through a series of partitions.

Hierarchical clustering can be either *agglomerative*, with fewer clusters at the higher level (by fusing clusters generated at the lower level), or *divisive*, which separate the n objects into more and finer groups in sequential steps. Agglomerative hierarchical clustering, in particular, starts with n clusters, each of which contains a single object in the dataset. In the second step, the two clusters that have the closest between-cluster distance are fused and are then treated as a single cluster in the next step. As the procedure continues, it results in a single cluster containing all the n objects. Agglomerative methods vary in the ways of defining the distance between two clusters when more than one object is present in either of them. For example, the single linkage method considers the shortest pair-wise distance between objects in two different clusters as the distance between the two clusters. In contrast, with the complete linkage method, the distance between two clusters is defined as the distance between the most distant pair of objects. Here, we use average linkage clustering, in which the average of the pair-wise distances between all pairs of objects coming from each of two clusters is taken as the distance between the two clusters.

The number of clusters was estimated using the *gap* method (which is described in Reference 27, together with a short review on methods for estimating the optimal number of clusters).

6.3 Results

We applied this method to the trajectories of the 326 post-operative patients in order to find different patterns of physiological recovery from major surgery. For this, the Gaussian process posteriors (over the uniform grid of test points sampled every hour) of the physiological trajectories were used. Hierarchical clustering was used to group similar trajectories based on the modified GA kernel distance described earlier.

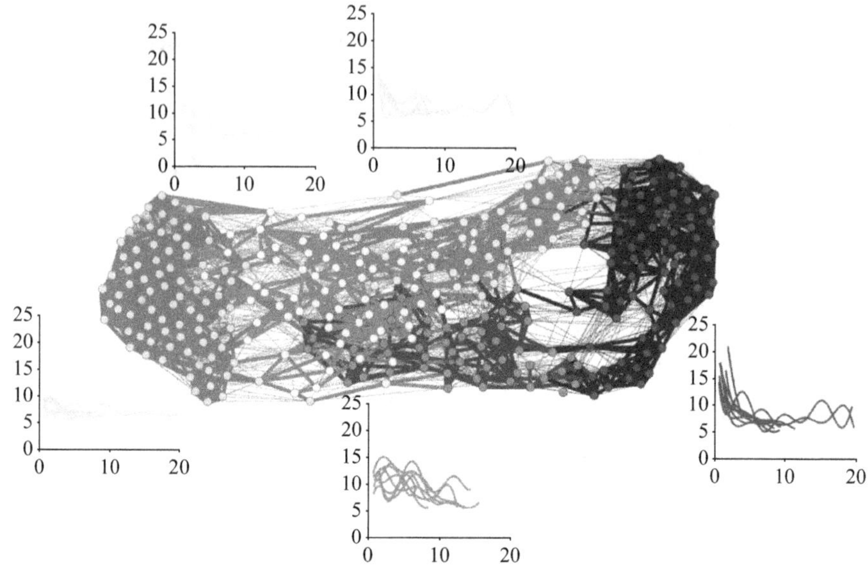

Figure 6.3 Representation of the clusters obtained during training using our patient-to-patient similarity approach: each node of the graph corresponds to a patient, and the edges connecting any two nodes represent the similarity between them. In each sub-plot, 10 random mean trajectories from each cluster are represented

The number of clusters obtained, determined using the *gap* method, was 5 functional clusters. Figure 6.3[3] illustrates the clusters of patients obtained. Figure 6.4 shows examples of trajectories associated with each cluster of patient trajectories, as an overall representation of the results obtained in this experiment. From the 326 patients included in the normal group, 87 (27%) were part of the cluster represented in the left part of the network represented in Figure 6.3 (first row of Figure 6.4), 79 (24%) were part of the cluster coloured with the dark colour (represented in the right part of the network in Figure 6.3, and last row of Figure 6.4), and the remaining of the patients were part of the other clusters (58 or 17% in the cluster represented in the second row of Figure 6.4, and 51 or 16% in each of the other two clusters).

6.4 Discussion

As expected, different patients may exhibit different physiological trajectories during recovery. Although all patients included in this analysis did recover from surgery and

[3]The graph was obtained using the freely available software called *Gephi*; for that, the similarity matrix (as computed by the proposed approach) was provided to the software, and the *ForceAtlas 2* algorithm was used to reorganise the layout of the graph, which takes into account the degree of similarity between the nodes and their neighbourhood.

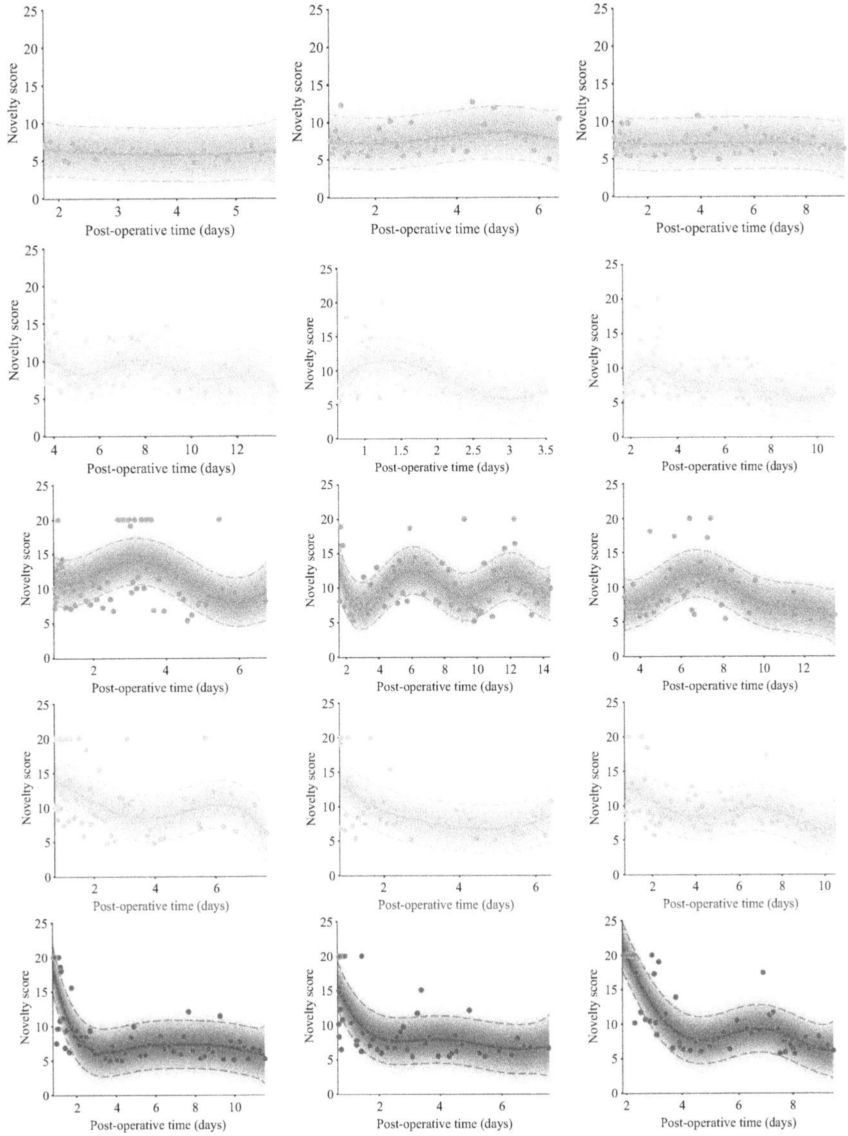

Figure 6.4 *Examples of the Gaussian process posteriors for three patients belonging to each cluster (each row represents patients from one cluster, which correspond to the clusters shown in Figure 6.3). Circles correspond to the raw data. Thick lines correspond to the posterior means, and dashed lines indicate the 95% confidence area for the posterior mean obtained. Shaded areas denote the uncertainty level of the mean (in darker areas, uncertainty is lower)*

were discharged home without any major adverse event in the course of their stay in the hospital, these results suggest that the physiological trajectories (based on the novelty scores) for these patients may be different from one another, as expected. While some patients exhibit a recovery trend with a pronounced decrease in the novelty score $z(\mathbf{x})$ in the first couple of days after surgery and a constant $z(\mathbf{x})$ for the remainder of their stay (Figure 6.4, bottom row), other patients present a relatively "stable" trajectory, with only small variations of $z(\mathbf{x})$ throughout their stay (e.g., Figure 6.4, top row). For other patients, a certain variation of $z(\mathbf{x})$ is manifested in their physiological trajectories.

Using the similarity metric and clustering procedure described earlier, the set of entities that are alike appear (visually) to be assigned to the same cluster, and entities from different clusters are also clearly less alike. There are many possible explanations for the different recovery patterns observed: the type of surgery that the patient underwent, the age of the patient, how fit the patient is at the time of operation and other possible underlying conditions. No direct and clear associations between the first two factors (surgery type and age) and the clusters of data were found, which may be due to the small number of patients included in this study and the variety of procedures that patients underwent, although there is room for exploring additional factors.

A few points should be made here regarding the analysis conducted and the results obtained. In the first place, we observe that small (daily) variations of the novelty scores were smoothed out in this analysis. The main goal of this approach was to capture the overall trajectory of recovery of post-operative patients, which motivated the selection of the covariance function (and hyperparameters priors) that was used to model the data with Gaussian processes. In order to also capture short-term variations, one could use a more complex covariance function derived by combining simple covariance functions. For example, the addition of two squared-exponential covariance functions, one to model the short-term variations in the novelty score, and one to model the long-term trends, could be used to provide a better fit to the data. Nevertheless, some additional work would be required to select the set of priors for each hyperparameter. A fully Bayesian approach would be advantageous in this case to better encode the level of uncertainty in the hyperparameters; i.e., rather than using an expensive grid-search optimisation procedure over all possible values for each hyperparameter, prior distributions could be set for each of the hyperparameters, which would be integrated out to obtain the Gaussian process posterior mean and variance.

It is also important to mention that, although we focused on the analysis using trajectories of novelty scores (resulting in "univariate" time-series data streams), the same approach could be used for multivariate time-series; for example, by considering all the vital signs, rather than the novelty score that combines them into a single score. As described earlier, the GA kernel distance is able to cope with multivariate time-series data. Nevertheless, the visualisation of the results for evaluating the performance of the method would be more challenging than that for the univariate case. Moreover, due to the increase of degrees of freedom in the multivariate case, a larger sample of data would be needed to derive a more representative set of trajectories for clustering.

We observe that the proposed approach may be used to recognise "normal" or previously observed physiological patterns and identify abnormal or "novel" physiological trajectories. For example, one may determine the distance (or similarity) between each test Gaussian posterior trajectory and the training Gaussian process posterior trajectories. According to this distance, the test trajectory may be either assigned to one of the five clusters of trajectories or classified as a "novel" trajectory (that is, it is substantially different from the trajectories computed during training). A similar approach has been described in Reference 28.

Finally, we also note that the comparison of our method with other approaches proposed in the literature (such as those proposed in References 9, 8, 6) may be difficult due to the characteristics of our observational dataset. The work described in this chapter may be more advantageous and provide promising results, as the described method includes a direct quantification of the uncertainty in the trajectory estimation (provided by the Gaussian process model), handling incompleteness, noise and artefact in a robust manner.

6.5 Conclusion

We have described a method by which unevenly sampled time-series data may be analysed to better understand the overall recovery trajectories of post-operative patients. Using a similarity metric, which is based on the concepts of DTW and GA kernel, and a hierarchical clustering method, different groups of physiological behaviours of recovery from surgery were revealed. The majority of patients were found to belong to one of two functional clusters: one group of patients who exhibited a recovery trend with a pronounced decrease in the novelty score in the first couple of days after surgery and a constant score for the remainder of their stay on the ward; and a group of patients who presented a relatively "stable" trajectory, with only small variations of the novelty score throughout their stay post-operatively.

The proposed approach may provide a new tool for studying and better understanding the recovery phase of patients post-operatively, which is known to be heterogeneous. As electronic medical records continue to collect data from other interventions (e.g., elective surgery), there will be a growing need for such tools based on machine learning to refine the characterisation of what constitutes a "normal" and an "abnormal" recovery from a major intervention, and quantify the effects of variability in treatment protocols across individuals in these groups.

Acknowledgements

Marco A. F. Pimentel was supported by a Health Innovation Challenge Fund by the Wellcome Trust and the Department of Health. David A. Clifton was supported by a Royal Academy of Engineering Research Fellowship; Balliol College, Oxford; and the Centre of Excellence in Personalised Healthcare funded by the Wellcome Trust and EPSRC [Grant WT 088877/Z/09/Z].

References

[1] J. Baker. The DRAGON system – an overview. *IEEE Transactions on Acoustics Speech and Signal Processing*, 23(1):24–29, 1975.

[2] J. A. Quinn, C. K. I. Williams, and N. McIntosh. Factorial switching linear dynamical systems applied to physiological condition monitoring. *IEEE Transactions on Pattern Analysis and Machine Intelligence*, 31(9):1537–1551, 2009.

[3] I. Stanculescu, C. K. I. Williams and Y. Freer. A hierarchical switching linear dynamical system applied to the detection of sepsis in neonatal condition monitoring. In *Proceedings of the 30th Conference on Uncertainty in Artificial Intelligence*, 2014.

[4] L. H. Lehman, S. Nemati, R. P. Adams, G. Moody, A. Malhotra and R. G. Mark. Tracking progression of patient state of health in critical care using inferred shared dynamics in physiological time series. In *Proceedings of the Annual International Conference of the IEEE Engineering in Medicine and Biology Society (EMBC)*, pages 7072–7075, 2013.

[5] A. S Willsky, E. B Sudderth, M. I. Jordan and E. B. Fox. Nonparametric Bayesian learning of switching linear dynamical systems. In *Advances in Neural Information Processing Systems*, pages 457–464, 2009.

[6] A. S. Willsky, E. B. Sudderth, M. I. Jordan and E. B. Fox. Sharing features among dynamical systems with Beta processes. In *Advances in Neural Information Processing Systems*, pages 549–557, 2009.

[7] L. H. Lehman, S. Nemati, R. P. Adams and R. G. Mark. Discovering shared dynamics in physiological signals: application to patient monitoring in ICU. In *Proceedings of the Annual International Conference of the IEEE Engineering in Medicine and Biology Society (EMBC)*, pages 5939–5942, 2012.

[8] S. Saria, D. Koller and A. Penn. Discovering shared and individual latent structure in multiple time series. *ArXiv preprint arXiv:1008.2028*, 2010.

[9] S. Saria, A. Duchi and D. Koller. Discovering deformable motifs in continuous time series data. In *Proceedings of the International Joint Conference on Artificial Intelligence (IJCAI)*, volume 22, page 1465, 2011.

[10] N. Lawrence. Probabilistic non-linear principal component analysis with Gaussian process latent variable models. *Journal of Machine Learning Research*, 6:1783–1816, Dec. 2005.

[11] C. E. Rasmussen and C. K. I. Williams. *Gaussian Processes for Machine Learning*. Cambridge, Massachusetts, MIT Press, 2006.

[12] L. Clifton, D. A. Clifton, M. A. F. Pimentel, P. J. Watkinson and L. Tarassenko. Gaussian processes for personalized e-health monitoring with wearable sensors. *IEEE Transactions on Biomedical Engineering*, 60(1):193–197, 2013.

[13] D. Wong, D. A. Clifton and L. Tarassenko. Probabilistic detection of vital sign abnormality with Gaussian process regression. In *IEEE 12th International Conference on Bioinformatics & Bioengineering (BIBE)*, pages 187–192, 2012.

[14] O. Stegle, S. V. Fallert, D. J. C. MacKay and S. Brage. Gaussian process robust regression for noisy heart rate data. *IEEE Transactions on Biomedical Engineering*, 55(9):2143–2151, 2008.

[15] D. Wong. *Identifying Vital Sign Abnormality in Acutely-ill Patients*. PhD thesis, University of Oxford, 2011.

[16] D. A. Clifton, L. Clifton, S. Hugueny, D. Wong and L. Tarassenko. An extreme function theory for novelty detection. *IEEE Journal of Selected Topics in Signal Processing*, 7(1):28–37, 2013.

[17] A. A. Kalaitzis and N. D. Lawrence. A simple approach to ranking differentially expressed gene expression time courses through Gaussian process regression. *BMC Bioinformatics*, 12(1):180, May 2011.

[18] M. A. F. Pimentel, D. A. Clifton, L. Clifton, P. J. Watkinson and L. Tarassenko. Modelling physiological deterioration in post-operative patient vital-sign data. *Medical & Biological Engineering & Computing*, 51(8):869–877, 2013.

[19] E. Parzen. On estimation of a probability density function and mode. *The Annals of Mathematical Statistics*, 33(3):1065–1076, 1962.

[20] M. A. F. Pimentel, D. A. Clifton, L. Clifton and L. Tarassenko. A review of novelty detection. *Signal Processing*, 99:215–249, 2014.

[21] H. Sakoe and S. Chiba. Dynamic programming algorithm optimization for spoken word recognition. *IEEE Transactions on Acoustics Speech and Signal Processing*, 26(1):43–49, 1978.

[22] C. Bahlmann, B. Haasdonk and H. Burkhardt. Online handwriting recognition with support vector machines – a kernel approach. In *Proceedings of the IEEE Eighth International Workshop on Frontiers in Handwriting Recognition*, pages 49–54, 2002.

[23] H. Shimodaira, H. S. K. -I. Noma, M. Nakai and S. Sagayama. Dynamic time-alignment kernel in support vector machine. *Advances in Neural Information Processing Systems*, 14:921, 2002.

[24] M. Cuturi. Fast global alignment kernels. In *Proceedings of the 28th International Conference on Machine Learning (ICML)*, pages 929–936, 2011.

[25] M. Cuturi, J. -P. Vert, Ø. Birkenes and T. Matsui. A kernel for time series based on global alignments. In *IEEE International Conference on Acoustics, Speech and Signal Processing (ICASSP)*, volume 2, pages 413–416, 2007.

[26] A. Takatsu. Wasserstein geometry of Gaussian measures. *Osaka Journal of Mathematics*, 48(4):1005–1026, 2011.

[27] R. Tibshirani, G. Walther and T. Hastie. Estimating the number of clusters in a data set via the gap statistic. *Journal of the Royal Statistical Society: Series B (Statistical Methodology)*, 63(2):411–423, 2001.

[28] M. A. F. Pimentel, D. A. Clifton and L. Tarassenko. Gaussian process clustering for the functional characterisation of vital-sign trajectories. In *IEEE International Workshop on Machine Learning for Signal Processing (MLSP)*, pages 1–6, 2013.

Chapter 7
A Bayesian model for fusing biomedical labels

Tingting Zhu, Gari D. Clifford and David A. Clifton

7.1 Background

In manual annotation of data, significant intra- and inter-observer disagreements exist [1,2]. Expert labelling (or 'reading' or 'annotating') of medical data by physicians or clinicians often involves multiple over-reads, particularly when an individual is under-confident of the diagnosis. However, experts are scarce and expensive and can create significant delays in labelling or diagnoses. Although medical training includes periodic assessment of general competency, specific assessments for reading medical data are difficult to be performed regularly. This data processing pipeline is further complicated by the ambiguous definition of an 'expert'. There is no empirical method for measuring level of expertise, even though label accuracy can vary greatly depending on the expert's experience. As a result, there exists a great deal of inter- and intra-expert variability among physicians depending on their experiences and level of training [1–8].

An effective probabilistic approach to aggregating expert labels which used an expectation–maximisation (EM) algorithm, was first proposed by Dawid and Skene [9]. They applied the EM algorithm to classify the unknown *true* states of health (i.e., fit to undergo a general anaesthetic) of 45 patients given the decision made by five anaesthetists. Raykar *et al.* [10] extended this approach to measure the diameter of a suspicious lesion on a medical image using a regression model. Their assumption was that the discrepancies of the lesion diameter estimates from different expert annotators were Gaussian distributed and noisy versions of the actual *true* diameter. The precision of each expert annotator and the underlying ground truth were jointly modelled in an iterative process using EM. More recently, Warby *et al.* [11] studied how to combine non-expert annotator's labels of sleep spindle location, a special pattern in human electroencephalography, through fusing annotations provided by non-experts. In that work, although naïve majority vote was used to aggregate the labels of the locations, they demonstrated that non-expert annotations were comparable to those provided by the experts (i.e., the by-subject spindle density correlation was 0.815).

Aggregating annotations (i.e., fusing multiple annotations for each piece of data from annotators with varying levels of expertise) from human and/or automated algorithms may provide a more accurate ground truth and reduce annotator inter- and

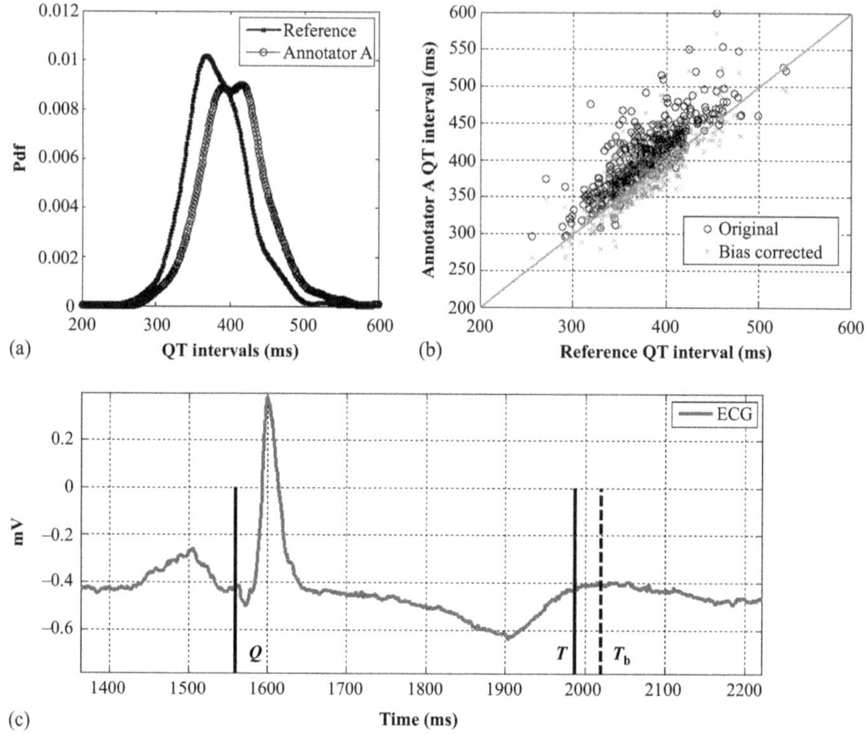

Figure 7.1 An example of bias in the context of electrocardiogram (ECG) QT interval labelling. (a) The probability density function of the QT intervals for the reference (supplied by the human experts) annotation and annotator A (such as an automated algorithm). (b) A plot of QT intervals across different recordings: the diagonal (grey) line indicates a perfect match of QT intervals between the reference and annotator A; the 'o' indicates the original QT intervals provided by annotator A; the 'x' indicates the bias-corrected QT intervals of annotator A, which fits closely to the diagonal line. (c) An example of bias that occurs in an ECG record for labelling QT interval. The reference QT interval on a single beat starts at the beginning of the Q wave and ends at the end of the T wave (denoted as Q and T), and the biased trend from annotator A is demonstrated as T_b

intra-variability. However, most annotators are likely to have some bias regardless of their expertise [12,13]. Bias is defined as the opposite of accuracy: it measures the average difference between the estimation and the *true* value, and it is annotator dependent. An example of bias is demonstrated in Figure 7.1 in the context of electrocardiogram labelling. In image segmentation, Warfield *et al.* [1] proposed a

Table 7.1 Survey of probabilistic techniques for fusing annotations to infer latent ground truth

Source	**Data Type**	**Feature Incorporation in the Model**	**Modelling of Annotator's Expertise**	**Modelling of Annotator's Bias**	**Dealing with Missing Annotations**
Wiebe *et al.* [18]	Categorical	✓	X	✓	N/A
Snow *et al.* [19]	Categorical, continuous	X	✓	✓	N/A
Warfield *et al.* [1]	Continuous	X	✓	✓	N/A
Commowick and Waefield [20]	Continuous	X	✓	✓	N/A
Raykar *et al.* [10]	Binary, ordinal, continuous	✓	✓	X	✓
Ipeirotis *et al.* [21]	Binary	X	✓	✓	N/A
Welinder and Perona [12]	Binary, multi-valued, continuous	X	✓	X	N/A
Welinder *et al.* [15]	Binary	✓	✓	✓	N/A
Baba and Kashima [22]	Categorical	X	✓	✓	N/A
Cabrera *et al.* [23]	Binary	✓	✓	✓*	N/A
Xing *et al.* [16]	Continuous	X	✓	✓	N/A
Xing *et al.* [24]	Continuous	X	✓	✓	N/A
Akhondi-Asl *et al.* [25]	Continuous	X	✓	✓	N/A
Ouyang *et al.*	Continuous	X	✓	✓	✓
Nasir *et al.* [26]	Continuous	X	X	✓	✓
Kamar *et al.* [27]	Categorical	✓	✓	✓**	N/A
Proposed model	Continuous	✓	✓	✓	✓

Notes: N/A—not available as it was not modelled or discussed in the publication. The values with * means the bias is modelled as observation-specific (i.e., dataset-specific) dependent, and the ** refers to both annotator- and dataset-specific.

model to estimate the annotator/labeller-generated segmentation by measuring the bias and variance of the distance between the segmentation boundary and a reference standard boundary. An EM algorithm was used to infer the boundary of a segmentation, and the bias and variance of each annotator in a jointly manner. A similar model was described by Ouyang *et al.* [14], which obtained the quantitative ground truth (such as count and percentage estimation) measure in crowd sensing. Welinder and Perona [12] designed a Bayesian EM framework for continuous-valued labels, which explicitly modelled the precision only of each annotator to account for their varying skill levels, without modelling the bias of annotators. A more specialised form of the Bayesian model of bias was detailed in a different study by Welinder *et al.* [15] but for binary classification tasks. Xing *et al.* had proposed using a Gaussian prior on the bias parameter for the identification of cardiac landmarks in two-dimensional images [16]. However, their model does not cater for missing annotations and the possibility of incorporating physiological features into the model to further improve the estimation of ground truth as shown in References 10, 17.

A more comprehensive survey of different approaches is listed in Table 7.1; the methodology proposed in this thesis particularly focuses on the improvement on these prior algorithms [1,10,12,15,16] by introducing the novelty of combining *continuous-valued annotations* to infer the underlying ground truth, while *jointly modelling the annotator's bias and precision* in an unified model using a Bayesian treatment.

In contrast to previous work [17], this article proposes a Bayesian framework for aggregating multiple continuous-valued annotations in medical data labelling, which takes into account the precision and bias of the individual annotators. Moreover, a generalised form is proposed, and can be extended to incorporate contextual features of the physiological signal, so that the weighting of each label can be adjusted based on the estimated bias and variance of the individual for different types of signal. To current knowledge, the proposed model for estimating continuous-valued labels in an unsupervised manner is novel in the medical domain.

7.2 A generative model of annotators

A generative model is commonly considered as a stochastic process that randomly simulates synthetic dataset(s) as observations, given some model parameter values. It is fully probabilistic as it models the joint probability of all parameters.

7.2.1 The ground truth model

Suppose that there are N records of physiological time-series data. The underlying ground truth (e.g., the *true* time or duration of an event or diameter of an object) for the ith record, z_i, can be assumed to be drawn from a Gaussian distribution[1] with mean a and variance $1/b$. The probability density function (denoted as pdf) of z_i is defined as follows:

$$p(z_i \mid a, b) = \mathcal{N}(z_i \mid a, 1/b), \tag{7.1}$$

where a can be expressed as a linear regression function $f(\mathbf{w}, \mathbf{x})$ with an intercept w_0 [10,17]: $\mathbf{w}$ are the coefficients of the regression that also includes w_0. $\mathbf{x}_i$ is a column feature vector for the ith record containing d features (i.e., d-dimensional design matrix, $\mathbf{X} = \left[\mathbf{x}_1^\top, ..., \mathbf{x}_N^\top\right]$). To cater for the modelling of w_0, a scalar value of one was added in the feature matrix (i.e., $\mathbf{x}_i = [1, \mathbf{x}_i]$)). w_0 models the overall offset predicted in the regression, which is different from the annotator-specific bias ϕ in the proposed model, which will be described in Section 7.2.2. Furthermore, the precision of the

[1] A univariate Gaussian distribution can be defined as $\mathcal{N}\left(z \mid \mu, \sigma^2\right) = \left(2\pi\sigma^2\right)^{(-1/2)} \exp\left(-(z-\mu)^2/2\sigma^2\right)$, where μ is the mean and σ^2 is the variance of the distribution.

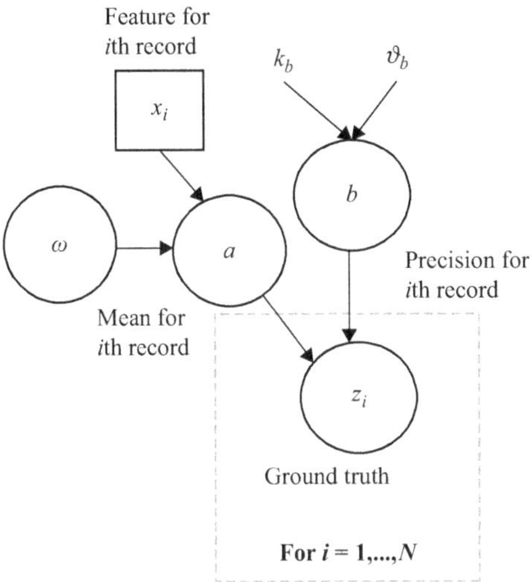

Figure 7.2 Graphical representation of the ground truth model: the z_i (the unknown underlying ground truth) corresponds to the true annotation for the ith record, from a total of N recordings. z_i is modelled by a Gaussian distribution with parameters mean a and variance $1/b$, where a can be a function of feature vector $\mathbf{x}_i$ as a linear regression function $f(\mathbf{w}, \mathbf{x})$ with an intercept, and $\mathbf{w}$ being the coefficients of the regression. The precision value, b, is drawn from a Gamma distribution with parameters k_b, ϑ_b

ground truth defined as the inverse-variance, b, is assumed to be modelled from a Gamma distribution[2] as follows:

$$p(b \mid k_b, \vartheta_b) = \text{Gamma}(b \mid k_b, \vartheta_b) \tag{7.2}$$

where k_b is the shape parameter and ϑ_b is the scale parameter. The graphical representation of the ground truth is shown in Figure 7.2. If one further assumes that the ground truth can be drawn independently from the N records, the conditional probability of $\mathbf{z}$ is given by:

$$p(\mathbf{z} \mid \mathbf{x}, \mathbf{w}, b) = \prod_{i=1}^{N} \mathcal{N}(\mathbf{x}_i^{\mathsf{T}}\mathbf{w}, 1/b) \tag{7.3}$$

[2]A Gamma distribution can be defined as $\text{Gamma}(x \mid k, \vartheta) = \frac{1}{\Gamma(k)\vartheta^k} x^{k-1} \exp\left(-\frac{x}{\vartheta}\right)$, where k is the shape of the distribution and ϑ is the scale of the distribution, $\Gamma(\cdot)$ is a gamma function. Gamma distribution is commonly used to model positive continuous values and it is therefore assumed that precision values are drawn from a Gamma distribution

7.2.2 The annotator model

Assuming for N recordings, there is a given dataset, $\mathbf{D} = [\mathbf{x}_i^\mathsf{T}, y_i^{j=1}, \cdots, y_i^{j=R}]_{i=1}^N$, where y_i^j corresponds to the annotation provided by the jth annotator for the ith record, and there are a total of R annotators. In this model, it is assumed that y_i^j is a noisy version of z_i, with a Gaussian distribution $\mathcal{N}(y_i^j \mid z_i, (\sigma^j)^2)$. The motivation for this comes from the central limit theorem: given the assumption that the annotations are independent and identically distributed, they will converge to a Gaussian distribution. In the absence of prior knowledge, this assumption allows for a robust and generalisable model for the given data. Here σ^j is the standard deviation of the jth annotator and represents his variance in annotation around z_i. Furthermore, the bias of each annotator, defined as the opposite of accuracy where it measures the average difference between the estimation and the *true* value, can be modelled as an additional term, denoted as ϕ^j [1]. The pdf of estimating y_i^j can then be written as:

$$p(y_i^j \mid z_i, (\sigma^j)^2) = \mathcal{N}(y_i^j \mid z_i + \phi^j, 1/\lambda^j) \tag{7.4}$$

where $(\sigma^j)^2$ is replaced with $1/\lambda^j$. λ^j is the precision of the jth annotator, defined as the estimated inverse-variance of annotator j. Note that λ^j and ϕ^j are considered to be constants for the jth annotator, i.e., all annotators are assumed to have consistent but usually different performances throughout records. It is assumed that $y_i^1, \cdots, y_i^R$ are conditionally independent given the ground truth z_i, and under the assumption that records are independent, the conditional pdf of $\mathbf{y}$ can be modelled as:

$$p(\mathbf{y} \mid \mathbf{z}, \boldsymbol{\phi}, \boldsymbol{\lambda}) = \prod_{i=1}^{N} \prod_{j=1}^{R} \mathcal{N}(z_i + \phi^j, 1/\lambda^j) \tag{7.5}$$

This may not be necessarily true, especially in cases where the annotations are generated by algorithms, some of which may be partially dependent variations of the same approach. Nevertheless, this choice was made to drastically simplify the model and subsequent derivation of the likelihood. Furthermore, it is assumed that the pdf of a given bias of annotator j, ϕ^j, drawn from a Gaussian distribution with mean μ_ϕ and variance $1/\alpha_\phi$ [16], is given by:

$$p(\phi^j \mid \mu_\phi, \alpha_\phi) = \mathcal{N}(\phi^j \mid \mu_\phi, 1/\alpha_\phi) \tag{7.6}$$

Although the biases of the annotators might be derived from other distributions, they are likely to be dataset dependent. In the absence of any knowledge of the underlying distribution of biases, they are assumed to be drawn from a Gaussian distribution. As described earlier that precision values can be modelled using a Gamma distribution, it is therefore assumed that precision values, such as λ^j and α_ϕ, were drawn from a Gamma distribution, with parameters k_λ, ϑ_λ, and k_α, ϑ_α, respectively:

$$p\left(\lambda^j \mid k_\lambda, \vartheta_\lambda\right) = \text{Gamma}\left(\lambda^j \mid k_\lambda, \vartheta_\lambda\right) \tag{7.7}$$

$$p\left(\alpha_\phi \mid k_\alpha, \vartheta_\alpha\right) = \text{Gamma}\left(\alpha_\phi \mid k_\alpha, \vartheta_\alpha\right) \tag{7.8}$$

The graphical representation of the annotator model is shown in Figure 7.3.

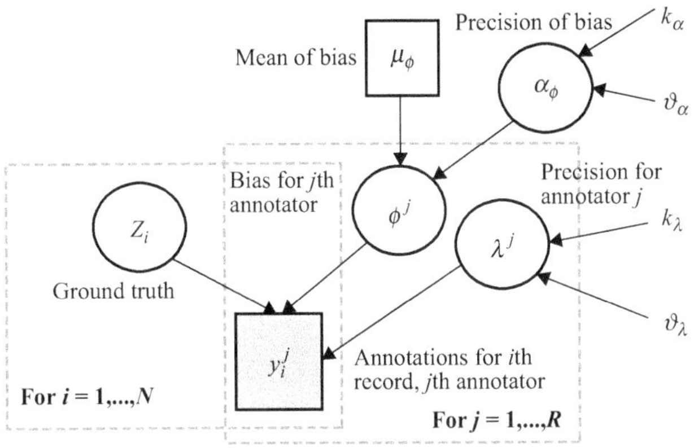

Figure 7.3 *Graphical representation of the annotator model: y_i^j corresponds to the annotation provided by the jth annotator for the ith record, and it is modelled by the z_i (the unknown underlying ground truth), the ϕ^j (bias), and the λ^j (precision). Furthermore, ϕ^j is modelled from a Gaussian distribution with mean μ_ϕ and variance $1/\alpha_\phi$. The λ^j and α_ϕ are drawn from a Gamma distribution with parameters k_λ, ϑ_λ, and k_α, ϑ_α, respectively*

7.3 Bayesian probability in parameter estimation

The generative models detailed in Section 7.2 describe how the data were produced given some parameter values. It is also possible to infer unknown or latent parameters in each model given the observations (i.e., annotations provided by annotators). Assuming there are observed data **D** and the parameter θ is to be estimated for a model, then Bayes' theorem can be used to evaluate the posterior probability of θ after **D** has been observed:

$$p(\theta \mid \mathbf{D}) = \frac{p(\mathbf{D} \mid \theta)\, p(\theta)}{\int_\theta p(\mathbf{D} \mid \theta)\, p(\theta)\, \mathrm{d}\theta} \tag{7.9}$$

where the quantity $p(\mathbf{D} \mid \theta)$ is the likelihood function of observing data **D** given different values of θ, and $p(\theta)$ is the prior probability distribution over θ. Prior knowledge of θ can be obtained from expert knowledge, contextual information, and previous observations before seeing the current data **D**. The denominator is the normalised constant described as the 'evidence' or marginal likelihood, which ensures that $p(\theta \mid \mathbf{D})$ is a probability density that integrates to one [28]. In many applications where the interest lies in estimating the posterior with various values of θ, the denominator is considered to be fixed, and hence the posterior is proportional to the product of the likelihood and the prior:

$$p(\theta \mid \mathbf{D}) \propto p(\mathbf{D} \mid \theta) p(\theta) \\ \propto \prod_{i=1}^{N} p(\mathbf{y}_i \mid \theta) p(\theta) \tag{7.10}$$

where $\mathbf{D}$ is assumed to have N independent observations, such as $\mathbf{D} = \{\mathbf{y}_{i=1}, \cdots, \mathbf{y}_{i=N}\}$, and $\mathbf{y}_i$ is a row vector for the ith observation.

In contrast to fully Bayesian methods, frequentist approaches can also be used to approximate the parameters of interest, where the posterior probability is determined entirely from the observations themselves. One of the most commonly used methods for this purpose is maximum likelihood (ML), which assumes the following:

$$p(\theta \mid \mathbf{D}) = \prod_{i=1}^{N} p(\mathbf{y}_i \mid \theta) \tag{7.11}$$

The ML approach obtains a point estimate for θ that maximises the likelihood function; i.e., $\underset{\theta}{\operatorname{argmax}} \left\{ \prod_{i=1}^{N} p(\mathbf{y}_i \mid \theta) \right\}$. An example of the ML approach for a given set of observation $\mathbf{y}_1$ is shown in Figure 7.4(a), where it estimates the most probable value of θ that best explains $\mathbf{y}_1$; i.e., $\underset{\theta}{\operatorname{argmax}} \{p(\mathbf{y}_1 \mid \theta)\}$. A similar example for two sets of observations $\{\mathbf{y}_1, \mathbf{y}_2\}$ is shown in Figure 7.4(b) where ML maximises the joint probability; i.e., $\underset{\theta}{\operatorname{argmax}} \{p(\mathbf{y}_1, \mathbf{y}_2 \mid \theta)\}$. Note that the prior $p(\theta)$ is missing in the ML approach, or equivalently, is assumed to have a uniform prior of one (i.e., there is equal probability for each value of θ). However, because the ML approach produces a point estimate, it can be heavily biased when only a small set of data is observed, and is sensitive to the choice of starting values where a local maximum (instead of the global maximum) may be found.

Beyond the ML approach, the maximum-a-posteriori (MAP) method incorporates a prior distribution over the data $\mathbf{D}$, which acts as a regularisation term to ensure that the posterior probability does not solely depend on a potentially small number of observations. The posterior of θ for MAP is written as:

$$p(\theta \mid \mathbf{D}) = \prod_{i=1}^{N} p(\mathbf{y}_i \mid \theta) p(\theta) \tag{7.12}$$

Figure 7.4 demonstrates the difference between the ML and the MAP approaches for one set or multiple sets of observations. The posterior of θ is estimated by the MAP approach as maximising the joint probability of the likelihood function and prior distribution (i.e., $\underset{\theta}{\operatorname{argmax}} \left\{ \prod_{i=1}^{N} p(\mathbf{y}_i \mid \theta) p(\theta) \right\}$). This is demonstrated as $\underset{\theta}{\operatorname{argmax}} \{p(\mathbf{y}_1 \mid \theta) p(\theta)\}$ for dataset $\mathbf{y}_1$ as shown in Figure 7.4(a), and $\underset{\theta}{\operatorname{argmax}} \{p(\mathbf{y}_1, \mathbf{y}_2 \mid \theta) p(\theta)\}$ for datasets $\{\mathbf{y}_1, \mathbf{y}_2\}$ as shown in Figure 7.4(b). The estimated posterior distribution of θ (i.e., $p(\mathbf{y}_1 \mid \theta)$ or $p(\mathbf{y}_1, \mathbf{y}_2 \mid \theta)$) using the ML approach differs from that obtained using MAP (i.e., $p(\mathbf{y}_1 \mid \theta) p(\theta)$ or

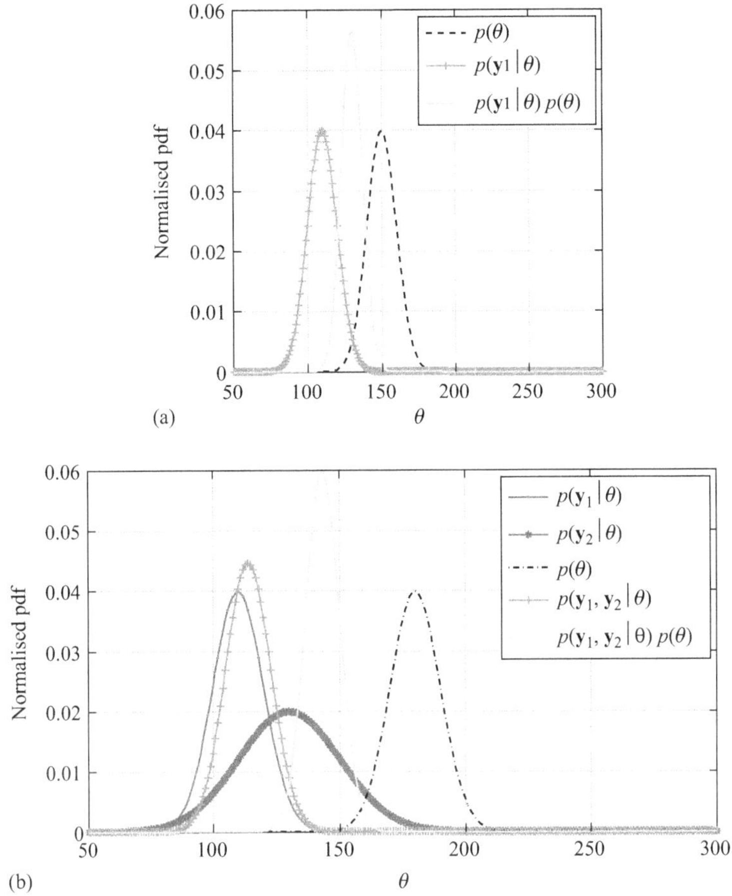

Figure 7.4 *Examples of the difference between the ML and the MAP approaches: (a) when there is a set of observations* $\mathbf{y}_1$*, the ML approach estimates the most probable value of* θ *that best explains these observations; i.e.,* $\underset{\theta}{\operatorname{argmax}}\{p(\mathbf{y}_1 \mid \theta)\}$*, whereas the MAP approach estimates the joint probability of the likelihood function and the prior by* $\underset{\theta}{\operatorname{argmax}}\{p(\mathbf{y}_1 \mid \theta)\, p(\theta)\}$*; (b) when there are two sets of independent observations,* $\mathbf{y}_1$ *and* $\mathbf{y}_2$*, the ML estimation of the* θ *maximises their joint probability; i.e.,* $\underset{\theta}{\operatorname{argmax}}\{p(\mathbf{y}_1, \mathbf{y}_2 \mid \theta)\}$*, while the MAP incorporates the prior as* $\underset{\theta}{\operatorname{argmax}}\{p(\mathbf{y}_1, \mathbf{y}_2 \mid \theta)\, p(\theta)\}$

$p(\mathbf{y}_1, \mathbf{y}_2 \mid \theta)\, p(\theta))$. The value for θ is chosen at the mode of its posterior distribution: it is 110 and 130 for dataset $\mathbf{y}_1$, 114 and 143 for datasets $\{\mathbf{y}_1, \mathbf{y}_2\}$ using ML and MAP, respectively. The BCLA model will be solved using the MAP approach and detailed in Section 7.4.

7.4 The Bayesian continuous-valued label aggregator

The Bayesian Continuous-Valued Label Aggregator (BCLA) model [29] was created to combine the ground truth and annotator models. It comprises two key contributions: (i) BCLA provides an unsupervised estimation of the continuous-valued annotations that are valuable for time-series-related data, as well as duration of events for physiological data; (ii) it introduces a unified framework for combining continuous-valued annotations to infer the underlying ground truth, while jointly modelling annotators' bias and precision values. The graphical form of BCLA is presented in Figure 7.5.

Under the assumption that records are independent, the likelihood of the parameter $\boldsymbol{\theta} = \{\mathbf{w}, \boldsymbol{\lambda}, \boldsymbol{\phi}, \alpha_{\phi}, b, z_i\}$ for a given dataset $\mathbf{D}$ can be formulated as:

$$p(\mathbf{D} \mid \boldsymbol{\theta}) = \prod_{i=1}^{N} p\left(y_i^1, \cdots, y_i^R \mid \mathbf{x}_i, \boldsymbol{\theta}\right) \tag{7.13}$$

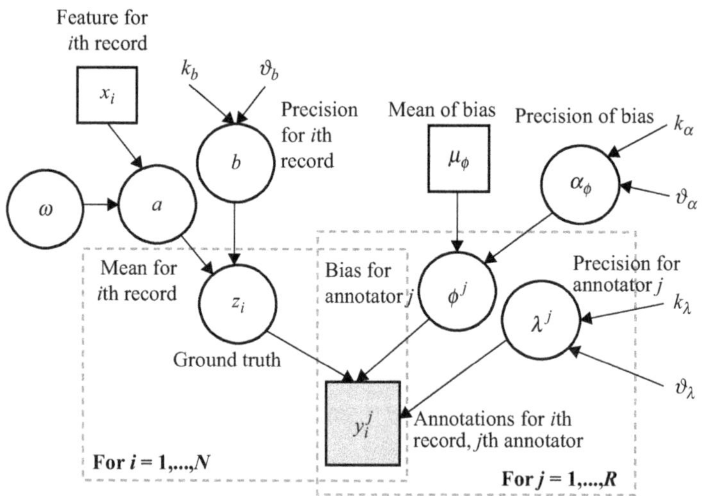

Figure 7.5 Graphical representation of the BCLA model: y_i^j corresponds to the annotation provided by the jth annotator for the ith record, and is modelled by the z_i (the unknown underlying ground truth), the ϕ^j (bias), and the λ^j (precision). Furthermore, z_i is drawn from a Gaussian distribution with parameters mean a and variance $1/b$, where a can be a function of feature vector $\mathbf{x}_i$ as a linear regression function $f(\mathbf{w}, \mathbf{x})$ with an intercept, and $\mathbf{w}$ being the coefficients of the regression. ϕ^j is modelled from a Gaussian distribution with mean μ_ϕ and variance $1/\alpha_\phi$. The b, λ^j, and α_ϕ are drawn from a Gamma distribution (denoted as Gamma*) with parameters k_b, ϑ_b, k_λ, ϑ_λ, and k_α, ϑ_α, respectively*

It is assumed that $y_i^1, \cdots, y_i^R$ are conditionally independent given the feature $\mathbf{x}_i$ (i.e., each annotator works independently to provide annotations). The likelihood of the parameter θ for a given dataset $\mathbf{D}$ can be written using Bayes' theorem as:

$$\begin{aligned}
p(\boldsymbol{\theta} \mid \mathbf{D}) &\propto p(\mathbf{D} \mid \boldsymbol{\theta})\, p(\boldsymbol{\theta}) \\
&= \text{Gamma}\left(\alpha_\phi \mid k_\alpha, \vartheta_\alpha\right) \text{Gamma}\left(b \mid k_b, \vartheta_b\right) \\
&\quad \times \left[\prod_{j=1}^{R} \mathcal{N}\left(\phi^j \mid \mu_\phi, 1/\alpha_\phi\right) \text{Gamma}\left(\lambda^j \mid k_\lambda, \vartheta_\lambda\right)\right] \\
&\quad \times \left[\prod_{i=1}^{N} \mathcal{N}\left(z_i \mid \mathbf{x}_i^{\mathsf{T}} \mathbf{w}, 1/b\right) \prod_{j=1}^{R} \mathcal{N}\left(y_i^j \mid z_i + \phi^j, 1/\lambda^j\right)\right]
\end{aligned} \tag{7.14}$$

7.4.1 The MAP approach of the BCLA model

The estimation of $\boldsymbol{\theta}$ can be solved using an MAP approach, which maximises the log-likelihood of the parameters, i.e., $\underset{\boldsymbol{\theta}}{\operatorname{argmax}} \{\log p(\boldsymbol{\theta} \mid \mathbf{D})\}$. The log-likelihood can be rewritten as:

$$\begin{aligned}
\log p(\boldsymbol{\theta} \mid \mathbf{D}) &= -\frac{1}{2} \sum_{i=1}^{N} \sum_{j=1}^{R} \left[\log\left(\frac{2\pi}{\lambda^j}\right) + \left(y_i^j - \phi^j - z_i\right)^2 \lambda^j\right] \\
&\quad -\frac{1}{2} \sum_{j=1}^{R} \left[\log\left(\frac{2\pi}{\alpha_\phi}\right) + \left(\phi^j - \mu_\phi\right)^2 \alpha_\phi\right] \\
&\quad -\frac{1}{2} \sum_{i=1}^{N} \left[\log\left(\frac{2\pi}{b}\right) + \left(z_i - \mathbf{x}_i^{\mathsf{T}} \mathbf{w}\right)^2 b\right] \\
&\quad + \left[(k_\lambda - 1)\log \lambda^j - \log\left(\Gamma(k_\lambda) \vartheta_\lambda^{(k_\lambda)}\right) - \frac{\lambda^j}{\vartheta_\lambda}\right] \\
&\quad + \left[(k_\alpha - 1)\log \alpha_\phi - \log\left(\Gamma(k_\alpha) \vartheta_\alpha^{(k_\alpha)}\right) - \frac{\alpha_\phi}{\vartheta_\alpha}\right] \\
&\quad + \left[(k_b - 1)\log b - \log\left(\Gamma(k_b) \vartheta_b^{(k_b)}\right) - \frac{b}{\vartheta_b}\right]
\end{aligned} \tag{7.15}$$

Parameters $\boldsymbol{\theta}$ can be derived by estimating the gradient of the log-likelihood, respectively:

$$\frac{\mathrm{d} \log p(\boldsymbol{\theta} \mid \mathbf{D})}{\mathrm{d}\lambda^j} = -\frac{1}{2} \sum_{i=1}^{N} \left[\left(y_i^j - \phi^j - z_i\right)^2 - \frac{1}{\lambda^j}\right] + \frac{k_\lambda - 1}{\lambda^j} - \frac{1}{\vartheta_\lambda}.$$

$$\frac{\mathrm{d} \log p(\boldsymbol{\theta} \mid \mathbf{D})}{\mathrm{d}\mathbf{w}} = \frac{1}{b} \sum_{i=1}^{N} \left(z_i \mathbf{x}_i - \mathbf{x}_i^{\mathsf{T}} \mathbf{w} \mathbf{x}_i\right)$$

$$\frac{\mathrm{d}\log p\,(\boldsymbol{\theta}\mid\mathbf{D})}{\mathrm{d}\phi^j}=\sum_{i=1}^{N}\lambda^j\left(y_i^j-\phi^j-z_i\right)-\phi^j\alpha_\phi+\mu_\phi\alpha_\phi$$

$$\frac{\mathrm{d}\log p\,(\boldsymbol{\theta}\mid\mathbf{D})}{\mathrm{d}\alpha_\phi}=\frac{R}{2\alpha_\phi}-\frac{1}{2}\sum_{j=1}^{R}\left(\phi^j-\mu_\phi\right)^2+\frac{k_\alpha-1}{\alpha_\phi}-\frac{1}{\vartheta_\alpha}$$

$$\frac{\mathrm{d}\log p\,(\boldsymbol{\theta}\mid\mathbf{D})}{\mathrm{d}b}=\frac{N}{2b}-\frac{1}{2}\sum_{i=1}^{N}\left(z_i-\mathbf{x}_i^{\mathsf{T}}\mathbf{w}\right)^2+\frac{k_b-1}{b}-\frac{1}{\vartheta_b}$$

By equating derivatives to zero, the parameters in $\boldsymbol{\theta}$ can be derived as

$$\frac{1}{\lambda^j}=\frac{1}{N+2(k_\lambda-1)}\left[\sum_{i=1}^{N}\left(y_i^j-\phi^j-z_i\right)^2+\frac{2}{\vartheta_\lambda}\right] \tag{7.16}$$

$$\mathbf{w}=\left(\sum_{i=1}^{N}\mathbf{x}_i\mathbf{x}_i^{\mathsf{T}}\right)^{-1}\sum_{i=1}^{N}\mathbf{x}_i z_i \tag{7.17}$$

$$\phi^j=\frac{1}{N+\frac{\alpha_\phi}{\lambda^j}}\left[\sum_{i=1}^{N}\left(y_i^j-z_i\right)+\mu_\phi\left(\frac{\alpha_\phi}{\lambda^j}\right)\right] \tag{7.18}$$

$$\frac{1}{\alpha_\phi}=\frac{1}{R+2(k_\alpha-1)}\left[\sum_{j=1}^{R}\left(\phi^j-\mu_\phi\right)^2+\frac{2}{\vartheta_\alpha}\right] \tag{7.19}$$

$$\frac{1}{b}=\frac{1}{N+2(k_b-1)}\left[\sum_{i=1}^{N}\left(z_i-\mathbf{x}_i^{\mathsf{T}}\mathbf{w}\right)^2+\frac{2}{\vartheta_b}\right] \tag{7.20}$$

This parameter estimation can be performed using the EM algorithm in a two-step iterative process:
(i) The E-step estimates the expected *true* annotations for the ith record, $\hat{z}_i$, in our MAP formulation as being a weighted sum of the provided annotations, and which can be estimated as:

$$\hat{z}_i=\frac{\sum_{j=1}^{R}\left[\left(y_i^j-\phi^j\right)\lambda^j\right]+\left(\mathbf{x}_i^{\mathsf{T}}\mathbf{w}\right)b}{\sum_{j=1}^{R}\lambda^j+b} \tag{7.21}$$

(ii) The M-step is based on the current estimation of $\hat{\mathbf{z}}$ and the dataset $\mathbf{D}$. The model parameters, $\mathbf{w}$, $\boldsymbol{\phi}$, α_ϕ, b, and $\boldsymbol{\lambda}$ can be updated using (7.17), (7.18), (7.19), (7.20), and (7.16) accordingly in a sequential order until convergence, which is now described.

7.4.2 Convergence criteria for the BCLA-MAP model

Extreme Value Theorem

Extreme value theorem (EVT) is generally used to describe the modelling of the distribution of extreme values (being either maxima or minima): if a function is continuous and contained in a closed interval, then it has a maximum and a minimum value. According to Fisher–Tippett theorem, given that there are m independent, identically distributed random values (i.e., $\mathbf{x} = [x_{i=1}, \cdots, x_{i=m}]$) that are observed from a function $F(x)$, $x_{max} = \max(\mathbf{x})$ can be modelled using a family of extreme value distributions such as Gumbel, Fréchet, and Weibull distributions [30].

EVT for the BCLA-MAP Model

When using the EM algorithm for an MAP-based model, one may encounter a convergence problem, particularly when estimating a large number of parameters. The estimation of the precision λ^j may lead to values that tend to infinity because the model favours the annotator with the highest precision in each EM update step, while maximising the likelihood. Instead of incorporating an additional parameter for a regularisation penalty that increases with the complexity of the model, the generalised extreme value distribution (GEVD)[3] can be used to model the maxima of the precision distribution, denoted as λ_m, in order to restrict the upper bound of the precision values and guarantee convergence of the MAP algorithm. The pdf of the GEVD for λ_m is:

$$p(\lambda_m \mid k, \mu, \vartheta) = \exp\left\{ -\left[1 + k\frac{(\lambda_m - \mu)}{\vartheta}\right]^{-\frac{1}{k}} \right\} \frac{1}{\vartheta}\left[1 + k\frac{(\lambda_m - \mu)}{\vartheta}\right]^{\left(-1-\frac{1}{k}\right)} \tag{7.22}$$

where k is a shape parameter, ϑ is a scale parameter, and μ is a location parameter. These parameters can be derived by fitting a GEVD to the maximum values drawn randomly from the *prior* distribution of the precision, $\text{Gamma}(\lambda \mid k_\lambda, \vartheta_\lambda)$. An upper bound of the maximum precision value can then be obtained by estimating $F(\lambda_m) = 0.99$ probability on the inverse cumulative distribution function $F(\lambda_m)$ of the GEVD. Figure 7.6 demonstrates an example of drawing the maxima of the precision distribution using different sample size (denoted as m) values. Figure 7.6(a) shows the majority of the probability density described by the GEVDs is shifted toward higher values on the x-axis as m increases: it is expected to have higher value of λ_m as more samples are drawn from the Gamma distribution. The ideal sample size, however, is application-dependent [31]: As the threshold values are monotonically increasing with increasing m, the GEVD can become less sensitive as it includes ever more extreme values which might be outliers in a given dataset. In the context of measuring ECG QT/QTc prolongation due to drugs, such an effect is only pertinent when the difference in QT/QTc exceeds ± 5 ms of the mean QT/QTc at the 95% confidence interval [32]. Thereby following this intuition, and choosing the upper bound of the precision to be approximately $\lambda_m = 0.04$. This corresponds to the fact that the most accurate estimation of QT/QTc would have an error rate below ± 5ms of the ground truth. The optimal value for m can then be estimated through obtaining the 99% probability of exceeding such threshold (i.e., $P(\lambda > \lambda_m) = 1 - \int_{-\infty}^{\lambda_m} p(\lambda_m)\, d\lambda_m = 0.99$). In the case where there is no physiological constraint on the value of λ_m, the GEVD can still be used to define a sensible threshold for a given dataset.

[3]GEVD combines Gumbel, Fréchet, and Weibull distributions into a single form.

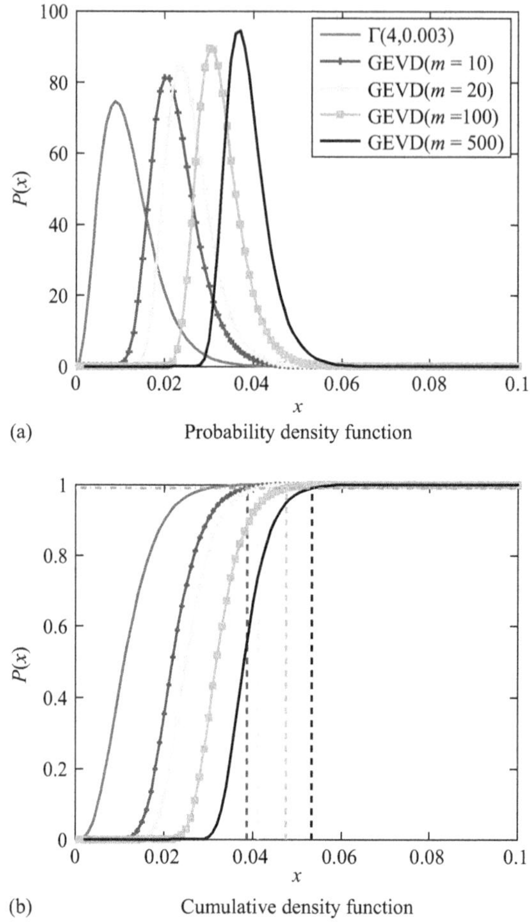

Figure 7.6 An example of estimating the $\lambda_m \sim \text{Gamma}(4, 0.003)$*: (a) shows the fitted GEVD corresponding to drawing m = 10, 20,100, and 500 samples from the Gamma distribution; (b) demonstrates the cumulative density function of the GEVDs with values (as dash vertical line) corresponding to the 99th percentile (as dotted horizontal line) for different m values*

7.4.3 Learning from incomplete data using the BCLA-MAP model

In the case where there exist missing labels from annotators, only the available annotations should be considered for inferring the ground truth. The expected z_i can be re-written as:

$$z_i = \frac{\sum_{j \in V_i} \lambda^j (y_i^j - \phi^j) + (\mathbf{x}_i^\top \mathbf{w}) b}{\sum_{j \in V_i} \lambda^j + b} \tag{7.23}$$

The precision of the jth annotator is as follows:

$$\frac{1}{\lambda^j} = \frac{1}{N_j} + 2(k_\lambda - 1)\left[\sum_{i \in U_j}\left(y_i^j - \phi^j - z_i\right)^2 + \frac{2}{\vartheta_\lambda}\right] \tag{7.24}$$

The bias value for the jth annotator can now be written as:

$$\phi^j = \frac{\sum\limits_{i \in U_j}\left(y_i^j - z_i\right) + \mu_\phi\left(\frac{\alpha_\phi}{\lambda^j}\right)}{N_j + \frac{\alpha_\phi}{\lambda^j}} \tag{7.25}$$

where U_j is the set of records with annotations provided by the jth annotator, and V_i is the set of annotators that provided annotations for the ith record. N_j is the number of records annotated by the jth annotator.

7.5 Data description

7.5.1 Simulated QT dataset with independent annotators

As described earlier, BCLA is created to explicitly model the precision and bias of each annotator in relation to the ground truth annotations. It can be applied to any continuous-valued labels with appropriate parameter values. As a demonstration of its application in the context of ECG QT interval annotations, a simulated dataset of the QT intervals was created. An example of a QT interval is demonstrated in Figure 7.1(c).

A total of 548 simulated records were generated, each with 20 independent annotators, thus providing a total of 10,960 annotations (see Figure 7.7). The simulated dataset assumed that annotators have precision values, $\boldsymbol{\lambda} \sim \text{Gamma}(4, 0.0003)$, with the assumption that the annotations provided by the best performing annotator are ±5ms from the ground truth. Annotators' biases, $\boldsymbol{\phi} \sim \mathcal{N}(10, 25)$, a Gaussian distribution with a mean 10 ms and a standard deviation $\alpha_\phi^{-1/2} = 25$ms, assuming that the automated annotations tend to overestimate manual annotations, as described in previous studies and discussed in Chapter 6 [33–35]. The *true* annotation for each record, $z_i \sim \mathcal{N}(400, 40)$ [36–38], a Gaussian distribution with a mean $a = 400$ms and with a standard deviation $b^{-1/2} = 40$ms. No particular features were considered in this case (i.e., $\text{x}_\text{i} = 1$) for the purpose of illustrating the general use of the model. Furthermore, an intercept term in $f(\mathbf{w}, \mathbf{x})$, w_0, was modelled in the feature (i.e., $\mathbf{x}_i = [1, \text{x}_\text{i}]$)). In addition, it was assumed that $\alpha_\phi \sim \text{Gamma}(3, 0.0005)$, ensuring the mean standard deviation where the biases drawn from is 25ms. The $b \sim \text{Gamma}(3, 0.0002)$, ensuring the mean standard deviation where the *true* annotations drawn from is 40 ms.

The generated 10,960 annotations were then provided to the model to evaluate its accuracy in estimating the *true* annotation in an unsupervised manner, as well as predicting the bias and precision of each simulated annotator. The goal of this synthetic experiment is to determine if the BCLA model can recover the true bias and

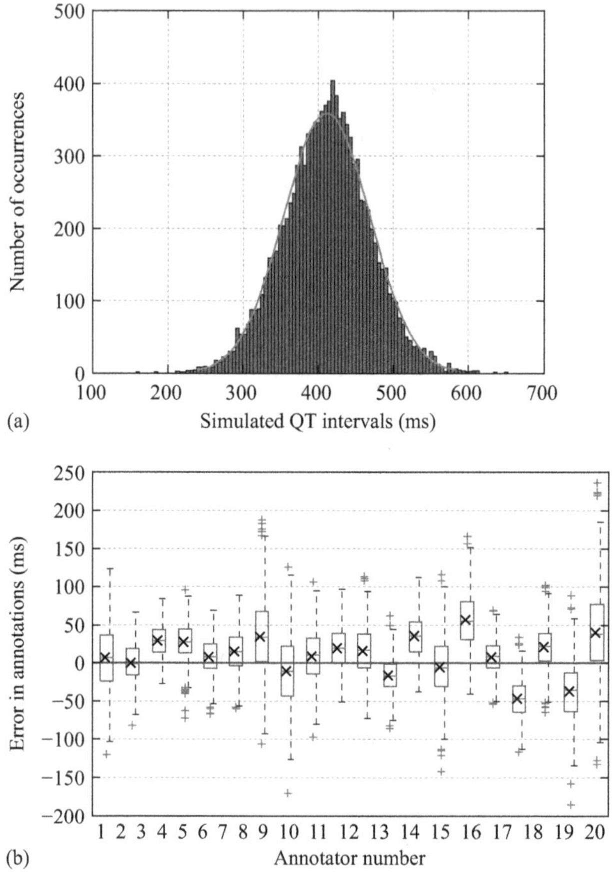

Figure 7.7 (a) The histogram of the simulated QT interval annotations for 548 records, with 20 annotations each provided by 20 simulated annotators. A fitted Gaussian distribution is superimposed. (b) Box plot of the error between the generated and true annotations for each of the 20 simulated annotators. The 'x' indicates the bias of each annotators. The span of each box represents the precision of the annotations over all annotations for each annotator

precision of each annotator, that are known in this experiment, and which were used to generate the synthetic data.

7.5.2 The 2006 PhysioNet challenge QT dataset

The 2006 PhysioNet/Computing in Cardiology (PCinC) Challenge QT database [39] provides an excellent opportunity to assess the feasibility of crowd-sourced

Table 7.2 Summary of the diagnostic conditions of subjects in the PTBDB

Diagnosis	**Number of subjects**
Healthy controls	52
Myocardial infarction	148
Cardiomyopathy/heart failure	18
Bundle branch block	15
Dysrhythmia	14
Myocardial hypertrophy	7
Valvular heart disease	6
Myocarditis	4
Miscellaneous	4
N/A	22

Note: N/A refers to subjects included in the PTBDB but their clinical summaries are missing.

annotations with large amounts of human or algorithmic annotations. Each participant in the Challenge was required to submit a Q onset with accompanying T offset for one 'representative' beat in lead II of each of the 549 recordings in the Physikalisch-Technische Bundesanstalt Diagnostic ECG Database (PTBDB) [40]. Each ECG Lead II (up to 2 min) in length was digitised at 1,000 samples per second, with 16-bit resolution, over a range of $\pm$16.384mV. The records were obtained from 290 subjects (209 men with mean age of 55.5 and 81 women with mean age of 61.6), each represented by between one and five recordings. About 20% of the subjects were healthy controls. The PTBDB contained records of patients with a variety of ECG morphologies having different QT intervals ranging from 256 to 529ms. Diagnostic classifications are detailed in Reference 40 and summarised in Table 7.2.

There were two categories of annotations: manual and automated (see Table 7.3). Eighty-nine entries to the competition were submitted, including revised submissions for a total of 38,621 annotations sourced from: 20 human annotators in Division 1; 48 automated algorithms in Division 2 (closed-source); and 21 in Division 3 (open-source). An additional division, Division 4, was created so as to combine all automated algorithms from Divisions 2 and 3, and to infer a potentially better estimation of QT intervals. The distribution of QT annotations for each division is shown in Figure 7.8, where it may be seen that QT annotations from all entries are not approximately Gaussian-distributed (Jarque–Bera test [41] with $p < 0.01$). A single record, 'patient285/s0544re', was excluded as it did not contain any recognisable ECG signals. Annotations for 548 records of the PTBDB were processed using different voting strategies. The maximum number of annotators per division and averaged number of annotations per record are listed in Table 7.3. As not all annotators had provided complete annotations (i.e., 548 annotations for all recordings), the histogram of the percentage of annotations per annotator in each division is shown in Figure 7.9. Note that 95% (i.e., 19 out of 20) manual annotators had labelled at least 50% of the

Table 7.3 Performance by competition entrants for each division of the PCinC QT dataset

	Manual annotators		Automated algorithms	
	Division 1	**Division 2 (closed-source)**	**Division 3 (open-source)**	**Division 4 (closed- & open-source)**
Number of annotators	20	48	21	69
Average annotations per 5-s segment	18	39	15	54
Average annotations per 2-min segment	18⋆	41⋆	21⋆	62⋆
RMSE of 5-s segment (ms)	6.65	16.36	17.46	16.36
RMSE of 2-min segment (ms)	6.67⋆	16.34⋆	17.33⋆	16.34⋆

Note: The manual/automated annotator having the lowest RMSE over a 5-s segment was selected to represent the best score. The results annotated ⋆ were published in the competition for a 2-min segment.

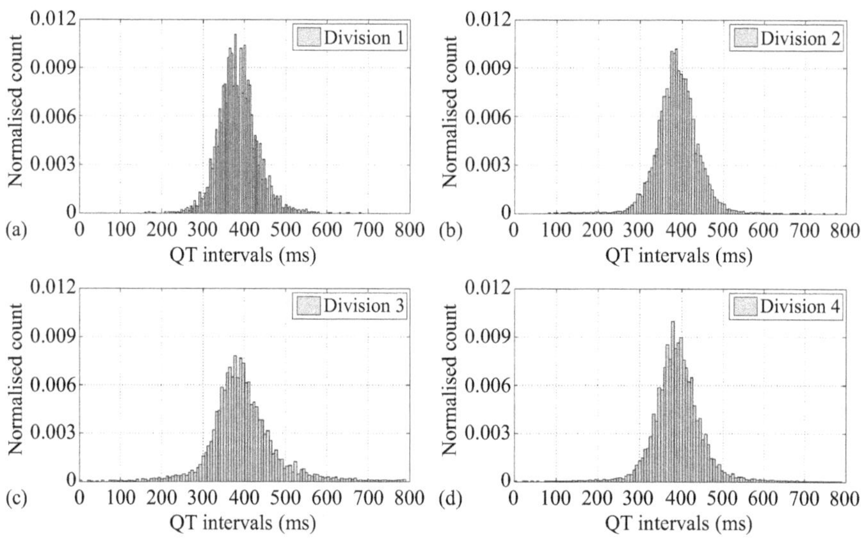

Figure 7.8 Histograms of the QT annotations for all entries including (a) human annotators (Division 1) and (b–d) automated algorithms (Divisions 2–4). QT annotations from all entries are not Gaussian-distributed (Jarque–Bera test [41] with $p < 0.01$)

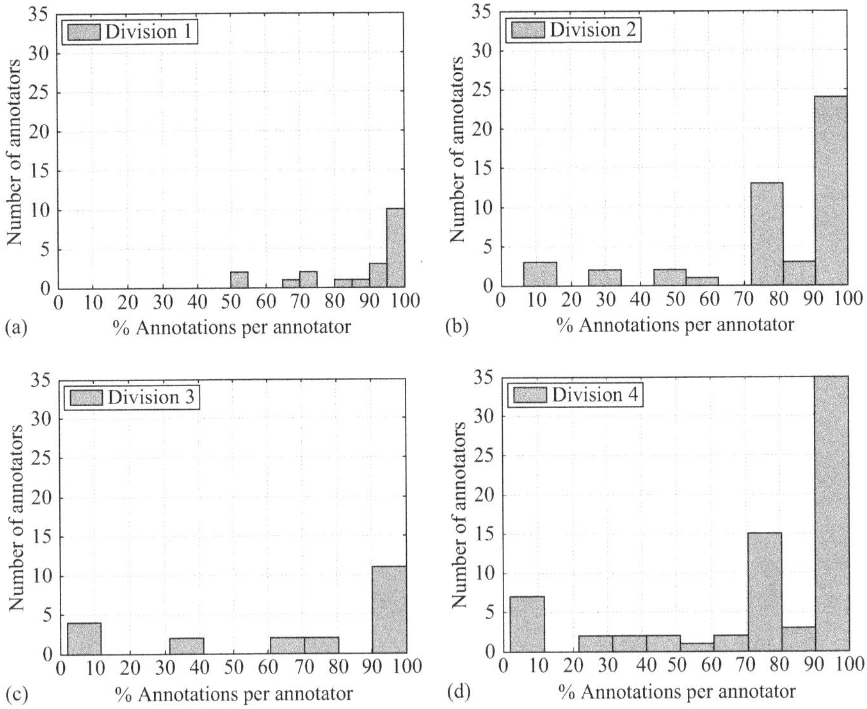

Figure 7.9 Histograms of the percentage of QT annotations per individual annotator for (a) manual annotators in Division 1 and (b–d) automated algorithms in Divisions 2, 3, and 4, where Division 4 is a combination of Divisions 2 and 3

recordings, but only 81.2% of the automated algorithms had done so in Division 4. The percentage of annotators per recording is also plotted for each division (see Figure 7.10). There are at least 33.3% and 28.6% of the annotators labelled one recording in the automated entry and the manual entry, respectively. Thus, we have a substantial 'missing data' condition that a fusion strategy must accommodate.

The competition score for each entry was calculated from the root-mean-square error (RMSE) between the submitted and the reference QT intervals. The reference annotations were generated from Division 1 entries using a maximum of 15 participants by taking the 'median self-centring approach' as detailed in Reference 42. The best-performing algorithm with least RMSE score for each division is also listed in Table 7.3. Furthermore, the majority of the QT annotations of each 2-min record occurred within the first 5s period, and the best scores in the first 5-s segment were similar to those of the 2-min segment (denoted by ⋆ in Table 7.3). To reduce any possible inter-beat variations, only the annotations within the first 5s segment of each record were chosen, ensuring that all annotators had approximately labelled the

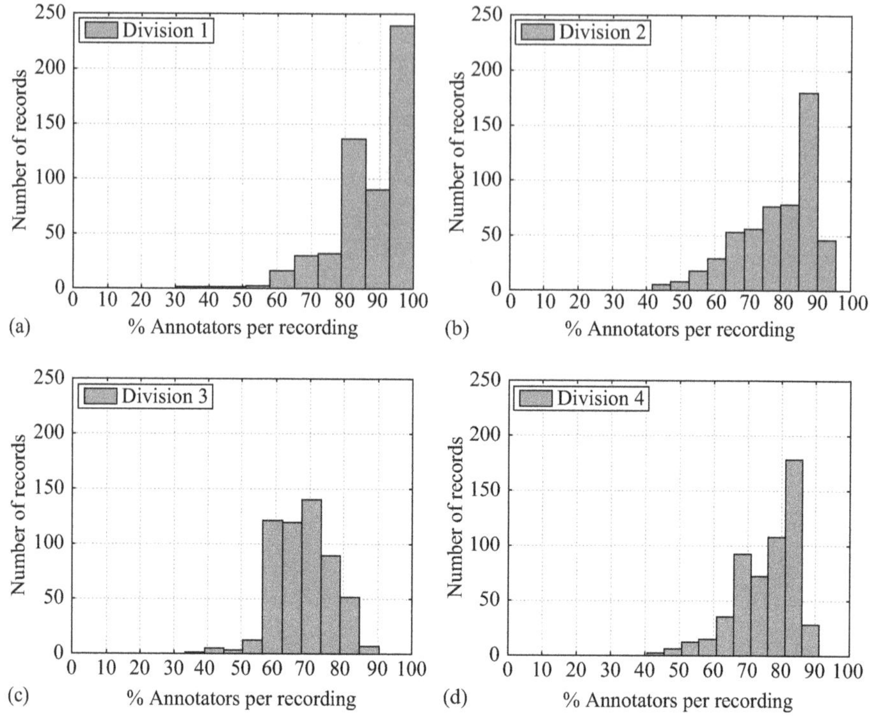

Figure 7.10 Histograms of the percentage of annotators per individual recording for (a) manual annotators in Division 1 and (b–d) automated algorithms in Divisions 2, 3, and 4

same region of a record, with similar QT morphologies. Therefore, the motivation for choosing the first 5s segment of each record was to consider a short segment where the QT interval is not changing dramatically (with respect to any particular beat that an annotator chose to view), while retaining the highest number of annotations. Those that fell outside this segment were considered to be missing information and discarded in the process of the QT estimation.

Although the QT annotations were provided in the PCinC QT dataset, the source code of the algorithms is not in the public domain. Furthermore, the reference QT intervals provided for the dataset were based on bootstrapping the median of 15 human annotators, which can be biased because humans tend to underestimate the QT interval [38]. A generative model is therefore proposed due to the need to provide an unbiased estimate of ground truth of the QT intervals.

The set of manual entry (i.e., Division 1) was used to generate the reference annotations, and so we therefore focused on the analysis of the sets of automated labels (i.e., Divisions 2, 3, and 4). In terms of parameter setting (see Table 7.4),

Table 7.4 The parameters of BCLA for modelling the 2006 PCinC dataset

Symbol	Definition	Value
k_b	Shape of Gamma distribution for b	3*
ϑ_b	Scale of Gamma distribution for b	0.0002*
μ_ϕ	Mean of the bias distribution	10†
k_α	Shape of Gamma distribution for α_ϕ	3†
ϑ_α	Scale of Gamma distribution for α_ϕ	0.0005†
k_λ	Shape of Gamma distribution for $\boldsymbol{\lambda}$	4‡
ϑ_λ	Scale of Gamma distribution for $\boldsymbol{\lambda}$	0.003‡

Note: b is the precision parameter for the model of the ground truth. α_ϕ is the precision parameter for the model of the bias. $\boldsymbol{\lambda}$ refers to annotators' precision values. The values denoted by * are determined with the assumption that the annotations provided by the best performing algorithm is ± 5 ms away from the dataset reference. The values denoted with † are derived from References 33–35. The values with ‡ are derived from References 36–38.

annotator-specific precision values, we chose $\boldsymbol{\lambda} \sim \text{Gamma}(k_\lambda, \vartheta_\lambda)$, with the assumption that the annotations provided by the best-performing algorithm are ± 5ms from the reference. Annotators' biases were set via $\boldsymbol{\phi} \sim \mathcal{N}(\mu_\phi, \alpha_\phi^{-1/2})$, with $\mu_\phi = 10$ms and $\alpha_\phi \sim \text{Gamma}(k_\alpha, \vartheta_\alpha)$, assuming that the automated annotations tend to overestimate manual annotations as described previously. The *true* QT interval for each record is $z_i \sim \mathcal{N}(a, b^{-1/2})$, where $b \sim \text{Gamma}(k_b, \vartheta_b)$ [36–38]. Instead of assuming the mean a of the underlying ground truth to be a fixed scalar, it was updated using a linear regression function, $f(\mathbf{w}, \mathbf{x})$, where the coefficients, $\mathbf{w}$, were estimated using (7.17). An intercept was included in $\mathbf{w}$ for modelling the overall offset predicted in f, and no particular features were considered for this example case (i.e., $x_i = 1$) as sole interest lies in the performance of the model.

7.5.3 Methodology of validation and comparison

The precision values $\boldsymbol{\lambda}$ inferred by BCLA-MAP were compared with those estimated using the EM algorithm proposed by Raykar *et al.* [10] (denoted as EM-R), which serves as one of our benchmarking algorithms. As EM-R does not explicitly model the bias of each annotator, the scalar Simultaneous Truth and Performance Level Estimation (denoted as sSTAPLE) model proposed by Warfield *et al.* [1] serves as the second benchmarking algorithm for comparison. Furthermore, the mean and standard deviation ($\mu \pm \sigma_\mu$ms) of 1,000 bootstrapped samples (i.e., random sampling with replacement) across records from the BCLA-MAP model were compared with the best algorithm (i.e., the 'theoretical best' algorithm with the least RMSE which can only be determined with knowledge of the true labels), the two benchmarks, and the traditional naïve mean and median voting approaches. The mean absolute error (MAE) of the annotations was calculated, which provides a measure of the difference between the estimated and the reference annotations (with a resolution of 1ms). A two-sided Wilcoxon rank-sum test ($p < 0.0001$) was applied to the 1,000 bootstrapped RMSEs and MAEs, to provide a comparison between the various methods. In assessing the performance of BCLA-MAP as a function of the number of annotators, a random number of annotators was selected 1,000 times. This was repeated with the number of the annotators varied from 3 to the maximum number in the division. The minimum number of annotators was chosen to be 3 to allow for obtaining results from the median voting approach.

7.6 Results and discussion

The convergence of the BCLA-MAP model is guaranteed by providing a threshold using the GEVD as a stopping criteria (see Equation (7.22)). In the PCinC QT dataset, the upper bound of the precision derived from the GEVD was 0.0418, which was based on the assumption that the best performing annotator is ±5ms away from the reference. The number of iteration is dependent on the number of records and the number of annotations. To illustrate the practical utility of the proposed model, it took 7.55 s for BCLA-MAP to perform 5,000 iterations when considering a total of 20,712 annotations (Division 2 in the PCinC QT dataset) using MATLAB® R2011a on a 3.3GHz Intel Xeon processor. Approximately 2,500 iterations were required to stabilise all the parameters. In comparison, both EM-R and sSTAPLE took similar amount of time on the same processor to run the same amount of annotations.

7.6.1 Simulated dataset

Figure 7.11(a) shows an example of the inferred results estimated using EM-R, sSTAPLE, and BCLA-MAP. As the EM-R algorithm modelled jointly the precision of each annotator and the noise of the underlying ground truth, its estimated σ cannot represent the real precision of each annotator. Furthermore, the EM-R algorithm does not consider the bias of each annotator, and it is observed that its estimated values of σ were well above the line of identity, indicating a consistent overestimation. By way of contrast, the BCLA-MAP and sSTAPLE models inferred values for σ that lie closely to the line of identity in the plot, indicating that both models can provide a reliable estimation of the *true* precision in the simulated results. In addition to precision, BCLA-MAP modelled the bias of each annotator accurately, which is superior to those estimated using sSTAPLE. The results are shown in Figure 7.11(b): the estimated biases from BCLA-MAP are very close to the *true* biases, whereas the sSTAPLE underestimated all the biases values. Although not all the estimated precisions and biases of each annotator were identical to the simulated values, the BCLA-MAP model inferred annotations without any prior knowledge of which annotator was the best and did so in an unsupervised manner.

In order to compare the accuracy of the inferred labels using the BCLA-MAP model, the simulated 548 annotations were bootstrapped 100 times with replacement. Each time, RMSE and MAE were calculated and compared to the best annotator, mean, EM-R, sSTAPLE, and median voting strategies. The results are shown in Table 7.5, which demonstrate that BCLA-MAP significantly outperformed the mean, median, EM-R, sSTAPLE, and best annotator when compared with the simulated *true* annotations.

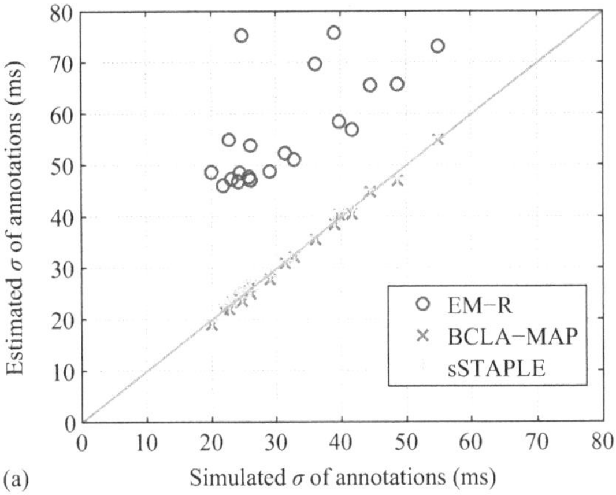

(a)

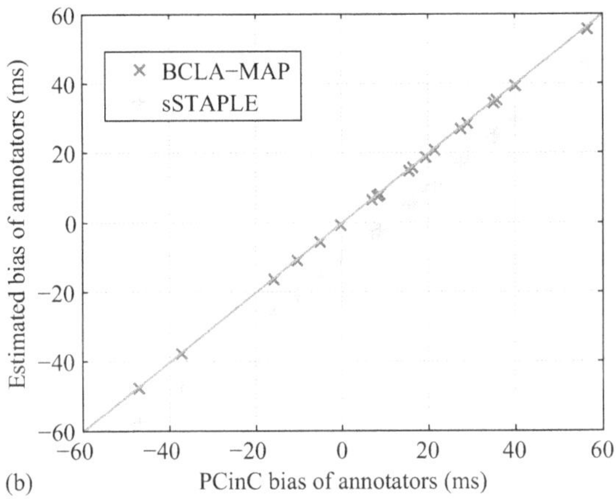

(b)

Figure 7.11 *A comparison of the simulated and inferred σ in (a) and bias in (b) of each annotator in the simulated dataset. The precision can be estimated by taking $1/(\sigma)^2$. The diagonal (grey) line indicates a perfect match between simulated and estimated results. Note that the EM-R significantly overestimates the σ values and the sSTAPLE significantly underestimates the bias values in all simulations*

7.6.2 PCinC QT dataset

Figure 7.12(a)–(g) shows the inferred precision and bias results estimated using EM-R, sSTAPLE, and BCLA-MAP for different divisions in the PCinC QT dataset. As mentioned previously, the EM-R algorithm does not directly model the precision of each annotator; its estimated σ of each annotator produces an offset from the values provided by the reference annotations. In contrast, BCLA-MAP and sSTAPLE inferred σ results that lie much closer to the line of identity, in Figure 7.12 (a), (c),

Table 7.5 RMSEs and MAEs of inferred labels using different strategies in the simulated dataset

	Best annotator	Median	Mean	EM-R	sSTAPLE	BCLA-MAP
RMSE (ms)	23.79 ± 0.63*	14.84 ± 0.38*	13.11 ± 0.31*	14.21 ± 0.36	12.45 ± 0.32†	6.27 ± 0.19*‡
MAE (ms)	18.99±0.58*	12.60 ± 0.36	11.26 ± 0.30*	12.64 ± 0.36	10.94 ± 0.33†	4.97 ± 0.16*‡

Results significantly different from others ($p < 0.0001$) as shown in ‡ for BCLA-MAP, † for sSTAPLE, and * (columns 2–4, and columns 6 and 7 only) for EM-R using the two-tailed Wilcoxon rank-sum test.

and (e); this indicates that the BCLA-MAP and sSTAPLE models can provide a reliable estimation of the *true* precision of each annotator. In terms of the bias estimation (see Figure 7.12 (b), (d), and (f)), which is considered in the sSTAPLE model, it does not model the mean of the biases, hence consistently produced an underestimation of bias values. In comparison, BCLA-MAP modelled the bias of each annotator accurately (see Figure 7.12(b), (d), and (f)). Although automated annotators 3 and 15 were predicted by BCLA-MAP to have lower bias values than those provided by the reference, they are considered to be outliers due to the assumption made in the model: annotators' biases were drawn from a Gaussian distribution with a mean 10 ms and with a standard deviation 25 ms. As Figure 7.13 shows, the biases of annotators 3 and 15 lie outside the 95% of the area (i.e., $\pm 1.96\sigma$ of the mean under the normal distribution) predicted by BCLA-MAP. In the case of annotator 7, its precision was underestimated (see Figure 7.12 (c) and (e)), which also affected BCLA-MAP's estimation of its bias value. It was observed that only 3.47% of records were annotated by annotator 7, making it harder for BCLA-MAP to provide a reliable estimation of precision and bias values for that annotator. It is a similar case for annotator 4, where only 2.74% of annotated records were provided, and which likewise affects the BCLA estimation of the bias value for that annotator.

In the evaluation of the inferred labels, the 548 records were bootstrapped 1,000 times, the RMSEs and MAEs of the BCLA-MAP model were generated and compared to the best annotator, mean, EM-R, sSTAPLE, and median voting approaches for the given reference. The results are displayed in Table 7.6: for Division 2 using 48 algorithms, BCLA-MAP achieved an RMSE of 12.65 ± 0.64ms, which significantly outperformed other approaches and provides an improvement of 15.78% over the next-best approach (EM-R with an RMSE of 15.02 ± 0.52ms); in the closed source entry Division 3 using 21 algorithms, BCLA-MAP again exhibited a superior performance over the other methods with an RMSE of 14.19 ± 0.87, and a 15.28% improved error rate over the next-best method (RMSE of 16.75 ± 1.81ms). When considering all automated entries (Division 4), BCLA-MAP provided an even more accurate performance than with the other two datasets (Divisions 2 and 3), as well as over other methods tested, with an RMSE of 11.89 ± 0.66ms. Note that as the PCinC QT dataset contains

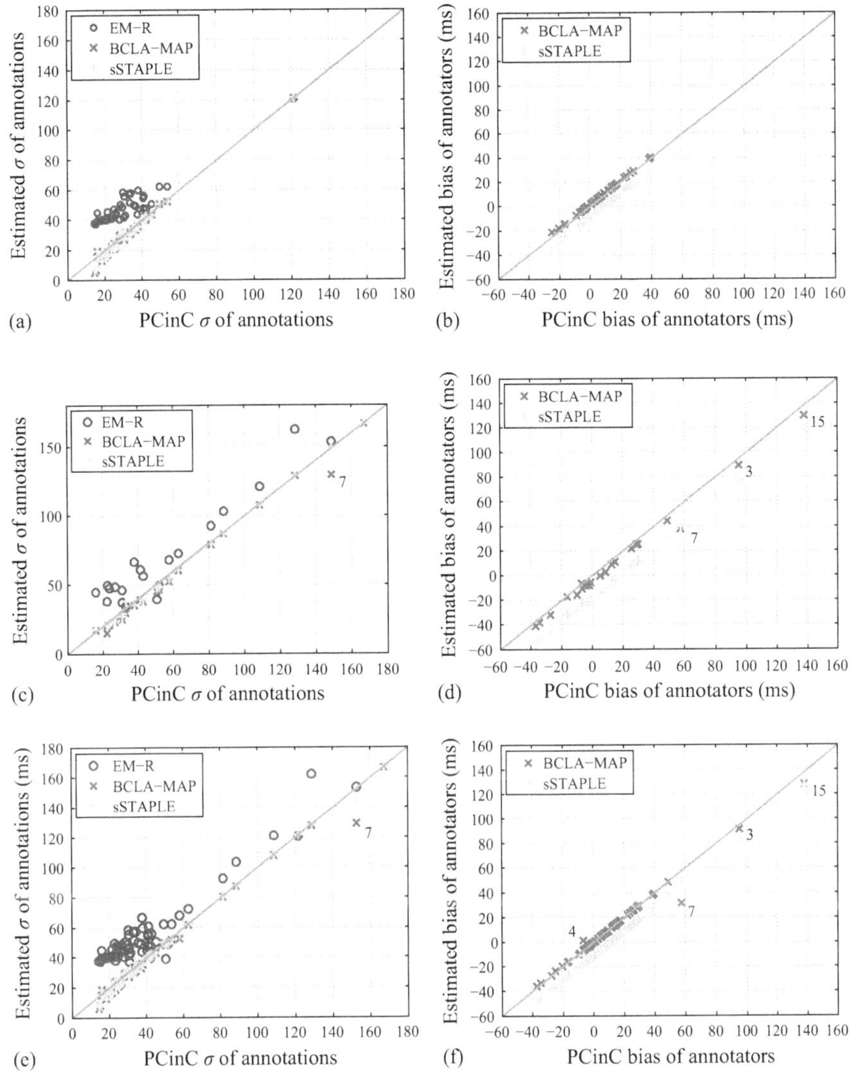

Figure 7.12 A comparison of the PCinC QT reference and inferred σ and bias of each annotator for Division 2 in (a) and (b), Division 3 in (c) and (d), and Division 4 in (e) and (f), respectively. The precision can be estimated by taking $1/(\sigma)^2$*. The leading diagonal line of each plot indicates a perfect matched between the Challenge reference and the estimated results. Note the annotators 3, 4, 7, and 15 are labelled in the corresponding plots*

Table 7.6 RMSEs and MAEs of inferred labels using different voting approaches in the PCinC QT dataset

Division	Best Annotator	Median	Mean	EM-R	sSTAPLE	BCLA-MAP
RMSE (ms)						
2(48)	$15.36 \pm 0.66*\dagger\ddagger$	$15.29 \pm 0.56*\dagger\ddagger$	$16.17 \pm 0.57*\dagger\ddagger$	$15.02 \pm 0.52\dagger$	$15.20 \pm 0.99\dagger$	$\underline{12.65 \pm 0.64}*\ddagger$
3(21)	$16.75 \pm 1.81*\dagger\ddagger$	$19.13 \pm 0.83*\dagger\ddagger$	$30.68 \pm 1.46*\dagger\ddagger$	$18.89 \pm 0.83\dagger\ddagger$	$22.33 \pm 1.08*\dagger$	$\underline{14.19 \pm 0.87}*\ddagger$
4(69)	$15.12 \pm 1.22*\dagger\ddagger$	$14.44 \pm 0.52*\dagger\ddagger$	$17.66 \pm 0.57*\dagger\ddagger$	$14.75 \pm 0.54\dagger\ddagger$	$16.32 \pm 0.61*\dagger$	$\underline{11.89 \pm 0.66}*\ddagger$
MAE (ms)						
2(48)	$10.80 \pm 0.57*\dagger\ddagger$	$11.75 \pm 0.42\dagger$	$12.64 \pm 0.44*\dagger\ddagger$	$11.80 \pm 0.43\dagger$	$11.64 \pm 0.65\dagger$	$\underline{9.34 \pm 0.43}*\ddagger$
3(21)	$10.62 \pm 1.14*\ddagger$	$14.05 \pm 0.55\dagger\ddagger$	$22.99 \pm 0.83*\dagger\ddagger$	$14.10 \pm 0.61\dagger\ddagger$	$19.15 \pm 1.78*\dagger$	$\underline{10.60 \pm 0.69}*\ddagger$
4(69)	$10.73 \pm 0.86*\dagger\ddagger$	$11.23 \pm 0.39*\dagger\ddagger$	$14.22 \pm 0.45*\dagger\ddagger$	$11.50 \pm 0.43\dagger\ddagger$	$13.23 \pm 0.49*\dagger$	$\underline{8.60 \pm 0.44}*\ddagger$

Results significantly different from others ($p < 0.0001$) as shown in † (columns 2–6 only) for the BCLA-MAP model, ‡ (columns 2–5, and 7 only) for the sSTAPLE, and * (columns 2– 4, and 6–7 only) for the EM-R using the two-tailed Wilcoxon rank-sum test. Note that the 'Best' annotator is defined as the single annotator with the least RMSE.

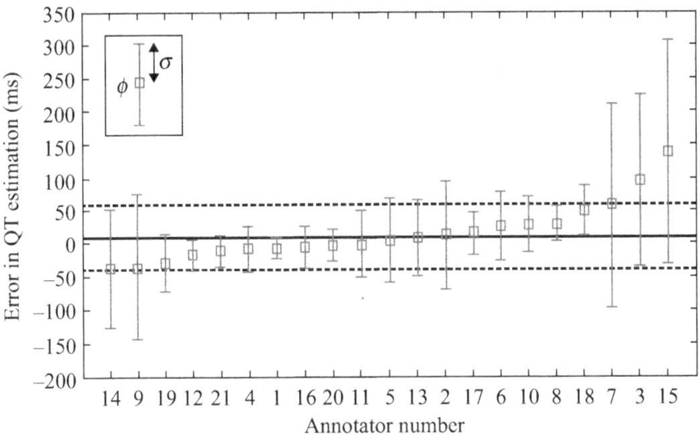

Figure 7.13 The mean (i.e., bias), ϕ, and σ of the difference in annotations for Division 3. The annotators were ranked based on their bias values. The solid line indicates the mean of the biases, whereas the dotted lines indicate 1.96σ of the mean assumed in BCLA-MAP

missing annotations, BCLA-MAP might produce a different error when different recordings are selected, even though the differences should become insignificant as the frequency of bootstrapping increases. Nevertheless, the BCLA-MAP model always outperformed the other voting strategies in our experiments.

A further evaluation of the accuracies in terms of RMSE were made as a function of the number of annotators (see Figure 7.14). The results were generated by subsampling annotators 1,000 times. EM-R, as a benchmarking algorithm, outperformed mean and median approaches initially, but then underperformed when compared to the median approach after 43 algorithms are used. The performance of sSTAPLE was worse, and only outperformed the mean voting approach. The BCLA-MAP model outperformed the other methods being tested with any number of annotators considered. In practice, it is rare to have more than three to five independent algorithms for estimating a label or predicting an event. In the case where only three automated algorithms were randomly selected, BCLA-MAP had on average 3.99%, 13.20%, 16.11%, and 20.41% improvement over the EM-R, sSTAPLE, median, and mean voting approaches, respectively. A further analysis was conducted to compare the difference in RMSE of the inferred ground truth between the BCLA-MAP and the EM-R algorithm for Division 4 (see Figure 7.15). The results in the figure show that the mean and median of the RMSEs of BCLA-MAP are always smaller than those of the EM-R out of the 1,000 runs. The frequency that BCLA-MAP outperformed EM-R (i.e., with smaller RMSE) is shown as a percentage in the lower part of Figure 7.15 for selecting different numbers of annotators.

Although the lowest BCLA-MAP RMSE (11.89 ± 0.66ms) in the automated entry is larger than the best-performing human annotator in the Challenge (RMSE =

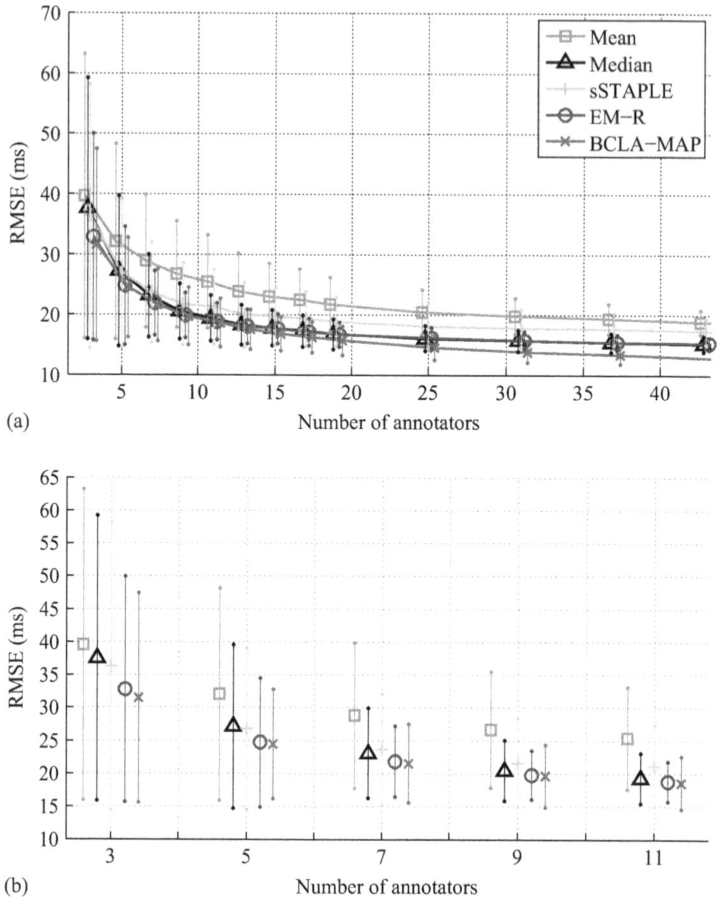

Figure 7.14 Mean and standard deviation of the RMSE results of using different voting approaches are shown as a function of the number of automated annotators. The plot was generated by randomly sampling the annotators 1,000 times. (a) Random sample of 3–69 annotators. (b)Inset: A close-up of the RMSE results when using 11 annotators or less

6.65ms), there were only two other human annotators who achieved a score below 10ms. Furthermore, as the annotations of automated algorithms were independently determined from the reference, whereas the reference includes the best human annotators, it is unsurprising that a combination of the automated algorithms would have worse performance. In comparison to the best-performing algorithms selected in the PCinC Challenge (see Table 7.3), BCLA-MAP has an improvement of 22.68%, 18.73%, and 27.32% RMSE for Divisions 2, 3, and 4, respectively.

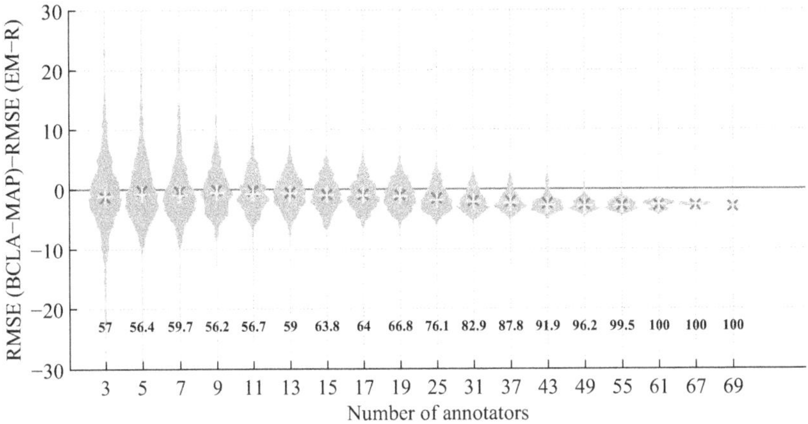

Figure 7.15 *The difference in the RMSE results between BCLA-MAP and EM-R as a function of the number of automated annotators. A probability density estimate of the sub-sampled 1,000 RMSE differences is calculated for selecting number of annotators from 3 to 69. The mean and the median of the density estimate are labelled as × and + respectively. The differences in RMSE that are less than zero were also computed as percentages as shown in the bottom of the plot. They indicate the percentage of times that the BCLA-MAP outperformed the EM-R algorithm from a total of 1,000 sub-sampled RMSEs*

7.7 Conclusion and future work

This chapter has proposed a generative Bayesian Continuous-Valued Label Aggregation framework incorporating the ground truth and annotator models. Furthermore, an MAP approach was proposed for the BCLA (i.e., BCLA-MAP) to infer the ground truth of continuous-valued labels where accurate and consistent expert annotations are not available. As a proof-of-concept, BCLA-MAP was applied to the QT interval estimation from the ECG using labels from the 2006 PCinC Challenge database, and it was compared to the mean, median, EM-R, and sSTAPLE methods. While accurately predicting each labelling algorithms's bias and precision, the root-mean-square error of BCLA-MAP outperformed the best Challenge entry, as well as other voting strategies. BCLA-MAP operates in an unsupervised Bayesian learning framework; no reference data were used to train the model parameters, and separate training and validation test sets were not required. Importantly, BCLA-MAP does guarantee a performance better than the best annotator without any prior knowledge of who or what is the best annotator.

Novel contextual features were introduced in our previous study [17] which allowed an algorithm to learn how varying physiological and noise conditions affect each annotator's ability to accurately label medical data. The inferred result was shown to provide an improved 'gold standard' for medical annotation tasks even when the ground truth is not available. As the next step, if we incorporate the context into the weighting of annotators, BCLA is expected to have an even larger impact for noisy datasets or annotators with a variety of specialisations or skill levels. The current model assumed consistent performance of each annotator throughout the records: i.e., his/her performance is time-invariant. Although this might not be true over an extended period of time where an annotators performance might improve through learning, or their performance might drop due to inattention or fatigue, the nature of the datasets being considered in this work are such that we can assume that performance across records is approximately consistent for each annotator. Future work will include modelling the performance of each annotator varying across records and through time to provide a more reliable estimation of the aggregated ground truth for datasets in which intra-annotator performance is highly variant.

Our model of the annotators currently does not factor in the possible dependency/correlation between individual annotators, which might not be the case for automated algorithms. Incorporating a correlation measure into the annotator's model could possibly allow for a better aggregation of the inferred ground truth. Annotators who are considered to be anomalous (i.e., those that are highly correlated to other experts but which have large variances and biases) should be penalised with lower weighting for their labels; expert annotators (i.e., those that are highly correlated to other experts but which have small variances and biases) should have their labels weighted more heavily in the model. Finally, combining annotations derived from reliable experts using the BCLA model could potentially lead to improved training for supervised labelling approaches.

Acknowledgement

TZ acknowledges the support of the RCUK Digital Economy Programme grant number EP/G036861/1 and an ARM Scholarship in Sustainable Healthcare Technology through Kellogg College. DAC is supported by the Royal Academy of Engineering and Balliol College.

References

[1] S. K. Warfield, K. H. Zou, and W. M. Wells, "Validation of image segmentation by estimating rater bias and variance," *Philosophical Transactions of the Royal Society A: Mathematical, Physical & Engineering Sciences,* vol. 366, pp. 2361–2375, 2008.

[2] O. S. Ofer Dekel, "Good Learners for Evil Teachers," in *Proceedings of the 26th Annual International Conference on Machine Learning,* 2009.

[3] S. M. Salerno, P. C. Alguire, and H. S. Waxman, "Competency in interpretation of 12 – lead electrocardiograms: a summary and appraisal of published evidence," *Ann Intern Med,* vol. 138, no. 9, pp. 751–760, 2003.

[4] J. P. Metlay, W. N. Kapoor, and M. J. Fine, "Does this patient have community-acquired pneumonia?: Diagnosing pneumonia by history and physical examination," *Journal of the American College of Cardiology,* vol. 278, no. 17, pp. 1440–1445, 1997.

[5] F. Molinari, L. Gentile, P. Manicone, *et al.*, "Interobserver variability of dynamic MR imaging of the temporomandibular joint," *La Radiologia Medica*, vol. 116, no. 8, pp. 1303–1312, 2011.

[6] H. Valizadegan, Q. Nguyen, and M. Hauskrecht, "Learning Medical Diagnosis Models from Multiple Experts," in *American Medical Informatics Association Annual Symposium Proceedings.* AMIA, 2012, pp. 921–930.

[7] I. Neamatullah, M. Douglass, L. Lehman, *et al.*, "Automated deidentification of free-text medical records," *BMC Medical Informatics and Decision Making,* vol. 8, no. 1, p. 32, 2008.

[8] R. R. Bond, T. Zhu, D. D. Finlay, *et al.*, "Assessing Computerised Eye Tracking Technology for Gaining Insight into Expert Interpretation of the 12-lead Electrocardiogram: An Objective Quantitative Approach," *Journal of Electrocardiology,* vol. 47, no. 6, pp. 895–906, 2014.

[9] A. P. Dawid and A. M. Skene, "Maximum likelihood estimation of observer errorrates using the EM algorithm," *Journal of the Royal Statistical Society Series C Applied Statistics,* vol. 28, no. 1, pp. 20–28, 1979.

[10] V. C. Raykar, S. Yu, L. H. Zhao, *et al.*, "Learning from crowds," *Journal of Machine Learning Research,* pp. 1297–1322, 2010.

[11] S. C. Warby, S. L. Wendt, P. Welinder, *et al.*, "Sleep – spindle detection: crowd-sourcing and evaluating performance of experts, non – experts and automated methods," *Nature Methods,* vol. 11, no. 4, pp. 385–392, 2014.

[12] P. Welinder and P. Perona, "Online crowdsourcing: Rating annotators and obtaining cost-effective labels," in *Computer Vision and Pattern Recognition Workshops (CVPRW), 2010 IEEE Computer Society Conference on,* 2010, pp. 25–32.

[13] T. Zhu, J. Behar, T. Papastylianou, and G. D. Clifford, "CrowdLabel: A crowd-sourcing platform for electrophysiology," in *Computing in Cardiology Conference,* Sept 2014, pp. 789–792.

[14] R. W. Ouyang, L. Kaplan, P. Martin, A. Toniolo, M. Srivastava, and T. J. Norman, "Debiasing crowdsourced quantitative characteristics in local businesses and services," in *Proceedings of the 14th International Conference on Information Processing in Sensor Networks*. New York, NY: ACM, 2015, pp. 190–201.

[15] P. Welinder, S. Branson, P. Perona, and S. J. Belongie, "The Multidimensional Wisdom of Crowds," in *Advances in Neural Information Processing Systems,* 2010, pp. 2424–2432.

[16] F. Xing, S. Soleimanifard, J. L. Prince, and B. A. Landman, "Statistical fusion of continuous labels: identification of cardiac landmarks," in *International Society for Optics and Photonics Medical Imaging,* 2011, pp. 7962–796 206.

[17] T. Zhu, A. E. Johnson, J. Behar, and G. D. Clifford, "Crowd-Sourced Annotation of ECG Signals Using Contextual Information," *Annals of Biomedical Engineering,* vol. 42, no. 4, pp. 871–884, 2014.

[18] J. M. Wiebe, R. F. Bruce, and T. P. O'Hara, "Development and Use of a Goldstandard Data Set for Subjectivity Classifications," in *Proceedings of the 37th Annual Meeting of the Association for Computational Linguistics on Computational Linguistics*, ser. ACL '99. Stroudsburg, PA: Association for Computational Linguistics, 1999, pp. 246–253.

[19] R. Snow, B. O'Connor, D. Jurafsky, and A. Y. Ng, "Cheap and Fast-but is It Good?: Evaluating Non-expert Annotations for Natural Language Tasks," in *Proceedings of the Conference on Empirical Methods in Natural Language Processing.* Stroudsburg, PA: Association for Computational Linguistics, 2008, pp. 254–263.

[20] O. Commowick and S. Warfield, "A Continuous STAPLE for Scalar, Vector, and Tensor Images: An Application to DTI Analysis," *IEEE Transactions on Medical Imaging,* vol. 28, no. 6, pp. 838–846, June 2009.

[21] P. G. Ipeirotis, F. Provost, and J. Wang, "Quality Management on Amazon Mechanical Turk," in *Proceedings of the ACM SIGKDD Workshop on Human Computation,* ser. HCOMP '10. New York, NY: ACM, 2010, pp. 64–67.

[22] Y. Baba and H. Kashima, "Statistical quality estimation for general crowdsourcing tasks," in *Proceedings of the 19th ACM SIGKDD International Conference on Knowledge Discovery and Data Mining*, ser. KDD '13. New York, NY: ACM, 2013, pp. 554–562.

[23] G. Cabrera, C. Miller, and J. Schneider, "Systematic labeling bias: Debiasing where everyone is wrong," in *Pattern Recognition (ICPR), 2014 22nd International Conference on,* Aug 2014, pp. 4417–4422.

[24] F. Xing, A. J. Asman, J. L. Prince, and B. A. Landman, "Finding seeds for segmentation using statistical fusion," in *International Society for Optics and Photonics Medical Imaging,* 2012, pp. 831430-831437.

[25] A. Akhondi-Asl, A. Hans, B. Scherrer, J. Peters, and S. Warfield, "Whole brain group network analysis using network bias and variance parameters," in *9th IEEE International Symposium on Biomedical Imaging (ISBI),* May 2012, pp. 1511–1514.

[26] M. Nasir, B. Baucom, P. Georgiou, and S. Narayanan, "Redundancy analysis of behavioral coding for couples therapy and improved estimation of behavior from noisy annotations," in *IEEE International Conference on Acoustics, Speech and Signal Processing*, April 2015, pp. 1886–1890.

[27] E. Kamar, A. Kapoor, and E. Horvitz, "Identifying and accounting for taskdependent bias in crowdsourcing," *Human Computation and Crowdsourcing,* 2015.

[28] C. M. Bishop, *Pattern recognition and machine learning.* Secaucus, NJ: Springer, 2006.

[29] T. Zhu, N. Dunkley, J. Behar, D. A. Clifton, and G. D. Clifford, "Fusing Continuous-Valued Medical Labels Using a Bayesian Model," *Annals of Biomedical Engineering,* vol. 43, no. 12, pp. 2892–2902, 2015.

[30] R. A. Fisher and L. H. C. Tippett, "Limiting forms of the frequency distribution of the largest or smallest member of a sample," in *Mathematical Proceedings*

of the Cambridge Philosophical Society, vol. 24, no. 2. Cambridge University Press, 1928, pp. 180–190.

[31] D. A. Clifton, "Novelty Detection with Extreme Value Theory in Jet Engine Vibration Data," Ph.D. dissertation, University of Oxford, 2009.

[32] International Conference on Harmonization of Technical Requirements for Registration of Pharmaceuticals for Human Use, "Guidance for Industry E14: Clinical Evaluation of QT/ QTc Interval Prolongation and Proarrhythmic Potential for Non-Antiarrhythmic Drugs," 2014.

[33] N. P. Hughes, "Probabalistic Models for Automated ECG Interval Analysis," Ph.D. dissertation, University of Oxford, 2006.

[34] J. P. Couderc, C. Garnett, M. Li, R. Handzel, S. McNitt, X. Xia, *et al.*, "Highly Automated QT Measurement Techniques in 7 Thorough QT Studies Implemented under ICH E14 Guidelines," *Annals of Noninvasive Electrocardiology,* vol. 16, no. 1, pp. 13–24, 2011.

[35] W. Andrew, V. Michael, D. Jeff, *et al.*, "Variability of QT Interval Measurements in OpioidDependent Patients on Methadone," *Canadian Journal of Addiction Medicine,* vol. 2, pp. 10–16, 2014.

[36] M. Malik, P. Fãrbom, V. Batchvarov, K. Hnatkova, and A. J. Camm, "Relation between QT and RR intervals is highly individual among healthy subjects: implications for heart rate correction of the QT interval," *Heart,* vol. 87, no. 3, pp. 220–228, 2002.

[37] I. Goldenberg, A. J. Moss, W. Zareba *et al.*, "QT interval: how to measure it and what is "normal"," *Journal of Cardiovascular Electrophysiology,* vol. 17, no. 3, pp. 333–336, 2006.

[38] G. D. Clifford, F. Azuaje, and P. E. McSharry, *Advanced Methods and Tools for ECG Analysis,* ser. Engineering in Medicine and Biology. Norwood, MA: Artech House, October 2006.

[39] G. B. Moody, H. Koch, and U. Steinhoff, "The PhysioNet/ Computers in Cardiology Challenge 2006: QT interval measurement," in *Computing in Cardiology Conference,* 2006, pp. 313–316.

[40] S. A. Bousseljot R, Kreiseler D, "Nutzung der EKG-Signaldatenbank CARDIODAT der PTB uber das Internet," *Biomedizinische Technik,* vol. 40(1), pp. 317–318, 1995.

[41] C. M. Jarque and A. K. Bera, "A Test for Normality of Observations and Regression Residuals," *International Statistical Review / Revue Internationale de Statistique,* vol. 55, no. 2, pp. 163–172, 1987.

[42] J. Willems, P. Arnaud, J. van Bemmel, *et al.*, "Assessment of the performance of electrocardiographic computer programs with the use of a reference data base." *Circulation,* vol. 71(3), pp. 523–534, 1985.

Chapter 8

Incorporating end-user preferences in predictive models

Suchi Saria and Daniel P. Robinson

8.1 Introduction

Many industries—for example, retail, manufacturing, and medicine—are recognizing the advantages of using predictive models to make key decisions. From an end-user's perspective, the cost of obtaining the input measurements should often be balanced with their effectiveness for aiding in prediction when choosing which model to deploy. In many important applications, the ability to efficiently control and take advantage of this trade-off is crucial to the end-user because resources are finite. In this chapter, we discuss a new scientific technology for providing users great flexibility in choosing the model that best fits their budget when faced with problems that have a complicated cost structure.

Consider the problem of rapid screening in medicine where predictive models are used to assess the risk of complications and appropriately triage patients. If the predicted risk is high, then the individual may be triaged to a higher intensity care protocol compared to when their risk is low. In this case, the caregiver orders the necessary battery of tests to acquire the measurements needed by the risk prediction model. Features computed from these measurements are then integrated by the model to predict risk. A private hospital, especially one with wealthy clientele, may have a higher tolerance for using costly screening tools compared to a community-based hospital. Similarly, a hospital with a smaller staff may be less willing to implement models that require additional new time-intensive measurements. However, the cost structure in healthcare is complicated, a fact that we expand upon with an example.

Consider the cost structure for deploying a predictive model in an intensive care unit (ICU). The set of measurements, tests used for ordering these measurements, and their costs are shown in Figure 8.1. The associated cost-dependency graph is shown in Figure 8.2. In such a setting, the following hold: (i) costs may be defined for tests, measurements, or activities and these costs may be of different types (e.g., the financial cost of acquiring a blood test versus the staff time taken to draw blood); (ii) features are obtained using one or more measurements which in turn are obtained by ordering a test (e.g., the creatinine trend feature is derived from the creatinine measurements obtained using the basic metabolic panel or BMP test); (iii) a test may

<table>
<tr><th>Test</th><th>Measurement</th><th>Routinely collected</th><th colspan="3">Cost (USD)</th><th>Wait time (minutes)</th><th>Measurement time (minutes)</th></tr>
<tr><td rowspan="13">Vitals and clinical history</td><td>Age, weight</td><td>Y</td><td rowspan="13" colspan="3">0</td><td>0</td><td>0</td></tr>
<tr><td>Temperature</td><td>Y</td><td>0</td><td>0</td></tr>
<tr><td>Heart rate</td><td>Y</td><td>0</td><td>0</td></tr>
<tr><td>Heart rhythm</td><td>Y</td><td>0</td><td>0</td></tr>
<tr><td>Respiratory rate</td><td>Y</td><td>0</td><td>0</td></tr>
<tr><td>Non-invasive blood pressure</td><td>Y</td><td>0</td><td>0</td></tr>
<tr><td>Blood oxygen (SpO_2)</td><td>Y</td><td>0</td><td>0</td></tr>
<tr><td>FiO_2</td><td>Y</td><td>0</td><td>0</td></tr>
<tr><td>Riker score</td><td>Y</td><td>0</td><td>0</td></tr>
<tr><td>Glasgow Coma Scale</td><td>Y</td><td>0</td><td>0</td></tr>
<tr><td>On dialysis</td><td>Y</td><td>0</td><td>0</td></tr>
<tr><td>On pacemaker</td><td>Y</td><td>0</td><td>0</td></tr>
<tr><td>Admission diagnoses</td><td>Y</td><td>0</td><td>0</td></tr>
<tr><td rowspan="5">Complete blood count (CBC)</td><td>White blood cell count</td><td>OD</td><td rowspan="3" colspan="3">CBC
24</td><td rowspan="13">50</td><td rowspan="13">20 mins of nursing time for a blood draw</td></tr>
<tr><td>Red blood cell count</td><td>OD</td></tr>
<tr><td>Platelets</td><td>OD</td></tr>
<tr><td>Hemoglobin</td><td>OD</td><td colspan="3">35</td></tr>
<tr><td>Hematocrit</td><td>OD</td><td colspan="3">9</td></tr>
<tr><td rowspan="8">Metabolic panel</td><td>Blood urea nitrogen (BUN)</td><td>OD</td><td>14</td><td rowspan="6">BMP
24</td><td rowspan="8">CMP
30</td></tr>
<tr><td>Creatinine</td><td>OD</td><td>14</td></tr>
<tr><td>Glucose</td><td>OD</td><td>11</td></tr>
<tr><td>Sodium</td><td>OD</td><td rowspan="3"></td></tr>
<tr><td>CO_2</td><td>OD</td></tr>
<tr><td>Potassium</td><td>OD</td></tr>
<tr><td>Calcium</td><td>OD</td><td rowspan="2" colspan="2"></td></tr>
<tr><td>Bilirubin</td><td>OD</td></tr>
<tr><td rowspan="3">Blood gases</td><td>$PaCO_2$</td><td>OD</td><td rowspan="3" colspan="3">Blood gas
72</td><td rowspan="3">50</td><td rowspan="3">0</td></tr>
<tr><td>PaO_2</td><td>OD</td></tr>
<tr><td>pH</td><td>OD</td></tr>
<tr><td rowspan="2">Coagulation</td><td>Prothrombin time (PT) and international normalized ratio (INR) test</td><td>OD</td><td colspan="3">14</td><td rowspan="2">50</td><td rowspan="2">20 mins of nursing time for a blood draw</td></tr>
<tr><td>Partial PT test</td><td>OD</td><td colspan="3">23</td></tr>
<tr><td>Urine</td><td>Urine volume</td><td>OD</td><td colspan="3">0</td><td>10</td><td>10 mins of nursing time</td></tr>
<tr><td>Lactates</td><td>Lactate test</td><td>OD</td><td colspan="3">30</td><td>35</td><td>0</td></tr>
</table>

Figure 8.1 The cost structure for the application of risk prediction of adverse events in the ICU. The table shows measurements and associated costs. We denote measurements made on demand as OD, while the others are routinely collected

consist of a single measurement (e.g., lactate level) or a panel of measurements (e.g., the BMP yields six different measurements); (iv) a measurement can be ordered via multiple tests (e.g., creatinine can be ordered on its own, or as part of a basic or a comprehensive metabolic panel, each having a different financial cost); (v) multiple features can be derived from the same measurement (e.g., the heart rate variability

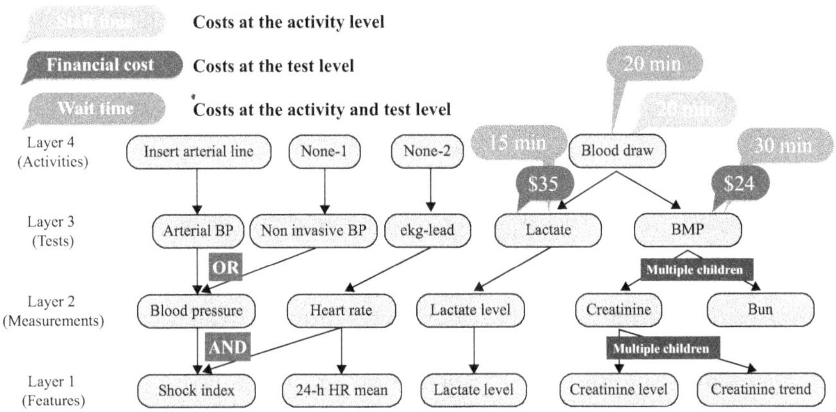

Figure 8.2 A portion of the dependency graph for the ICU example

and the heart rate trend can both be derived from the heart rate trace); (vi) some features may require multiple measurements (e.g., shock index is derived from blood pressure and heart rate measurements); and (vii) costs may be of more than one type (e.g., the monetary cost of a measurement versus the number of staff hours taken to make the measurement). These aspects make the cost structure complicated, which makes it difficult to incorporate users' preferences into the models that we seek.

The challenge of learning models in the presence of costs has been addressed extensively in recent years [1–5]. These solutions have typically used a framework based on empirical risk minimization with a sparsity inducing penalty based upon cost. However, these solutions have primarily focused on applications where the cost of a model is defined directly in terms of feature costs (e.g., the number of computational cycles required to compute that feature), making them inappropriate for some applications. This observation motivates our work and can be summarized as follows:

> *In many real-world applications, it is too restrictive to assume that the user can specify their cost preferences in terms of feature costs alone.*

We address this issue by designing a new regularizer that faithfully reflects the structure of the underlying cost graph. This regularizer may then be used to perform various prediction tasks via regularized risk minimization.

The complications associated with incorporating costs extend beyond healthcare. For example, in traffic prediction, a user may collect measurements such as past traffic patterns measured via sensors (e.g., pneumatic road tubes, piezo-electric sensors, cameras, and manual counting) at different locations, weather, neighborhood layout, and transient event information (e.g., games or live shows) [6]. Considerations in choosing which models to use include the cost of acquiring and deploying the sensors, the staff time to maintain the sensors, and the financial costs of acquiring weather and live event stream data. Depending on the availability and cost of resources, one may wish to deploy different models in different regions. Therefore, this application yields a complex cost structure, and the ability to effectively account for these costs is paramount.

8.1.1 Background and motivation

The mathematical setup for learning predictive models typically involves data formally represented by sets of pairs $\{(x_i, y_i)\}_{i=1}^N$ for some integer N, where $x_i \in \mathbb{R}^n$ for some integer n and $y_i \in \mathbb{R}$, for all $1 \leq i \leq N$. The vector x_i denotes the ith input (feature) vector and y_i represents the output (label) for the ith input vector x_i. The goal is then to predict the *unknown* output associated with a newly obtained input vector by using the knowledge one learns from the data $\{(x_i, y_i)\}_{i=1}^N$. Perhaps the most common approach for performing this task is to build predictive models via empirical regularized-loss minimization. This process involves five key steps: (i) obtaining the data pairs $\{(x_i, y_i)\}_{i=1}^N$ as mentioned above; (ii) choosing a data fidelity function L that is used to quantify the quality of a model; (iii) picking a regularizer R that is sensible for your application since the regularizer gives preference to the model selected; (iv) minimizing a weighted sum of the fidelity function and the regularizer, whose minimizer becomes the parameter vector that defines the predictive model; and (v) using the computed model to predict the output for new feature vectors.

In this chapter, we account for complex cost structures by focusing on the design of the *regularizer* used to define the optimization problem when performing regularized risk minimization. Specifically, the problem takes the form

$$\underset{\beta \in \mathbb{R}^n}{\text{minimize}} \; f(\beta) := \frac{1}{N} \sum_{i=1}^{N} L(\beta; (x_i, y_i)) + R(\beta) \tag{8.1}$$

where $\beta \in \mathbb{R}^n$ is the parameter vector—associated with the feature vector—that must be learned. Examples of commonly used regularizers include

$$R(\beta) := \lambda \|\beta\|_2^2 \tag{8.2a}$$

$$R(\beta) := \lambda \|\beta\|_1 \text{ and} \tag{8.2b}$$

$$R(\beta) := \lambda \|\beta\|_0 \tag{8.2c}$$

for some weighting parameter $\lambda > 0$, and frequently used loss functions include

$$L(\beta; (x_i, y_i)) := (y_i - \beta^T x_i)^2 \text{ and} \tag{8.3a}$$

$$L(\beta; (x_i, y_i)) := \log(1 + \exp^{y_i x_i^T \beta}) \tag{8.3b}$$

The function L in (8.3a) is often used in regression problems for which y_i may take on any value in $\mathbb{R}$, whereas the function in (8.3b) is frequently used to perform logistic regression when $y_i \in \{-1, 1\}$, i.e., binary classification.

As mentioned previously, the regularizer R should be sensibly chosen to reflect the demands of your application. For example, the ℓ_2 regularizer in (8.2a) is often used to prevent overfitting of the model to the acquired test data, which would often happen if the fidelity function L alone is used to define the optimization problem (8.1). On the other hand, the ℓ_1 regularizer given by (8.2b) is frequently used to promote sparsity (zero components) in the solution to (8.1). This choice is popular since it assists in selecting those features that are most important for prediction, which in turn allows for simpler models. The fact that the ℓ_1 regularizer promotes sparsity is now well understood [7] and is related to the fact that it is the best convex relaxation of the ℓ_0-norm defined in (8.2c).

The previous paragraph explains why the choice of regularizer amounts to giving preference to certain models, for example, the ℓ_1-norm (8.2b) prefers models defined by a sparse parameter vector β. Thus, in practice, the regularizer should be chosen to reflect the user's preference for the types of models they prefer, a task that is complicated by the complexity of application-specific cost graphs.

We often make reference to the cost of a model. The idea of cost may refer to hard-currency, but generally may refer to any measurable quantity that influences the users preference for one model over another. For example, the ℓ_0- and ℓ_1-norms reflect the importance of the number of non-zeros (i.e., the cost in these examples) to the user. If the ℓ_2-norm is chosen as the regularizer, then this reflects the users preference to prevent model overfitting (i.e., the cost in this case).

In many applications, combinations of the above fidelity functions L and regularizers R have been successful. We claim, however, that in these instances the costs associated with the applications were *directly* tied to the feature vectors themselves. For example, in compressed sensing, one wishes to find sparse solutions to a linear system of equations. Thus, the cost, i.e., the number of non-zeros in a prospective solution, is harmonious with the ℓ_1-regularizer, which promotes sparse solutions. It is then no surprise that one can recover a wealth of interesting and relevant models by systematically adjusting the weighting parameter λ appearing in (8.2b) and solving the optimization problem (8.1). The following claim further clarifies our motivation:

> *For many important big data applications, standard regularizers do not accurately capture the costs that are most relevant. Thus, new frameworks should be designed for defining structured regularizers that reflect the complex cost structures present in many real-life problems.*

How does one design an appropriate regularizer for problems with a complicated cost structure, such as for the ICU example above? In this work, we address that difficulty by designing structured regularizers that are in harmony with the complex cost structures in many big data applications. As a result, we can systematically adjust weighting parameters that define our structured regularizer to obtain a rich landscape of models that reflect the *true* costs of interest.

8.1.2 Related work

Learning models in the presence of costs have received significant attention in recent years (e.g., [1–3,5,8]). Existing work has primarily targeted applications where the cost of computation is the primary concern. Moreover, much of this work has focused on optimizing performance when information is acquired incrementally [1,2,9–11]. In Reference 2, they define the problem of cost-sensitive classification and use a partially observable Markov decision process to trade-off the cost of acquiring additional measurements with classification performance. While they apply their method to a medical diagnosis problem, their costs were approximated at the feature level. In Reference 1, stage-wise regression is used to learn a collection of regression trees in a manner that ensures that classifiers built from more trees are more accurate, but more expensive. For the task of ranking web page documents, they showed improved speed and accuracy by accounting for feature costs—simple lookups (e.g., word occurrences) versus those needing more computation (e.g., a document-specific BM25 score for measuring relevance to a query). For structured prediction, Weiss *et al.* [12] proposed a two-tier collection of models of varying costs and a model selector; for each new test example, their selector adaptively chooses a model. For vision applications (e.g., articulated pose estimation in videos), they showed gains in performance by adaptively selecting models of varying costs, which required a histogram of gradient features at a fine (expensive) versus a coarse (cheap) resolution. These solutions focused on applications with no dependencies between costs for the units being reasoned over (i.e., feature or model costs are independent) and provided upfront. As predictive models continue to find their way into many important real-world applications, a means for incorporating rich cost structures is needed.

Returning to our healthcare example, the challenge of incorporating costs arises from the dependencies between features, measurements, tests, and required activities. Measurements may be obtained from a singleton test or as a part of the test that yields multiple measurements. Tests may have different resource costs associated with them, while features may be derived from more than one measurement. These dependencies between features, measurements, and tests yield a complex dependence structure between the features. Moreover, various costs are specified at different levels of this hierarchy; therefore, the cost of a feature is not specified upfront, but rather is dependent on which other features, measurements, and tests are selected.

Cost imposed via a hierarchical dependency graph is reminiscent of past works utilizing structured sparsity penalties (see the survey [13,14]), especially those using tree-based regularizers [15] and penalties with overlapping groups and hierarchical structure [14,16]. Different from these past works, a key challenge for our task is that the structure of the group regularizer is not given and its construction is not straightforward. Specifically, we show that cost-dependency graphs are naturally captured via Boolean circuits—graphs where nodes share a combination of AND and OR connections with its parents. However, only leaf nodes (i.e., feature nodes) of this circuit are included in the regularizer while the internal nodes (e.g., measurements needed to obtain features) induce dependencies between the leaf nodes. The presence of mixed AND/OR relationships and the non-inclusion of internal nodes renders our application different from past works. Other regularizers such as OSCAR [17] and Laplacian Net [18] aim at discovering group structure when the features are highly correlated. In our setting, the groups are determined by the structure of the cost graph, not by the correlations between the features.

8.1.3 Key contributions

We develop a new framework for defining structured regularizers suitable for problems with complex cost structures by drawing upon a surprising connection to Boolean circuits. In particular, we represent the problem costs as a Boolean circuit, and then use properties of Boolean circuits to define the *exact cost penalty*. Based on our exact cost penalty, any standard convex relaxations may be employed for the purpose of computational efficiency, and here we choose a standard L_1-L_∞ norm relaxation. Our new regularizer may be used within an empirical risk minimization framework to trade-off cost versus accuracy. We focus on the one-shot setting (i.e., when all measurements are obtained upfront), although our regularizer is also applicable in the incremental setting. Since the cost-structure of many real-life applications may be represented as a Boolean circuit, the contribution of our work is substantial.

Our ideas are presented in the context of a challenging healthcare application—the development of a rapid screening tool for sepsis [19]—using data from patients in the ICU [20]. Our experiments show that our regularizer allows for a collection of models that are in harmony with a user's cost preferences. Numerical comparisons to a cost-sensitive $L1$—a natural competitor to our proposed regularizer that does not account for the complicated cost structure—shows that models obtained with our regularizer have a better prediction/cost trade-off. Compared to existing approaches in predictive modeling where cost preferences are often accounted for post hoc, our scheme provides a new way to account for complex cost preferences during model selection.

8.2 Regularizers for complex cost structures

Our scheme is general since it may be applied to any problem with a cost structure that may be represented as a finite-layer Boolean circuit. However, for clarity of exposition, we first focus on a particular healthcare application that also serves as the basis for the numerical results presented.

8.2.1 An example from the ICU

We formulate a structured regularizer for the cost structure associated with risk prediction applications for the in-hospital setting. These include a diverse set of problems such as the prediction of those at risk for death, the likelihood of readmission, and the early detection of adverse events such as shock and cardiac arrest.

In Figure 8.1, we list the measurements used in our study. Each measurement (e.g., lactate level or creatinine) is obtained by ordering a test; a test may comprise a single measurement (e.g., lactate level), a panel (e.g., CBC panel), or a more complex study (e.g., an imaging study). A measurement can be ordered via multiple tests; for example, creatinine can be ordered on its own, as part of a basic or a comprehensive metabolic panel, each having a different financial cost. Multiple features can be derived from the same measurement (e.g., the heart rate variability and the trend of the heart rate can both be derived from the heart rate trace). To make things even more complicated, the features that are used to make predictions are derived from measurements, and therefore some features may require multiple measurements (e.g., the shock index feature is derived from blood pressure and heart rate measurements). Finally, one is also interested in the time required by the caregivers to perform the activities required to obtain the necessary tests. These complicated dependencies between features, measurements, tests, and caregiver activities are represented as the (relatively simple) Boolean circuit given by Figure 8.2.

In Figure 8.2, the features are represented by nodes in layer-1, and their calculation requires a subset of measurements from layer-2, that is, nodes in layer-1 share an AND or OR relationship with those in layer-2. Measurements can be obtained in a number of ways by performing various tests, which are represented at layer-3, that is, nodes in layer-2 share an AND or OR relationship with those in layer-3. The caregiver activities are represented at layer-4 and are performed when a test is needed that requires that action, i.e., layer-3 shares an AND relationship with layer-4. Every relationship in this Boolean circuit is described using only logical AND and OR operations. Note that, without loss of generality, we include fictitious nodes "none-1" and "none-2" in layer-4 so that the collection of input nodes are in the same layer.

There are three relevant costs: the financial cost of ordering a test, the waiting time to obtain a test result, and the caregivers' time needed to perform the activities required for the tests. The ideal regularizer should account for the following: (i) obtaining a measurement may cost different amounts depending on which test(s) is ordered to obtain it; (ii) features share costs with other features derived from the same measurement; (iii) a feature may require multiple measurements so that its cost depends on more than one measurement; and (iv) caregiver time and financial costs are additive while wait time is the maximum of the separate wait times.

Our structured regularizer requires the following sets:

$$\mathscr{F} := \{f_1, \cdots, f_{n_f}\}, \qquad \mathscr{M} := \{m_1, \cdots, m_{n_m}\},$$

$$\mathscr{T} := \{t_1, \cdots, t_{n_t}\}, \qquad \mathscr{A} := \{a_1, \cdots, a_{n_a}\}$$

to be the sets of features (layer-1 nodes), measurements (layer-2 nodes), tests (layer-3 nodes), and caregiver activities (layer-4 nodes), with n_f, n_m, n_t, and n_a being the number of each, respectively. We use $f_i \hookleftarrow m_i$ to mean that there is a directed edge that links node m_j to node f_i. The relationships between the layers of our specific Boolean circuit allow us to interpret $f_i \hookleftarrow m_j$, $m_j \hookleftarrow t_k$, and $t_k \hookleftarrow a_l$ to mean that the ith feature requires the jth measurement, the jth measurement can be obtained by performing the kth test, and the kth test requires the lth activity.

We now define the set valued mappings $m(f_i) := \{m_j : f_i \hookleftarrow m_j\}$, $t(m_j) := \{t_k : m_j \hookleftarrow t_k\}$, and $t(a_l) := \{t_k : t_k \hookleftarrow a_l\}$, which represent the set of measurements required to obtain feature i, the set of tests that produce measurement j, and the set of tests that require action l. We have overloaded the definition of the function t above, that is, we have two different definitions for $t(m_j)$ and $t(a_l)$, but this should not lead to any confusion since the correct definition is always clear from the context.

Next, we address the fact that some features may be obtained in multiple ways by ordering various combinations of tests. If this is not considered, the cost of a feature may be over penalized by our regularizer. To deal with this issue, let w_i denote the numbers of ways feature i can be obtained. Then, for the ith feature, we define $\vec{f_i} := [f_{i,1}, \cdots, f_{i,w_i}]^T$ and $\vec{\beta_i} := [\beta_{i,1}, \cdots, \beta_{i,w_i}]^T$ so that $\beta_{i,p}$ represents the parameter associated with ordering feature f_i in the pth way. This allows us to define the *extended* feature and parameter vectors $\vec{f} := [\vec{f_1}, \ldots, \vec{f_{n_f}}]^T$ and $\vec{\beta} := [\vec{\beta_1}, \ldots, \vec{\beta_{n_f}}]^T$.

Modeling financial cost and caregiver time. To model the financial cost that is incurred at the test level, we introduce for each test t_k and feature f_i, the quantity $\vec{n}_{k,i} := [n_{k,i,1}, \cdots, n_{k,i,w_i}]^T$ with

$$n_{k,i,p} := \begin{cases} 1 \text{ if } t_k \text{ is used when } f_i \text{ is ordered in its } p\text{th way,} \\ 0 \text{ otherwise,} \end{cases}$$

for all $1 \leq k \leq n_t$, $1 \leq i \leq n_f$, and $1 \leq p \leq w_i$. Given the financial cost $C_k^{\mathcal{T}}$ of ordering test k and a weighting parameter $\lambda_\$$, the *exact* structured penalty for financial cost is

$$R^\$_{exact}(\vec{\beta}) := \lambda_\$ \sum_{k=1}^{n_t} \mathscr{C}_k^{\mathcal{T}} I\left(\sum_{i=1}^{n_f}\sum_{p=1}^{w_i} I(n_{k,i,p}\beta_{i,p})\right) \tag{8.4}$$

where the indicator function I satisfies $I(0) = 0$ and $I(z) = 1$ for all $z \neq 0$. It follows from (8.4) that a financial cost for test t_k is incurred only when instructed to order some feature f_i in the pth way ($\beta_{i,p} \neq 0$), and that the pth way requires test t_k ($n_{k,i,p} \neq 0$). The regularizer (8.4) is not computationally friendly, so we also consider the relaxed structured and convex regularizer

$$R^\$_{relax}(\vec{\beta}) := \lambda_\$ \sum_{k=1}^{n_t} \mathscr{C}_k^{\mathcal{T}} \Big\| \bigvee_{i=1}^{n_f} \vec{n}_{k,i} \odot \vec{\beta_i} \Big\|_\infty \tag{8.5}$$

where for a set of vectors $\{z_i\}_{i=1}^n$ and subset $S = \{i_1, i_2, \ldots, i_r\} \subseteq \{1, 2, \ldots, n\}$ we let

$$\bigvee_{i=1}^{n} z_i := [z_1^T \ldots z_n^T]^T \text{ and } \bigvee_{i\in S} z_i := [z_{i_1}^T \ldots z_{i_r}^T]^T.$$

Note that the formulation of (8.5) as a sum of group ℓ_∞-norms means that black-box software such as SPAMS may be used. Here, for concreteness we have introduced one particular relaxation of the exact regularizer (8.4), namely (8.5). Later we briefly discuss how other standard convex relaxations as well as less commonly encountered nonconvex relaxations may be used.

Similarly, for the caregivers time cost, we define $\vec{n}_{l,i} := [n_{l,i,1}, \cdots, n_{l,i,w_i}]^T$ with

$$n_{l,i,p} := \begin{cases} 1 \text{ if } a_l \text{ is used when } f_i \text{ is ordered in its } p\text{th way,} \\ 0 \text{ otherwise,} \end{cases}$$

for all $1 \leq l \leq n_a$, $1 \leq i \leq n_f$, and $1 \leq p \leq w_i$, where we have again overloaded notation. The ℓ_∞-norm relaxation regularizer associated with the caregiver activity time then becomes

$$R^{\circledcirc}_{relax}(\vec{\beta}) := \lambda_{\circledcirc} \sum_{l=1}^{n_a} \mathscr{C}_l^{\mathscr{A}} \| \bigvee_{i=1}^{n_f} \vec{n}_{l,i} \odot \vec{\beta}_i \|_\infty \tag{8.6}$$

with $\mathscr{C}_l^{\mathscr{A}}$ being the time cost associated with the lth activity and $\lambda_{\circledcirc} > 0$ a weighting parameter. Overall, the ℓ_∞-relaxation of our exact structured regularizer becomes

$$R_{relaxed}(\vec{\beta}) := R^{\$}_{relaxed}(\vec{\beta}) + R^{\circledcirc}_{relaxed}(\vec{\beta}) \tag{8.7}$$

By varying $\lambda_\$$ and $\lambda_{\circledcirc}$, we trade-off financial (\$) and caregiver activity time ($\circledcirc$) costs.

Remark 1. *If a scaled-ℓ_1-norm (a scaled version of* (8.2b)*) is adopted instead of our structured regularizer, the user chooses a weight for each feature by condensing the complex cost structure into a single number, necessarily in an ad hoc way.*

Remark 2. *Consider the following* 3*-layer Boolean circuit: let layer-*1 *contain the nodes $\mathscr{F}$, layer-*2 *contain the nodes $\mathscr{X} := \{f_{i,p} : 1 \leq i \leq n_f$ and $1 \leq p \leq w_i\}$, and layer-*3 *contain the nodes $\mathscr{A}$. Let the gate functions at layer-*1*, for each f_i, be*

$$g_{f_i}(\mathscr{X}) := \underset{1 \leq p \leq w_i}{\text{OR}} f_{i,p}$$

*for all $1 \leq i \leq n_f$, and the gate functions at layer-*2*, for each $f_{i,p}$, be*

$$g_{f_{i,p}}(\mathscr{A}) := \underset{\{l : n_{l,i,p} = 1\}}{\text{AND}} a_l$$

for all $1 \leq i \leq n_f$ and $1 \leq p \leq w_i$. In particular, only OR *gate functions are used in layer-*1 *and only* AND *gate functions are used in layer-*2*. The properties of this* 3*-layer circuit allows us to conclude that for a given caregiver activity a_l, we have*

$$\left\| \bigvee_{i=1}^{n_f} \vec{n}_{l,i} \odot \vec{\beta}_i \right\|_\infty \equiv \left\| \bigvee_{(i,p) \in S_l} \vec{\beta}_{i,p} \right\|_\infty$$

with the index set S_l defined as

$$S_l := \{(i,p) : n_{l,i,p} = 1\} \equiv \{(i,p) : \textit{ the output of } g_{f_{i,p}}(\,\cdot\,) \textit{ depends on } a_l\}$$

which allows us to define our regularizer (8.6) *directly from our knowledge of the* 3*-layer Boolean circuit. In fact, the only properties of the circuit that we used were (i) layer-*1 *was the feature layer; (ii) layer-*3 *contained the nodes whose costs we were modeling; (iii) layer-*1 *only contained* OR *gates; and (iv) layer-*2 *only had* AND *gates. This motivates the general case that we consider in the next section.*

Modeling testing wait time: Although not required, here we choose a simpler approach to address the time cost needed to obtain test results. Note that the wait time for a set of test results is the maximum of the wait times for each individual test (this assumes that tests can be ordered in parallel). Therefore, for a given upper bound, say W, on the tolerated testing wait time, we only allow tests to be used that have a wait time that is less than W. This amounts to selecting a reduced Boolean circuit containing only these allowed tests, the caregiver actions required to obtain these allowed tests, measurements that result from the allowed tests, and finally the features that may be calculated from the included measurements.

8.2.2 The structured regularizer for the general case

We show how to define our regularizer for any problem whose cost structure may be represented as a finite r-layer Boolean circuit; Figure 8.2 is such an instance.

An r-layer Boolean circuit consists of layers of finitely many nodes. The lowest layer (layer-1) consists of the set of output nodes, while the highest layer (layer-r) contains the input nodes. Additionally, we are given Boolean functions—defined on the basis $\mathscr{B} = \{\text{AND}, \text{OR}, \text{NOT}\}$—for all nodes. Formally, each Boolean function performs the basic logical operations from $\mathscr{B}$ on one or more logical inputs from the previous layer and produces a single logical output value. The healthcare example in Figure 8.2 is a 4-layer Boolean circuit with the features corresponding to layer-1, the measurements to layer-2, the tests to layer-3, and the activities to layer-4.

Let $\mathscr{N}_i := \{x_{i,1}, x_{i,2}, \ldots, x_{i,n_i}\}$ be the nodes in layer-i for some n_i. By removing double negations, and using the laws of distribution and De Morgan's laws, the r-layer circuit may be reduced to a 3-layer Boolean circuit in disjunctive normal form [21,22]. The nodes in the 3-layer circuit are then layer-3: $\{x_{r,1}, x_{r,2}, \ldots, x_{r,n_r}\}$, layer-2: $\{z_1, z_2, \ldots, z_m\}$, and layer-1: $\{x_{1,1}, x_{1,2}, \ldots, x_{1,n_1}\}$ for some m and set $\{z_i\}_{i=1}^m$ of nodes for layer-2. Moreover, the only logical operations used by the Boolean functions $g_{z_i}(\cdot)$ in layer-2 are AND and NOT operations, while the Boolean functions $g_{x_{1,i}}(\cdot)$ in layer-1 only use logical OR operations. (In Remark 2, we showed how a circuit of this form could be obtained for the healthcare example.) If we define the vectors $\vec{z} := [z_1, z_2, \ldots, z_m]^T$ and $\vec{\beta} := [\beta_1, \beta_2, \ldots, \beta_m]^T$, then we define our cost-driven structured regularizer as

$$R_{relax}(\vec{\beta}) := \lambda \sum_{k=1}^{n_r} \mathscr{C}_k \| \bigvee_{j \in S_k} \beta_j \|_\infty$$

with $S_k := \{j : g_{z_j}(\cdot) \text{ depends on the logical value of } x_{r,k}\}$. When this regularizer is used in model prediction, an optimal value for the extended vector $\vec{\beta}$ is obtained. Using this vector and the fact that layer-1 only has OR gates, we known that a node $x_{1,i}$ in layer-1 (i.e., the feature layer for the healthcare application) has the logical value of 1 (i.e., the feature should be computed) if $\beta_j \neq 0$ for some $j \in \{k : g_{x_{1,i}}(\cdot) \text{ depends on the logical value of } z_k\}$.

Remark 3. *Although our exact penalty takes the form of an overlapping group regularizer, what is non-trivial is determining which features belong to which groups* *for complex cost graphs. By relating the cost graph to a Boolean circuit, we can use properties of Boolean circuits to define the extended feature set and overlapping structure that is correct for arbitrary cost graphs. This connection also allows for the use of off-the-shelf software such as SymPy*[1] *to convert an arbitrary graph to the 3-layer circuit in disjunctive normal form used to define our exact regularizer.*

8.2.3 Relaxations of our exact structured regularizer

There are many computationally viable options for relaxing our exact structured regularizer given by (8.4). Here, mostly for simplicity, we chose to use the ℓ_∞-norm convex relaxation as shown in (8.5) so that we could use the off-the-shelf solver SPAMS. Of course, other convex relaxations based on the ℓ_1- and ℓ_2-norm are possible. If one is willing to forego the convenience of using a black-box solver, one can investigate more accurate *nonconvex* relaxations such as

$$R^{\$}_{relax}(\vec{\beta}) := \lambda_{\$}\sum_{k=1}^{n_t} \mathscr{C}_k^{\mathscr{T}} \cdot g_k(\vec{\beta}) \tag{8.8}$$

for functions g_k that approximate the indicator function. Thus, it is reasonable to select functions g_k that are nonnegative, monotonically increasing, and concave on the domain $[0, \infty)$. One attractive choice is the function $g_k(z) = 1/(1 + e^{-z})$, that is, the sigmoid function, although choices such as $g_k(z) = z/\sqrt{1 + z^2}$ and $g_k(z) = 1/(1 + |z|)$ are also possible. The concavity assumption on g_k means that the sum of the logistic function (a convex function) with the regularizer (8.8) is the difference of convex functions. Specialized algorithms for solving such structured problems have already been developed [23–25].

8.3 Numerical experiments

We present results from the numerical experiments performed with our cost-sensitive structured regularizer on an example from healthcare. In healthcare, rising costs present a significant new opportunity for the development of predictive models that are cost-sensitive. In 2014, the healthcare budget in the United States came to 17% of GDP with a total annual expenditure of \$3.1 trillion dollars [26]. It is estimated that between one-fourth and one-third of this amount is unnecessary, with most attributed to avoidable testing and diagnostic costs [26].

Here, we consider the goal of developing cost-sensitive predictive tools that may be used for automated screening [27] and triage [28,29] purposes. Specifically, we focus on the early detection of septic shock—an adverse event resulting from sepsis. Though many have tackled the task of early detection (see references within [30,31]), none have incorporated end-user cost preferences. Before presenting our numerical results, we give a brief background on sepsis.

[1] http://docs.sympy.org/0.7.6/modules/logic.html.

Sepsis is the 11th leading cause of patient mortality in the United States, with mortality rates between 30% and 50% in those who develop septic shock [32]. Although early treatment can reduce the patient mortality rate, less than one-third of the patients receive the appropriate therapy before onset. Therefore, an early warning system that accurately predicts a sepsis event will allow for appropriate treatment and result in a higher quality of care and patient outcome.

We combine the logistic-regression fidelity function L defined in (8.3b) with our structured regularizer R_{relax} given by (8.7) to predict the probability that a patient will develop septic shock. Note that other fidelity functions such as a time-to-event based objective, for example, [30], can also be used. We use MIMIC-II [33], a large publicly available dataset containing electronic health records from patients admitted to the ICU at the Beth Israel Deaconess Medical Center over a period of seven years. We constructed the full cost-graph in collaboration with domain experts, which resulted in 119 nodes and 294 edges. Using this data, we ran tests to answer the following two questions.

- Does our new structured regularizer produce diverse models?
- How does our structured regularizer perform compared to standard practices involving the ℓ_1-norm, which does not directly model the relevant costs?

We do not consider stage-wise alternatives because they are suboptimal to the proposed cost-sensitive ℓ_1-norm, which yields a global optimum. We also note that no other appropriate group sparsity-based methods exist to be compared to (see the discussion in Section 8.1.2).

8.3.1 Dataset

We processed the data in the MIMIC-II dataset from all adults (older than 15 years) with at least one measurement of blood urea nitrogen, hematocrit, and heart rate. This yielded data from 16,232 patients. Septic shock onset was identified using the 2012 Surviving Sepsis Campaign definitions [34], which resulted in 2,291 patients; we refer to these patients as positive cases. For patients with severe sepsis who never developed septic shock but received treatment, their outcome is confounded [35]. For these patients, it is unknown whether they would have developed shock without treatment and, therefore, they are excluded from the dataset [35]. Patients who never developed septic shock and were never treated to prevent shock are referred to as negative cases. Our final dataset contained 12,646 negative cases.

8.3.2 Experimental setup

We split the individuals in our dataset among training (75%) and test (25%) sets. From the training set, we process the data in a streaming fashion to extract positive and negative samples consisting of the features observed at a given time, and an associated label that is positive if septic shock was experienced within the following 48 hours and negative otherwise. Since the dataset is highly imbalanced, during training, we subsample the negative pairs to generate a balanced training set.

For individuals in our test set, we use the learned model to predict the risk of septic shock at each time point. This results in a trajectory of risk for septic shock over time for each individual. For a given threshold, an individual is said to be *identified* by the model as having shock if their risk trajectory ever rose above that threshold prior to shock onset. For this threshold, we calculate: (i) sensitivity as the fraction of patients who develop septic shock and are identified as having a high risk of septic shock; (ii) the false-positive rate (FPR) as the fraction of patients who never develop septic shock but are identified as high-risk patients by our model; and (iii) specificity as $1 - \text{FPR}$. The receiver operating characteristic (ROC) curve and the area under the curve (AUC) are obtained by varying the threshold value, with patients identified as at-risk if their predicted probability was above the threshold value. We use the bootstrap with 10 samples to estimate the confidence intervals for the AUC.

We used the SPAMS [36] suite of optimization routines to minimize the sum of the logistic function and our structured regularizer (8.7). Since our regularizer is a sum of group ℓ_∞-norms, we used their MATLAB® interface to their MEXFISTGRAPH routine. We changed the values of two default control parameters. We set the maximum allowed iteration limit to be 5,000 and the termination tolerance (duality gap) to be 10^{-3}. Overall, we found SPAMS to be reliable with termination usually resulting from meeting the termination tolerance, but occasionally the maximum allowed iteration limit was reached. In these latter cases, there did not appear to be any noticeable reduction in the predictive ability of the models obtained.

8.3.3 Model diversity

Three costs were considered: (i) the financial cost associated with ordering a test; (ii) the nursing-staff's time needed to perform the activities required for the tests; and (iii) the waiting time needed to obtain a test result. For a chosen maximum wait time, as well as chosen weighting parameters $\lambda_{\$}$ and $\lambda_{\text{⏱}}$, our algorithm minimizes the sum of the logistic function and the regularizer (8.7), which returns parameters that define a model from which we may compute an associated ROC, AUC, financial cost, nurse-time, and test result wait time. By sweeping over a range of values for the maximum allowed wait time, $\lambda_{\$}$, and $\lambda_{\text{⏱}}$, we obtain models with various costs that reflect preferences for different models. For our cost-dependency structure, there are three possible maximum wait times: 50 minutes, 10 minutes, and 0 minutes. For each of these scenarios, we select values for $\lambda_{\$}$ and $\lambda_{\text{⏱}}$ from an equally spaced grid over the interval $[10^{-3}, 10^{-7}]$, which yields a collection of models at the cost-accuracy frontier. Four models—denoted as $\mathscr{M}_1$, $\mathscr{M}_2$, $\mathscr{M}_3$, and $\mathscr{M}_4$—are represented in Table 8.1 to illustrate the trade-off achieved by our approach.

Model $\mathscr{M}_1$ is the most cost-effective. It uses existing measurements that are routinely collected and thus neither incurs a financial cost nor needs nursing-time to acquire new measurements. Since no additional tests are required, the wait time for the model is zero minutes. The model achieves a relatively high AUC of 82.79. The set of measurements that were most predictive include: clinical history (on ventilator, on pacemaker, has cardiovascular complications); vitals (shock index, raw and derived

Table 8.1 The costs for different models obtained from our structured regularizer. The sensitivity levels correspond to a specificity level of 0.85

Models	$\mathcal{M}_1$	$\mathcal{M}_2$	$\mathcal{M}_3$	$\mathcal{M}_4$
Sensitivity	0.61	0.66	0.65	0.72
AUC	82.79 ± 0.55	84.45 ± 0.64	84.75 ± 0.55	87.21 ± 0.46
Financial cost	$0	$0	$72	$170
Caregiver time	0 minutes	10 minutes	0 minutes	30 minutes
Result time	0 minutes	10 minutes	50 minutes	50 minutes
Tests needed	routine	Routine/urine	abg/routine	abg/cbc/cmp/hct/ hemoglobin/routine/urine
Activities needed	None	Urine	Arterial stick	Arterial stick/blood draw/urine

features of the heart rate, SpO_2, FiO_2, blood pressure, respiratory rate); and time since first presentation of systemic inflammatory response syndrome.

At the other extreme, model $\mathcal{M}_4$ has a financial cost of $170, requires a nurse-time of 30 minutes, and a total test result wait time of 50 minutes. It requires measurements attained from numerous additional tests such as the arterial blood gas, comprehensive metabolic panel, hematocrit, hemoglobin, and urine tests. By using these measurements, the accuracy increases to an AUC of 87.21, and shows a clinically significant gain in sensitivity compared to the performance of model $\mathcal{M}_1$.

Models $\mathcal{M}_2$ and $\mathcal{M}_3$ have cost and performance intermediate to models $\mathcal{M}_1$ and $\mathcal{M}_4$. It is interesting to see that $\mathcal{M}_2$ and $\mathcal{M}_3$ achieve similar performance in very different ways. Model $\mathcal{M}_2$ selects a urine measurement with a test result wait time of 10 minutes along with 10 minutes of nurse time, while $\mathcal{M}_3$ does not require any nurse time, but needs 50 minutes of wait time to receive test results.

For the specificity level of 0.85, the models vary significantly in terms of sensitivity. As expected, model $\mathcal{M}_1$ has the lowest sensitivity value of 0.61, followed by model $\mathcal{M}_3$ with a value of 0.65, then model $\mathcal{M}_2$ with a value of 0.66, and finally model $\mathcal{M}_4$ with a value of 0.72. Thus, when additional resources are available, $\mathcal{M}_4$ is significantly better at identifying patients that eventually did experience septic shock. The added sensitivity is useful in healthcare units that host vulnerable populations.

8.3.4 Comparison with the ℓ_1- and scaled ℓ_1-norm

Simple regularizers (e.g., the ℓ_1-norm) cannot capture the rich structure of the cost-dependencies in real-world domains such as healthcare. Figure 8.3 compares our structured group regularizer (Group) to the ℓ_1-norm (L1) and a scaled-ℓ_1-norm (L1-scaled). The L1 method is a straightforward implementation of logistic regression plus ℓ_1-norm minimization. The L1-scaled algorithm uses the same logistic function, but uses the scaled-ℓ_1-norm given by $R(\beta) := \lambda \|S\beta\|_1$ for some diagonal scaling matrix $S = \text{diag}(s_1, \ldots, s_n)$ and weighting parameter $\lambda > 0$. In our tests, we defined s_i as the maximum of 1 and the minimum cost required to obtain the ith feature. Although

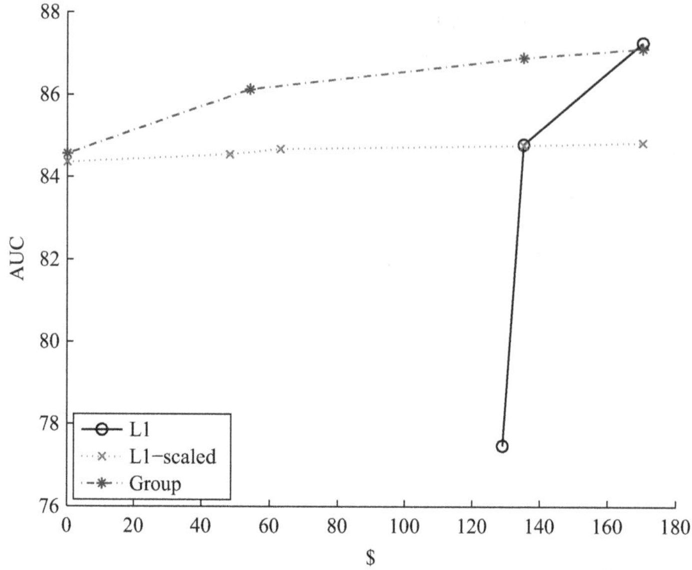

Figure 8.3 The cost in dollars ($) versus the area under the curve (AUC) for the ℓ_1 (L1), scaled-ℓ_1 (L1-scaled), and group regularizer (Group)

this choice is reasonable, it is also ad hoc, which is necessarily true for any choice of the scaling matrix S. This is a consequence of taking a complicated cost structure and representing it by n numbers, which is too simplistic.

Figure 8.3 compares the trade-off between financial cost and AUC values of Group, L1, and L1-scaled. (Similar plots could be constructed for test result time and nurse time.) The reported cost of a model is obtained by post-processing, whereby we sum the costs for the unique set of tests required. Each point in the plot represents a pair ($\$, \text{AUC}$) for some model. For algorithms L1 and L1-scaled, the points were obtained by varying λ over the interval $[10^{-3}, 10^{-7}]$. For algorithm Group based on the regularizer (8.7), we fixed $\lambda_{\text{⏱}} = 10^{-7}$ and let $\lambda_{\$}$ take on the same values as for λ; this placed different levels of emphasis on *only* the financial cost, which further illustrates the flexibility of our cost-driven structured regularizer. For all three algorithms, we only use tests that have a maximum allowed wait time of 50 minutes.

Algorithm L1 performs the worst. In particular, the cheapest model recovered by algorithm L1 costs $129 and had an AUC of approximately 77.5. At that same price-point, algorithms L1-scaled and Group were able to obtain AUC values of approximately 84.6 and 86.1. This is not surprising since the ℓ_1-regularizer employed by algorithm L1 causes the most predictive features to be chosen first, without any regard to the financial cost. This empirical evidence is not surprising and may be used to motivate algorithm L1-scaled. In essence, L1-scaled incorporates a primitive measure of the cost for each feature through the choice of s_i. Figure 8.3 also shows that our cost-sensitive regularizer significantly outperforms algorithm L1-scaled. Finally, observe that a surprisingly high AUC value (approximately 84.5) may be achieved by algorithms L1-scaled and Group using models that do not have a financial cost. For the prediction of sepsis, this means that although expensive tests produce measurements that allow for better prediction accuracy, one may still do well without incurring any (additional) financial costs. This observation should be leveraged when implementing screening tools or assessing risk stratification.

8.4 Conclusions and discussion

We designed a structured regularizer that captures the complex cost structure that exists in many applications. The feature, measurement, test, caregiver activity hierarchy in healthcare was used as an example, but we also showed how our method can be used anytime the cost structure can be represented as a finite-layer Boolean circuit. By building a regularizer that was in harmony with a user's application-specific cost preferences, our experimental tests produced a diverse collection of models. Moreover, our cost-sensitive regularizer achieved better prediction accuracy for the same (often lower) cost when compared to the ℓ_1 or weighted-ℓ_1 norms that are commonly used. Finally, we comment that the design of our regularizer must only be done once up-front for each application, and then may be used multiple times to answer a host of questions, for example, through model prediction.

Although our running example focused on implementing costs incurred by the institution—financial cost, staff time, and wait time—the penalty can be augmented to include patient-centered costs such as their tolerance for invasive tests and preference for certain tests. Furthermore, the model can be re-run (in real-time or cached) for different patients with contrasting preferences.

Beyond sepsis, our regularizer applies to early detection for potentially preventable conditions such as pneumonia, c-diff, and renal failure, which are estimated to cost the healthcare system 88 billion dollars [37]. More broadly, our regularizer is applicable to any cost-sensitive prediction problems whose cost-graph may be represented using the logical AND and OR structure associated with Boolean circuits. Returning to our example in traffic prediction, features (e.g., mean and trend) of the traffic velocity can be computed from streams acquired from one or more sources (e.g., querying crowdsourced GPS devices, pneumatic road tubes, piezoelectric sensors, cameras, and manual counting) at different locations including live event stream sources [6]. Considerations for which models to choose include the cost of acquiring and deploying the sensors, the staff time to maintain the sensors, and recurring costs of acquiring traffic, weather and live event stream data. Depending on the availability and cost of resources, one may wish to deploy different models in different regions.

Although our cost-sensitive regularizer may be used in many important applications, it has limitations. Its more accurate modeling of the cost-graph is achieved at the expense of requiring additional computation to construct. Converting a *general* r-layer Boolean circuit to a three-layer Boolean circuit has complexity $O(s^{fr})$, where s is the number of nodes and f is the fan (the largest number of allowed gate inputs/outputs) of the circuit. However, most cost-graphs are highly structured, thus dramatically reducing the computational cost. For example, constructing the regularizer for the ICU application took approximately 10 seconds on a MacBook Air laptop (1.8 GHz Intel Core i5 processor with 4GB of RAM). This modest additional cost is a consequence of the structure of the cost-graph: most nodes have relatively few connections to nodes in adjacent layers, and the logical gates mostly contain simple OR and AND constructs.[2] Since these properties hold for many cost-graphs of real-life problems, our approach is often practical.

It is possible that costs are nested, for example, a compound test may comprise ordering two tests at the level below, and the cost of the compound test is cheaper. In this case, we could augment the graph with edges from each of the two lower level tests to (replicated) tests at the compound test level, with associated Boolean OR gates. We may then apply the strategies described here to the augmented cost graph.

References

[1] Xu Z, Weinberger K, Chapelle O. The greedy miser: learning under test-time budgets. In: *Proceedings of the 29th international conference on machine learning*; 2012. p.1175–82.

[2] Ji S, Carin L. Cost-sensitive feature acquisition and classification. *Pattern Recogn* 2007;40(5):1474–85.

[3] Weiss DJ, Taskar B. Learning adaptive value of information for structured prediction. In: *Advances in neural information processing systems*. Lake Tahoe, CA; 2013. p. 953–61.

[4] Weiss D, Sapp B, Taskar B. Structured prediction cascades; 2012. arXiv preprint arXiv:1208.3279.

[5] Xu Z, Kusner M, Chen M, Weinberger KQ. Cost-sensitive tree of classifiers. In: *Proceedings of the 30th international conference on machine learning*; 2013. p. 133–41.

[6] Horvitz EJ, Apacible J, Sarin R, Liao L. Prediction, expectation, and surprise: methods, designs, and study of a deployed traffic forecasting service; 2012. arXiv:1207.1352.

[7] Candès EJ, Compressive sampling. In: *Proceedings of the international congress of mathematicians*, vol. 3, Madrid, Spain; 2006. p. 1433–52.

[8] Raykar VC, Krishnapuram B, Yu S. Designing efficient cascaded classifiers: tradeoff between accuracy and cost. In: *Proceedings of the 16th ACM SIGKDD. ACM*; 2010. p. 853–60.

[2]Patients in the ICU are critically ill and monitored intensely. This results in substantially more measurements compared to the ambulatory setting (typically five to six measurements are collected) and in-hospital setting (a smaller subset of measurements are collected compared to the ICU). Therefore, the cost-graph for the ICU example is larger than cost-graphs in other healthcare settings.

[9] Trapeznikov K, Saligrama V. Supervised sequential classification under budget constraints. In: *Proceedings of 16th international conference on artificial intelligence and statistics*. Scottsdale, AZ; 2013. p. 581–9.

[10] Kanani P, Melville P. Prediction-time active feature-value acquisition for cost-effective customer targeting. In: *Advances in neural information processing systems*. Vancouver, BC, Canada; 2008.

[11] Kapoor A, Horvitz E. Breaking boundaries: active information acquisition across learning and diagnosis. In: *Advances in neural information processing systems*. Vancouver, BC, Canada; 2009.

[12] Weiss D, Sapp B, Taskar B. *Dynamic structured model selection*. In: ICCV; 2013. p. 2656–63.

[13] Wainwright MJ. Structured regularizers for high-dimensional problems: statistical and computational issues. *Annu Rev Stat Appl* 2014;1: 233–53.

[14] Bach F, Jenatton R, Mairal J, Obozinski G. Optimization with sparsity-inducing penalties. *Found Trends Mach Learn* 2012;4(1):1–106.

[15] Kim S, Xing EP. Tree-guided group lasso for multi-task regression with structured sparsity. In: *Proceedings of the 27th international conference on machine learning*; 2010. p. 543–50.

[16] Zhao P, Rocha G, Yu B. Grouped and hierarchical model selection through composite absolute penalties. Department of Statistics, UC Berkeley, Tech. Rep. p. 703.

[17] Zhong LW, Kwok JT. Efficient sparse modeling with automatic feature grouping. *IEEE Trans Neural Netw Learn Syst* 2012;23(9):1436–47.

[18] Huang J, Ma S, Li H, Zhang C-H. The sparse laplacian shrinkage estimator for high-dimensional regression. *Ann Stat* 2011;39(4):2021.

[19] Angus DC, van der Poll T. Severe sepsis and septic shock. *N Engl J Med* 2013;369:850–1.

[20] Saeed M, Villarroel M, Reisner AT, Clifford G, Lehman L-W, Moody G, *et al.* Multiparameter intelligent monitoring in intensive care ii (mimic-ii): a public-access intensive care unit database. *Crit Care Med* 2011;39(5):952.

[21] Pfahringer B. Conjunctive normal form. In: *Encyclopedia of machine learning*. Springer; 2010. p. 209–10.

[22] Zeng X, Sun X, Yu Y, Wu L. The reduction generated algorithm of minimal disjunctive normal form based on discernibility matrix. In: *9th international conference on fuzzy systems and knowledge discovery (FSKD)*. IEEE; 2012. p. 265–9.

[23] Mairal J. Stochastic majorization-minimization algorithms for large-scale optimization. In: *Advances in neural information processing systems*; 2013. p. 2283–91.

[24] Tao PD, The dc (difference of convex functions) programming and dca revisited with dc models of real world nonconvex optimization problems. *Ann Operat Res* 2005;133(1–4):23–46.

[25] Tao PD, An LTH. Convex analysis approach to dc programming: theory, algorithms and applications. *Acta Math Viet* 1997;22(1):289–355.

[26] Smith M, Saunders R, Stuckhardt L, McGinnis JM. (eds.). *Best care at lower cost: the path to continuously learning health care in America.* National Academies Press, Washington D.C.; 2013.

[27] Raffle AE, Gray JM. *Screening: evidence and practice.* Oxford University Press; 2007.

[28] Wilson LO, Wilson FP, Wheeler M. Computerized triage of pediatric patients: automated triage algorithms. *Ann Emerg Med* 1981;10(12):636–40.

[29] Saria S, Rajani AK, Gould J, Koller D, Penn AA. Integration of early physiological responses predicts later illness severity in preterm infants. *Sci Transl Med* 2010;2(48):48ra65–48ra65.

[30] Henry KE, Hager DN, Pronovost PJ, Saria S. A targeted real-time early warning score (trewscore) for septic shock. *Sci Transl Med* 2015;7(299):299ra122.

[31] Ho JC, Lee CH, Ghosh J. Septic shock prediction for patients with missing data. *ACM Trans Manage Inf Syst* 2014;5(1):1:1–1:15.

[32] Angus DC, Linde-Zwirble WT, Lidicker J, Clermont G, Carcillo J, Pinsky MR. Epidemiology of severe sepsis in the united states: analysis of incidence, outcome, and associated costs of care. *Crit Care Med* 2001;29(7):1303–10.

[33] Saeed M, Lieu C, Raber G, Mark R. Mimic ii: a massive temporal ICU patient database to support research in intelligent patient monitoring. In: *Computers in cardiology, 2002*. IEEE; 2002. p. 641–4.

[34] Dellinger RP, Levy MM, Rhodes A, Annane D, Gerlach H, Opal SM, et al. Surviving sepsis campaign: international guidelines for management of severe sepsis and septic shock, 2012. *Intensive Care Med* 2013;39(2):165–228.

[35] Paxton C, Niculescu-Mizil A, Saria S. Developing predictive models using electronic medical records: challenges and pitfalls. In: *AMIA Annual Symposium Proceedings*, vol. 2013. American Medical Informatics Association; 2013. p. 1109.

[36] Mairal J, Jenatton R, Bach FR, Obozinski GR. Network flow algorithms for structured sparsity. *Adv Neural Inf Process Syst* 2010;1558–66.

[37] Fuller R, McCullough E, Bao M, Averill R. Estimating the costs of potentially preventable hospital acquired complications. *Health Care Financ Rev* 2009;30(4):17–32.

Chapter 9

Variational Bayesian non-parametric inference for infectious disease models

James Hensman and Theodore Kypraios

9.1 Introduction

9.1.1 Infectious disease modelling

The past two decades have seen a significant growth in the field of mathematical modelling of communicable diseases and this has led to a substantial increase in our understanding of infectious disease epidemiology and control. Although this growth was stimulated initially by the appearance of HIV in the early 1980s, it has been maintained due to other important events such as, for example, Foot-and-Mouth [1–3], SARS outbreaks [4], healthcare-associated infections (such as MRSA and *Clostridium difficile*) [5,6], Avian, H1N1 and H3N2 influenza [7–9], and more recently, Ebola [10]. Understanding the spread of communicable infectious diseases is of great importance to prevent major future outbreaks and therefore it remains high on the global scientific agenda, including contingency planning for the threat of a possible influenza pandemic. It has been widely recognised that mathematical and statistical modelling has become a valuable tool in the analysis of infectious disease dynamics by supporting the development of control strategies, informing policymaking at the highest levels, and in general playing a fundamental role in the fight against disease spread [11].

9.1.2 Why non-parametric inference?

Despite the enormous attention given to the development of methods for efficient parameter estimation in infectious disease models, there has been relatively little activity in the area of *non-parametric* inference. That is, drawing inference for the quantities which govern transmission, (i) the *force of infection* and (ii) the period during which an individual remains infectious, without making certain modelling assumptions about the force's (parametric) functional form or that the period belongs to a certain family of parametric distributions, respectively.

The first motivation for fitting non-parametric models is that *it helps to avoid erroneous conclusions* and biased results arising from the use of parametric models with inappropriate assumptions either about the functional form of the force of infection and/or the distribution that the infectious period is assumed to follow. Second, inferring the force of infection via a non-parametric framework *offers great modelling flexibility*. One of most common assumptions in epidemic modelling is that the net rate of spread of infection at some time t ($\lambda(t)$) is assumed to be proportional to the density of susceptible individuals ($S(t)$) multiplied by the density of infectious individuals ($I(t)$) at time t, known as the *mass-action principle*. Despite the attempts that have been made to relax this assumption motivated by certain applications (e.g. sexually transmitted diseases), they have been concerned with the assignment of different (parametric) functional forms to $\lambda(t)$ such as $S(t)I(t)^{\alpha}$ and $S(t)I(t)/(1+\alpha I(t))$ for some unknown parameter α which needs to be estimated from the data.

Finally, Markov Chain Monte Carlo (MCMC) methods are generally applicable and, to some extent straightforward, to implement and this has resulted in the analysis of disease outbreak data often using complex parametric models. It is often questionable whether or not such model complexity is needed or if there is sufficient information in the data to estimate all the model parameters accurately. Hence, issues such as over- or under fitting are of major concern. Non-parametric inference methods allow the data to speak for themselves without the need for questionable parametric assumptions.

9.1.3 Previous work

Not only has there been very little work to date concerning non-parametric inference for epidemic models, but until recently, it had also been solely focused within the classical (frequentist) framework. Becker and Yip [12] have considered non-parametric estimation of the person-to-person infection rate using martingale methods. Additionally, similar methods have been used by Huggins *et al.* [13] to estimate the unknown number of initially susceptible individuals in the population [14]. Although martingale methods are very elegant, they are rather specialised methods and not as widely applicable as most other approaches to fitting epidemic models to data and are restricted to frequentist rather than Bayesian inference. Recently, a novel non-parametric method for the survival analysis of outbreak data has been proposed [15], but currently, the developed framework suffers from some rather unrealistic assumptions. Recently, Xu *et al.* [16] and Knock and Kypraios [17] developed Bayesian non-parametric methods for stochastic epidemic models which are partially observed through time. In particular they focused on models of the *Susceptible–Infective–Removed* (SIR) type in which only the times at which individuals were removed from the population are observed. The main idea behind these papers is to relax the usual mass-action assumption under which new infections occur at rate $\beta S_t I_t$ and replace it with a function that depends on time say, for example, $g(t)$ and infer $g(t)$ within a Bayesian framework. That involved assigning a flexible prior on $g(t)$ such as a second-order B-spline, piecewise constant, and a Gaussian process (GP) prior and estimating it using MCMC algorithms. Although it has been demonstrated that Bayesian non-parametric inference for epidemic models can be achieved, one practical challenge with these methods is that the computational complexity increases with the size of the population as well as with model complexityis some nonlinear function of time t, the number of susceptibles S_t and I_t infectives, i.e. replacing $\beta S_t I_t$ by $g(t, S_t, I_t)$. In this chapter, we show that one can overcome these difficulties by adopting a framework using Variational Bayesian inference.

9.2 Background

Before describing the models of interest, we provide some background material on GPs and variational Bayes (VB). GPs form the non-parametric core of our methodology, allowing for non-parametric modelling of functions. VB forms the computational core of our ideas, allowing for rapid approximate inference in the proposed models.

9.2.1 *Gaussian processes*

GPs were presented in a statistical context by O'Hagan and Kingman [18], but appear across the sciences under different guises. For example, Brownian motion is an example of a GP [19] and the Kalman filter[1] [20–22] is another. The popularity of GP methods as machine learning tools is more recent and is perhaps due to increases in computational power.

GP models are widely used in machine learning as they provide a non-parametric model of functions. The model may be used directly in regression, or used through via a link function in classification [23], or in a variety of other models such as robust regression [24]. A tutorial and overview is given by Rasmussen and Williams [25].

The main definition and key property of a GP is that it is an infinite collection of variables, any finite sub set of which has a multivariate Gaussian distribution. We write

$$f(t) \sim \mathcal{GP}(m(t), k(t, t')) \tag{9.1}$$

to indicate that the function $f(t)$ is drawn from a GP, and the key property is represented as

$$\mathbf{f} \sim \mathcal{N}(\mathbf{m}, \mathbf{K}) \tag{9.2}$$

where $\mathbf{f}$ is a vector collecting N evaluations of the function f at time points of interest $\mathbf{f} = [f(t_i)]_{i=1}^N$, and $\mathbf{m}$ and $\mathbf{K}$ are a mean vector and covariance matrix, respectively, built as

$$\mathbf{m} = [m(t_i)]_{i=1}^N \qquad \mathbf{K}_{ij} = k(t_i, t_j) \tag{9.3}$$

The properties of the GP and the functions $f(t)$ drawn from it are defined by the mean function $m(t)$ and the covariance function $k(t, t')$. The mean function is usually assumed to be zero, or a suitable constant, and the covariance function must be positive definite: for our purposes, we will assume that $k(t, t')$ produces a positive definite matrix $\mathbf{K}$.

[1]The term 'Kalman filter' has become popular for a model we would prefer to call a 'linear dynamical system': the Kalman filter is a method for inference on such a model.

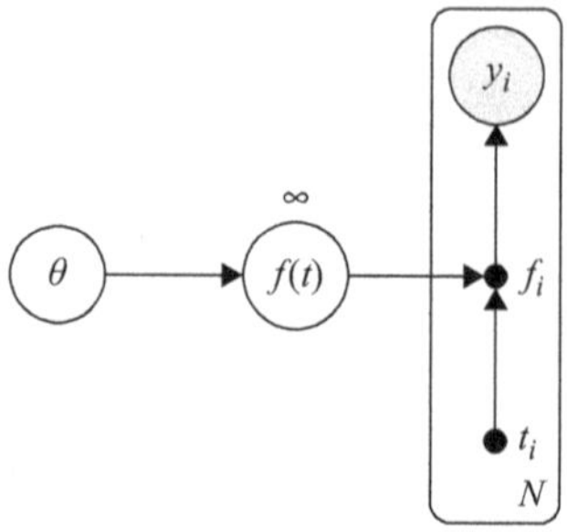

Figure 9.1 A graphical model of a GP model. Here, θ represents parameters of the covariance function, the infinite node $f(t)$ represents a draw from the GP, and the shaded (observed) node y represents the data. We have used small solid nodes to represent deterministic relations, i.e. the values of the function at the data points f_i are fixed given the function $f(t)$. Confer Figure 9.2

A popular choice of covariance function is the Matern family, which corresponds to autoregressive systems [25]. There are several kernels in the family, and here we use the Matern-3/2 kernel, which corresponds to a second-order system:

$$k(t,t') = \sigma^2 \left(1 + \frac{\sqrt{3}}{\ell}|t - t'|\right) \exp\left(-\frac{\sqrt{3}}{\ell}|t - t'|\right) \tag{9.4}$$

The parameters σ^2 and ℓ control the vertical and horizontal scale (wiggliness) of the function: we fit these parameters by (approximate) maximum likelihood (see below).

It is possible to build rich models using GPs by manipulating the covariance function: a small family of existing covariance functions can be combined by addition and multiplication (which both preserve positive definiteness) to provide complex distributions over functions. For example, Lloyd *et al.* [26] built an 'Automatic statistician' which searched over combinations of kernel functions, and Alvarez *et al.* [27] used linear operations on kernels to build models of complex dynamical interactions.

To turn a GP into a statistical model, we consider it to be a distribution of some unobserved, or *latent*, function, and conditionally model the data using some simple parametric model (i.e. noise). For example, in a classification task the likelihood is usually a Bernoulli draw conditioned on a sigmoidal transformation ϕ of the process: $p(y_i|f(t_i)) = \phi(f(t_i))^{y_i}(1 - \phi(f(t_i)))^{(1-y_i)}$, with $y \in \{0, 1\}$, or for Poisson regression of (which we make use below), the rate of the Poisson is given by the exponent of the process: $p(y_i|f_i) = e^{f_i y_i} e^{-e^{f_i}} / y_i!$. We illustrate this general GP model in Figure 9.1.

The usefulness of GPs as statistical models hinges on the ability to compute at only the data points: it is hard to imagine how one might represent entire arbitrary random functions (or distributions on them) using a computer otherwise. Inference thus focuses on the latent vector $\mathbf{f}$, but it is important to remember that the model contains the whole process: this come into play when making predictions, when we

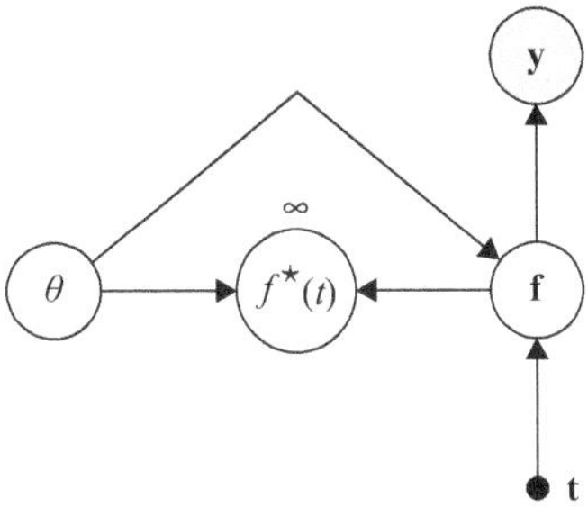

Figure 9.2 A graphical model of a GP model, with the conditioning property of the process emphasised. Here, θ and y are as Figure 9.1, but the function $f(t)$ has been split into the function values at the data points **f** *and the remaining function values $f^\star(t)$. It is this conditional property that allows inference in a GP model*

would like to represent uncertainty over a latent function value (or unseen data) located at a new point $f(t^\star)$. Conditioned on the function values at the data **f**, the remainder of the GP is distributed according to the conditional process:

$$f^\star(t) \mid \mathbf{f} \sim \mathcal{GP}(m(t) + k(t, \mathbf{t})\mathbf{K}^{-1}(\mathbf{f} - \mathbf{m}), k(t, t') - k(t, \mathbf{t})\mathbf{K}^{-1}k(\mathbf{t}, t')) \tag{9.5}$$

where we have used $k(t, \mathbf{t})$ to represent a vector containing evaluations of the kernel function at time t and all observed times $\mathbf{t} = [t_i]_{i=1}^N$. Figure 9.2 emphasises the conditional property of the GP that is used for inference. This construction will also prove important when deriving our VB approximation.

9.2.2 Variational Bayes

VB is a method for inference, which stands as an alternative to MCMC. A contemporary review is given by Blei *et al.* [28], and we provide here a more focussed introduction, directing our attention towards inference in GP models. The central idea is to approximate the posterior distribution by choosing from a pre-defined family of distributions in such a way as to minimise the Kullback–Leibler (KL) divergence between the approximation (q) and the true posterior (p). For a general model with latent variables **x** and data **y**, the key expression is

$$\begin{aligned} \mathrm{KL}[q(\mathbf{x};\eta) \,||\, p(\mathbf{x}|\mathbf{y})] &= -\mathbb{E}_{q(\mathbf{x};\eta)}\left[\log \frac{p(\mathbf{y}|\mathbf{x})p(\mathbf{x})}{q(\mathbf{x};\eta)}\right] + \log p(\mathbf{y}) && (9.6) \\ &= -\mathrm{ELBO} + \log p(\mathbf{y}) && (9.7) \end{aligned}$$

Having specified a family of approximating distributions $q(\mathbf{x};\eta)$ with free parameters η, the (intractable) KL (left-hand side) is minimised by maximising the 'Evidence Lower BOund' or ELBO with respect to the free parameters η (note that $p(\mathbf{y})$ can be considered a constant).

VB has been popular for semi-conjugate exponential family models: for these models a VBEM (Variational Bayesian Expectation Maximisation) algorithm exists which iterates between variables in a similar way to a Gibbs sampler [29–31]. The difference is that rather than sampling forms the conditional distribution for each variable (as in the Gibbs sampler), VBEM updates a factorising marginal distribution for each variable in turn, i.e. $q(\mathbf{x};\eta) = q(\mathbf{x}_1;\eta_1)q(\mathbf{x}_2;\eta_2)\ldots$. The popularity of these methods lies perhaps in their algorithmic elegance rather than statistical accuracy or computational efficiency: the approximate posterior is assumed to factorise, which is often deemed too strong an assumption; the algorithm is a coordinate ascent method which touches all the data at each step. The efficiency of the method can be improved by either geometric-gradient-based methods [32,33] or using mini-batches of the data [34].

Recent research in VB has focussed on two main directions: first, to increase the flexibility of the approximating distribution (and thus the accuracy of the method), for example, using mixture-distributions [35], complex reparametrisations [36], or recognition models [37,38]. Another interesting direction has been to make the method applicable to a wider variety of models [39].

In the case of GP models, there are some model-specific properties that may be exploited. Opper and Archambeau [40] described, how for many GP models, the posterior may be approximated with a Gaussian distribution, and how the factorising nature of the likelihood leads to a reduced number of parameters for the approximate covariance. Nguyen and Bonilla [41] described a scheme where the GP posterior was approximated by a mixture of Gaussians, and Hensman *et al.* [42] detailed connections between the variational approach and Expectation Propagation.

In the following section, we describe in detail a variational approach to inference in GP models, and demonstrate the effective fitting of these models to some simple epidemiological datasets.

9.3 Modelling framework

9.3.1 SIR model definition

We first describe the principles and basic assumptions of the most well-studied stochastic epidemic model, the so-called SIR model. Consider a closed population of N individuals, each of whom, at any given time $t \in \mathbb{R}$, is in one of three states: susceptible, infective, or removed. The epidemic is initiated by one infective in an otherwise entirely susceptible population. For $t \geq 0$ and $i = 1, \ldots, k$ denote by $S(t)$ and $I(t)$ the numbers of susceptibles and infectives at time t, respectively. The epidemic process $\{S(t), I(t)\}$ can be defined as a bivariate Markov chain with the following transition rates:

$$\begin{aligned}(i,j) &\rightarrow (i-1,j+1) : \beta S(t)I(t)\\ (i,j) &\rightarrow (i,j-1) : \gamma I(t)\end{aligned}$$

and the corresponding transition probabilities to an infection and removal:

$$\mathbb{P}[X(t+\delta t)-S(t)=-1, Y(t+\delta t)-I(t)=1 \mid \mathscr{H}_t] = \beta S(t)\, I(t)+o(\delta t)$$
$$\mathbb{P}[X(t+\delta t)-S(t)=0, Y(t+\delta t)-I(t)=-1 \mid \mathscr{H}_t] = \gamma I(t)+o(\delta t)$$

All other transitions having probability $o(\delta t)$ and $\mathscr{H}_t$ is the sigma-algebra generated by the history of the process up to time t. The form of the transition probabilities shows that the probability of infection at time t is proportional to the total number of infectives and susceptibles at time t. The constant of proportionality, β, is referred to as the *infection rate*. The transition probability of a removal shows that the length of the infectious periods is independent, identically distributed exponential random variables with mean $1/\gamma$, and therefore γ is referred as the removal rate for each individual. Furthermore, a removed individual plays no further part in the epidemic and the epidemic ends when there are no more infectives in the population. All of the infectious periods and the infection process are assumed to be independent of each other.

Under the assumption of an Exponential infectious period distribution the SIR model is often called the *general stochastic epidemic* and is the most widely studied version of the removal rate. Although one may assume a different distribution for the infectious period, one key reason for the Exponential distribution is that the epidemic model is Markov which in turns makes it possible to analyse certain aspects of the model using techniques from Markov Chain theory.

Despite the mathematical advantages, one practical drawback with the choice of exponentially distributed infectious period is that it is not very realistic for most diseases. Therefore, other common choices are (i) *constant* which corresponds to the assumption that an individual who becomes infective remains so for exactly d time units before becoming removed, and (ii) Gamma or Weibull distribution which unlike the Exponential has two parameters which enable separate specification of the mean and the variance of the infectious period distribution.

In this chapter, we are concerned with the infection mechanism (i.e. the rate at which new infections occur) and therefore, for simplicity, we will assume that the infectious period distribution is Exponential.

9.3.2 Approximating the SIR model with a log Gaussian Cox process

It follows from the above definition of the SIR model in Section 9.3.1 that while there is at least one susceptible and at least one infective, new infections in the population as a whole occur at the points of a time inhomogeneous Poisson process with an rate $\lambda(t)=\beta S(t)I(t)$.

The Poisson process is a widely used model for point data in temporal settings. The inhomogeneous variant of the Poisson process allows the rate at which events occur to vary in time. Although in some applications one may have a preconceived idea of the appropriate parametric functional form for this variation, it is often the case that one does not want to impose a particular functional form. In this case, it is often desirable to use another stochastic process to describe non-parametrically the variation intensity function in a Poisson process. This construction is called a *doubly stochastic* Poisson process, or a Cox process [43]. One variant of the Cox process is the Gaussian Cox process, where the intensity function is a transformation (to ensure positivity) of a random realisation from a GP.

9.3.3 Relaxing the parametric assumptions of the SIR model

Returning to the SIR model, one therefore can replace the overall incidence rate of new infections, $\lambda(t) = \beta S(t)\, I(t)$, by $\lambda(t) = \beta(t)S(t)I(t)$, relaxing the assumption of homogeneity (i.e. that each individuals aims to infect other at the same rate) while retaining the mass-action assumption. On the other hand, it is very natural to consider, alternatively, that the rate at which new infections occur is an arbitrary function $\lambda(t) > 0\,(t \in \mathbb{R})$ that only depends on time and estimate $\lambda(t)$ within a Bayesian framework given some observed disease outbreak data. If we assume that *a priori* $\log(\lambda)$ follows a GP distribution, we have a log Gaussian Cox process (LGCP).

9.3.4 Bayesian inference for an LGCP

Likelihood-based inference for an LGCP model is generally intractable, due to the need to integrate an infinite-dimensional random function. However, approximate inference can be performed by discretising time into bins and assuming that the width of the bin is small enough that the intensity may be considered constant across each bin [44].

Likelihood. Denote by $\mathbf{y} = (y_i)_{i=1}^N$ the number of counts (cases) in each bin i, $i = 1, \ldots, N$. We have that $y_i \sim Po(\lambda(t_i)\Delta t)$ where Δt is the width of each bin, and $\lambda(t_i)$ denotes the intensity in bin i. This gives rise to likelihood of the observed data

$$p(\mathbf{y} \mid \lambda(t)) = \prod_{i=1}^{n} \frac{(\lambda(t_i)\,\Delta t)^{y_i} \exp\{-\lambda(t_i)\,\Delta t\}}{y_i!} \tag{9.8}$$

Prior. Since we shall be modelling the log-intensity with a GP, the latent variables are $f(t_i) = \log \lambda(t_i)$, collected into the vector $\mathbf{f} = (f(t_i))_{i=1}^N$. As described in Section 9.2.1, the prior density is then

$$p(\mathbf{f}) = |2\pi \mathbf{K}|^{-1/2} \exp\left\{-\frac{1}{2}(\mathbf{m} - \mathbf{f})^\top \mathbf{K}^{-1}(\mathbf{m} - \mathbf{f})\right\} \tag{9.9}$$

Posterior. Combining the likelihood function with the prior distribution we can derive the density of the posterior distribution up to a normalising constant:

$$p(\mathbf{f} \mid \mathbf{y}) \propto \exp\left\{\mathbf{y}^\top \mathbf{f} - \Delta t \sum_{i=1}^{n} \exp\{f(t_i)\} - \frac{1}{2}(\mathbf{m} - \mathbf{f})^\top \mathbf{K}^{-1}(\mathbf{m} - \mathbf{f})\right\} \tag{9.10}$$

Posterior computation. One method for inference in this problem is to draw samples from $p(\mathbf{f} \mid \mathbf{y})$ using MCMC [45]. Inference in latent Gaussian models such as this one is known to be challenging because of the high dimensionality and strong dependencies between the variables [46,47]. Any MCMC method will be computationally intensive when the dimension of $\mathbf{f}$ is large since we have to solve the system of equations $(\mathbf{m}-\mathbf{f})^{\top}\mathbf{K}^{-1}(\mathbf{m}-\mathbf{f})$, which costs $\mathcal{O}(N^3)$ operations. The LGCP exacerbates this problem since we wish to discretise the time into as many bins as possible to improve the accuracy of (discrete) approximation to the continuous model. For that reason, we employ a VB framework to infer the posterior over f.

9.3.5 Sparse variational approximations to GPs

A particular feature of GP models is that the covariance matrix grows with the number of data (or in our case, the number of bins). On the one hand, this is a reflection of the non-parametric nature of the model: more data lead to more latent variables and so more model flexibility. On the other hand, this feature is a nuisance because in order to evaluate the posterior (or approximate it with VB) one must decompose a large, potentially dense matrix. A simple approach to reduce the computational burden is to use only a sub set of the data [48]: hence the name 'sparse' approximation.

An improved idea which has gained much traction in the literature is to approximate the covariance matrix $\mathbf{K}$ with another matrix whose decomposition is easier. The projected process approximation [49] and the FITC (Fully Independent Training Conditional [50]) models provide alternative GP priors [51] which give rise to covariance matrices which can be decomposed more easily. An issue with this approach is that we have fundamentally *changed the model* from the original specification, and have no guarantee that the model will fit in the same way as the original. For example, FITC exhibits heteroscedastic behaviour [52], which whilst interesting, is not a part of the original model.

VB provides an opportunity to make a more pleasing approximation, in the sense that the posterior is approximated, not the model. An important property of the approximation that we will describe is that the complexity of the approximation is increased, we are guaranteed to move closer to the true posterior in the KL sense. The key idea is that the family of approximating distributions q is a GP, but with lower complexity than the original: the ELBO can be computed with complexity $\mathcal{O}(NM^2)$, where N is the number of data, and M is the 'effective' number of data in the approximation ($M < N$). This idea was first studied by Titsias [53], who studied the special case of Gaussian noise. Further work was done by Hensman *et al.* [54] to make the idea scale to larger datasets and non-Gaussian likelihoods [55]. Finally these ideas were made more formal by Matthews *et al.* [56] and Hensman *et al.* [57].

We begin by defining the form of the variational approximation. Following the idea of pseudo-inputs (or inducing inputs) as first introduced by [50], let $\mathbf{z} = (z_m)_{m=1}^{M}$ be a series of points that live in the time domain, and let the variables $\mathbf{u} = (u_m)_{m=1}^{M}$ represent the value of the GP function at those times, so $u_m = f(z_m)$, where f is our GP object. The remainder for the GP variables (including those at the data points $\mathbf{f}$) will be represented by the GP conditional

$$f^{\star}(t) \mid \mathbf{u} \sim \mathcal{GP}(k(t,\mathbf{z})k(\mathbf{z},\mathbf{z})^{-1}\mathbf{u}, k(t,t') - k(t,\mathbf{z})k(\mathbf{z},\mathbf{z})^{-1}k(\mathbf{z},t')) \tag{9.11}$$

where we have denoted the $M \times M$ covariance matrix evaluated at all inducing points as $k(\mathbf{z},\mathbf{z})$. This approximation to the posterior is represented graphically in Figure 9.3.

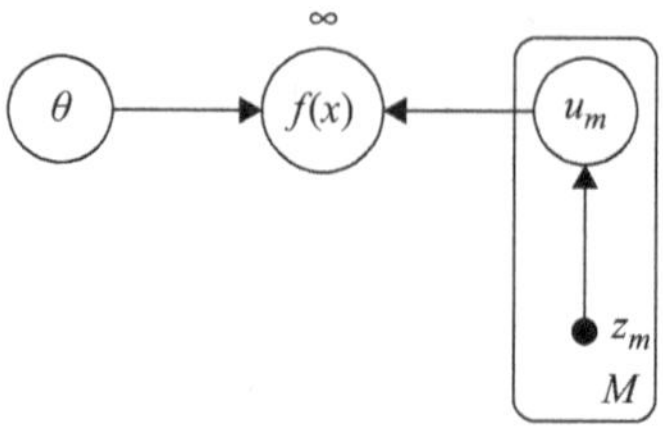

Figure 9.3 A graphical model of a sparse GP approximation

It remains to define an approximation for the crucial variables $\mathbf{u}$, which play a similar role in the sparse approximation as the variables $\mathbf{f}$ do when computing using, for example, MCMC as described above. We assume a Gaussian distribution for $\mathbf{u}$, with variational parameters $\boldsymbol{\mu}$ and $\mathbf{L}$.

$$q(\mathbf{u}) = \mathcal{N}(\boldsymbol{\mu}, \mathbf{L}\mathbf{L}^\top) \tag{9.12}$$

where $\mathbf{L}$ is a lower triangular matrix. The variational parameters are then $\eta = \{\mathbf{z}, \boldsymbol{\mu}, \mathbf{L}\}$, and we optimise the ELBO with respect to these parameters.

To deal with the covariance function parameters, we make an approximate maximum-likelihood estimate. Note that if the KL divergence in (9.7) is small, then the ELBO is a good approximation to the likelihood. We thus maximise the ELBO with respect to the covariance function parameters alongside η.

Substituting the proposed definitions for the approximate distribution into (9.7), we have

$$\text{ELBO} = \mathbb{E}_{q(f^\star,\mathbf{f},\mathbf{u})}\left[\log \frac{p(\mathbf{y} \mid \mathbf{f})p(\mathbf{f} \mid \mathbf{u})p(\mathbf{u})p(f^\star \mid \mathbf{f},\mathbf{u})}{q(\mathbf{f} \mid \mathbf{u})q(\mathbf{u})q(f^\star \mid \mathbf{f},\mathbf{u})}\right] \tag{9.13}$$

$$= \mathbb{E}_{q(\mathbf{f})}[\log p(\mathbf{y} \mid \mathbf{f})] - \text{KL}[q(\mathbf{u}) || p(\mathbf{u})] \tag{9.14}$$

Because the form of the conditionals $\mathbf{f} \mid \mathbf{u}$, $f^\star \mid \mathbf{f}, \mathbf{u}$ is the same for both the model (nominator) and approximation (denominator), the terms $p(f^\star \mid \mathbf{f}, \mathbf{u})$ and $p(\mathbf{f} \mid \mathbf{u})$ cancel, resulting in a simpler expression. It is fortuitous that the cancellation occurs because these terms either have an infinite number of variables ($f^\star$), or cost $\mathcal{O}(N^3)$ to compute ($\mathbf{f}$). For more details, see References 55, 57. An important note is that the values $f^\star$ are infinite, and so the notation $p(f^\star)$ is inaccurate, since we cannot place a probability measure on an infinite object in this way. Nonetheless, the intuition is correct and a more rigorous derivation [56] gives the same result.

Finally, a note about computation and optimisation. The expression for the ELBO can be computed in $\mathcal{O}(NM^2)$ and we intend to optimise it with respect to the variational parameters $\eta = \{\boldsymbol{\mu}, \mathbf{L}, \mathbf{z}\}$. For the purposes of this chapter, we considered a grid of $\mathbf{z}$ over the time domain of interest, and fixed $\mathbf{z}$ to these values. The remaining parameters were optimised using a gradient-based optimiser. The models were implemented in GPflow,[2] which is capable of automatically computing derivatives, simplifying the implementation.

[2]Available at github.com/gpflow.

9.4 Results

We will now illustrate our framework via some examples. First we use simulated data to show that method works well in practice and highlight the flexibility that it offers. In addition, we also will use our framework to analyse a classic dataset of an outbreak of Smallpox in a village in Nigeria.

We are primarily concerned with inferring non-parametrically the force of infection. Given that we assume that the times at which individuals become infected and then recovered (removed) from the population are both observed, estimation of the parameters governing the infectious period distribution is straightforward in either a frequentist or Bayesian framework. Furthermore, this estimation is independent of the estimation of the force of infection; see, for example, Reference 3 for more details. Therefore, from now on, we shall concentrate only on estimating the force of infection. We will do that by employing the framework of sparse variational approximation to GP as described in Section 9.3.5.

9.4.1 Dataset 1: Synthetic data from a homogeneously mixing mass-action SIR model

We first simulate some synthetic data from a Markovian homogeneously mixing SIR model (see Section 9.3.1) with the incident rate of new infections being $\beta S(t)I(t)$. We set $\beta = 0.0002$ and $\gamma = 1$ with the epidemic starting with one infective among a population of $N = 10,000$ susceptibles. The number of individuals who were ever infective was $n = 8,089$. The epidemic started at time 0 and the last removal occurred at time $T = 18.95$. We discretise the interval $[0, 18.95]$ into 635 bins each of them having width 0.03 and the number of cases in each bin are shown in Figure 9.4.

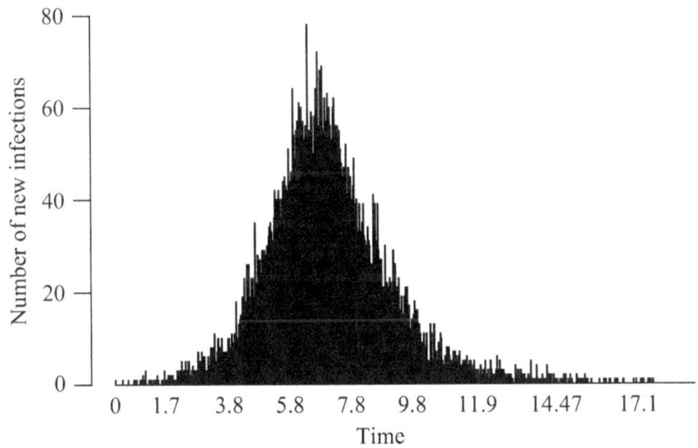

Figure 9.4 Observed number of new infections; data were generated from a homogeneously mixing mass-action SIR model with an overall force of infection $\beta S(t)I(t)$, where $\beta = 0.0002$

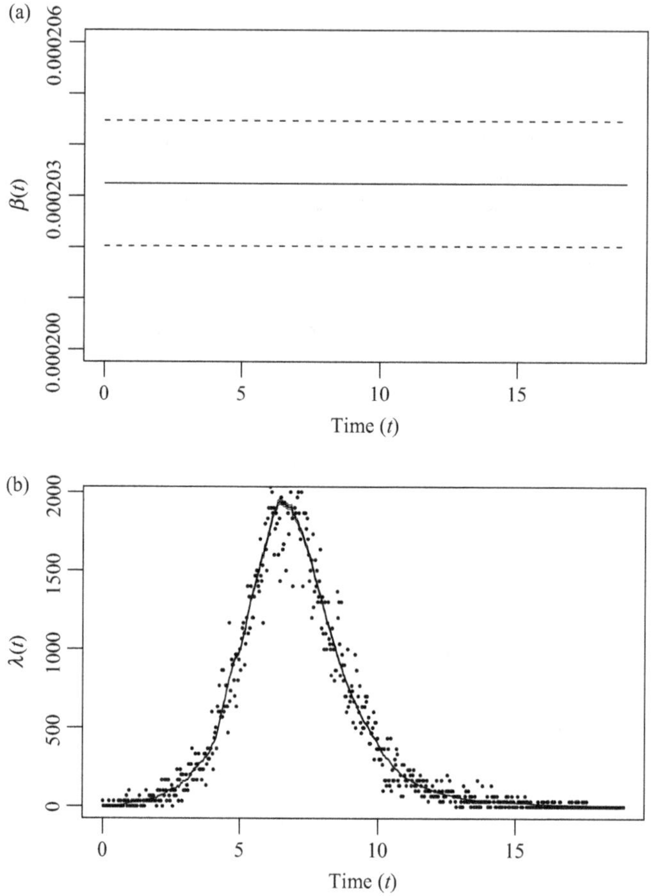

Figure 9.5 *(a) The (exponentiated) GP posterior of the person-to-person infection rate $\beta(t)$ for the simulated mass-action data. The model for the force-of-infection is $\lambda(t) = \beta(t)S(t)I(t)$, where $\beta(t) = \exp(f(t))$, and $f(t)$ is modelled with a GP. The black line represents the posterior mean, the dashed lines represent 95% credible intervals. The GP represent a constant function, which is in agreement with the model ($\beta = 0.0002$). (b) The corresponding estimated overall force of infection $\lambda(t)$*

As mentioned earlier, a natural starting point for non-parametric inference is to retain the usual natural mass-action assumption for the incidence of new infections, but assume that the person-to-person infection rate is not constant but instead time-dependent. The model was fitted using a sparse variational approximation as outlined in Section 9.3.5. Figure 9.5 (a) shows the posterior mean of the person-to-person infection rate $\beta(t)$ as well as the corresponding 95% credible intervals.

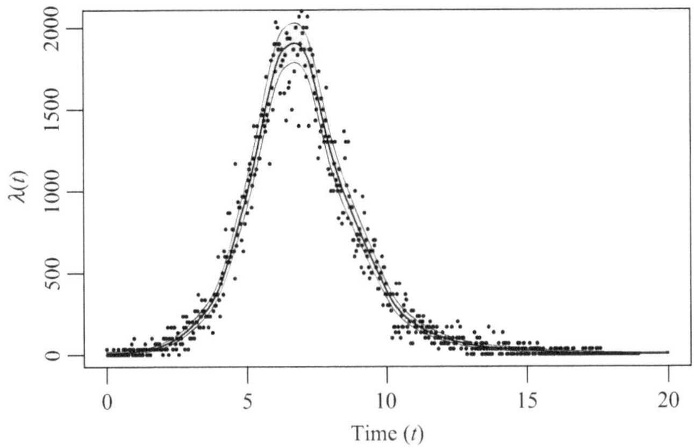

Figure 9.6 *The estimated overall force of infection $\lambda(t)$ for the simulated mass-action data when modelled as a log Gaussian Cox process, $\lambda(t) = \exp(f(t))$, with $f(t)$ modelled as a GP. The black line represents the posterior mean, the shaded area represents the 95% credible interval, and the dots represent the observed (new) infections per bin*

The proposed algorithm estimates $\beta(t)$ to be flat with fairly high precision which is of course consistent with the truth since the data were generated by $\beta(t) = 0.0002$. Figure 9.5(b) shows the corresponding estimated overall force of infection $\lambda(t)$ since $S(t)$ and $I(t)$ can be calculated from the data. Next, we relax totally the mass-action assumption and assume that the overall force of infection $\lambda(t)$ is a function of time only. Figure 9.6 reveals that the estimated function matches very well the observed data.

Assuming that the force of infection is either $\beta S(t)I(t)$ or $\lambda(t)$ represents two extreme situations. In the former case, it is assumed that the transmission dynamics are governed by a mass-action term in homogeneously mixing population, whilst in the latter any information about the number of susceptible $S(t)$ and infectives $I(t)$ in the population at any given time t is ignored. Hence, it is natural to introduce a model in which the force of infection is assumed to be a function of the product of $S(t)I(t)$, and model the logarithm of that function as a GP, i.e. $\lambda(t) = \exp(f(S(t)I(t))$. Figure 9.7(b) shows the posterior distribution of $\lambda(t)$ versus $S(t)I(t)$. Figure 9.7(a) indicates we successfully recover the (true) linear relationship between $\lambda(t)$ and product of the susceptibles and infectives over time, while the corresponding estimate for $\lambda(t)$ is very similar to the one derived when fitting the model where $\lambda(t) = \exp(f(t))$ and shown in Figure 9.6.

9.4.2 Dataset 2: Synthetic data from a seasonal SIR model

We now generate data from a modified mass-action model with time-varying contact rate giving the overall rate of infection $\frac{1.7}{10{,}000}(1 + \cos(t))S(t)I(t)$ where $\gamma = 1$ with

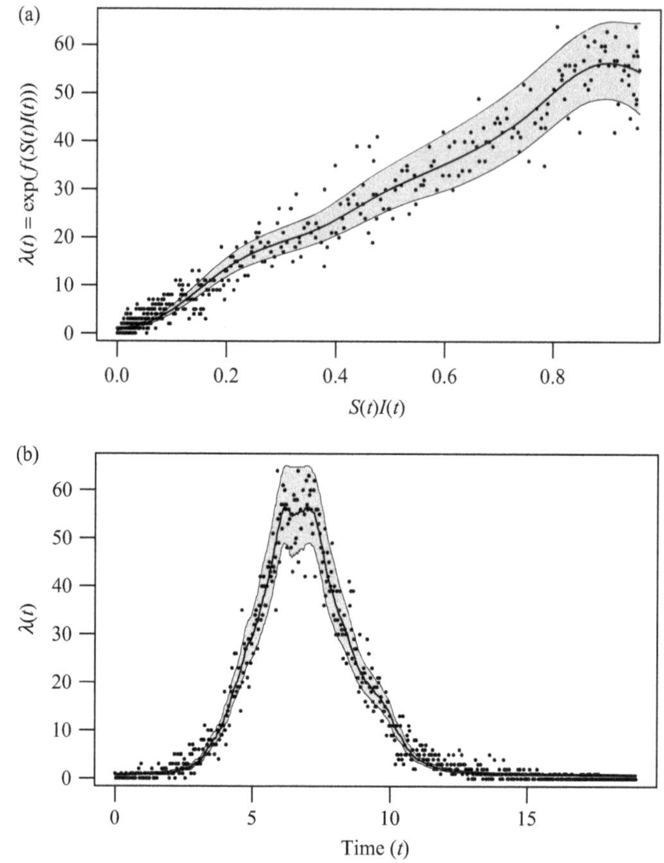

Figure 9.7 *(a) Here, the mass-action data are modelled using* $\lambda(t) = \exp\{f(S(t)* I(t))\}$*, with f modelled using a GP. The ground truth is that the response is linear, but the very flexible GP model manages to capture the simple linear behaviour well. The posterior mean (black line) and 95% credible intervals (shaded area) of the overall force of infection* $\lambda(\cdot)$ *are shown along with the data. (b) A temporal view of the corresponding posterior distribution of* $\lambda(t)$ *under this model*

the epidemic started by one infective among a population of 10,000 susceptibles. The number of individuals who were ever infective was $n = 6,111$. We discretise the interval $[0, 27.85]$ to 931 bins each of them of them having width 0.03. Figure 9.8 shows the observed number of cases per bin, whilst Figure 9.9 shows the estimated force of infection $\lambda(t)$ when it is assumed to depend on time only. Again, a very good much between the fitted curve and the observed data are revealed.

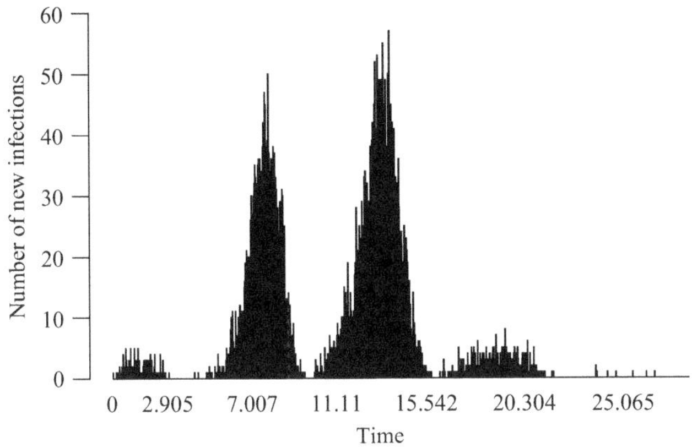

Figure 9.8 *Observed number of new infections. Data were generated from a seasonal mass-action SIR model with an overall force of infection* $\beta(1 + \cos(t))S(t)I(t)$, *where* $\beta = 0.00017$

9.4.3 Application to the Abakaliki Smallpox data

We now consider a classic Smallpox dataset taken from Reference 58 (p. 125). The data were originally reported in a World Health Organisation report and consist of a time series of 30 case detection times. The data have been analysed by numerous authors [59–61] and the references therein] assuming a homogeneously mixing population of 120 individuals. On the other hand, Eichner and Dietz [62] took into account the populations' mixing structure as well as other important factors and fitted a more elaborate epidemic model.

First, we assume that the detection times correspond to removal times following, for example, Reference 61. Furthermore, we assume a constant infectious period of 11 days [63] and that allows to count the number of infected and susceptible individuals per day. The data are modelled as log Gaussian Cox process and we consider three different models for the overall force of infection $\lambda(t)$:

- M_1: $\lambda(t) = \exp(f(t))$
- M_2: $\lambda(t) = \beta(t)S(t)I(t) = \exp(f(t))S(t)I(t)$
- M_3: $\lambda(t) = \exp(f(S(t)I(t)))$

where $f(\cdot)$ is modelled a GP. In other words, the incidence rate of new infections is assume to be a function of time only under model M_1 and a function of the product of $S(t)I(t)$ under M_3. Model M_2 retains the mass-action assumption but allows the person to person infection rate to be non-constant but instead time dependent.

Figure 9.10 shows our estimated force of infection and reveals some oscillations over time. This is in agreement with the work of Becker and Yip [12] who analysed the Abakaliki data by also assuming known infection times and latent periods and used a kernel smoothing method to estimate the infection rate as a function of time. They also concluded that the infection rate displays some oscillation over time.

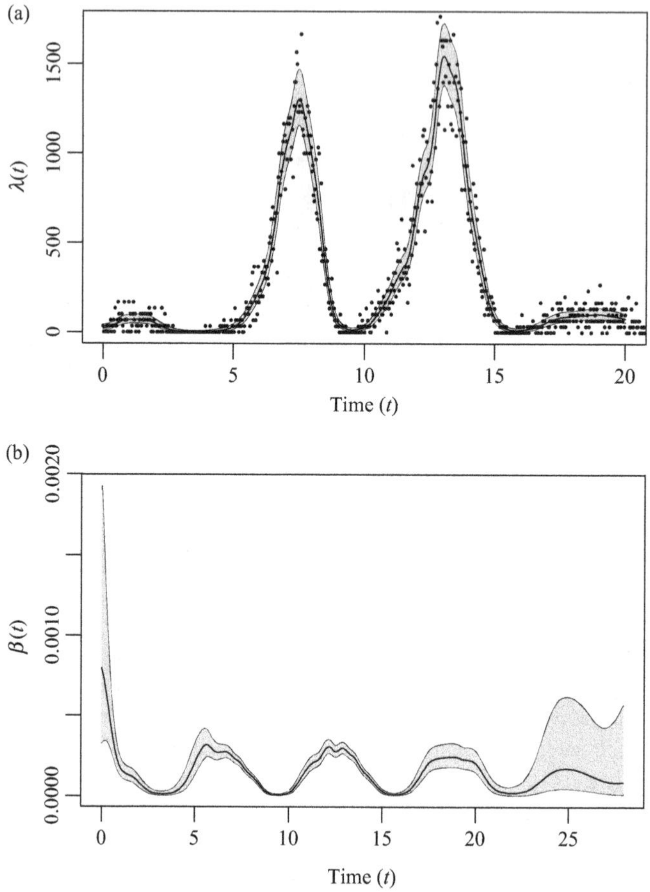

Figure 9.9 *(a) The estimated overall force of infection $\lambda(t)$ for the simulated seasonal data when modelled as a log Gaussian Cox process, $\lambda(t) = \exp(f(t))$, with $f(t)$ modelled as a GP. The black line represents the posterior mean, the shaded area represents the 95% credible interval, and the dots represent the observed (new) infections per bin. (b) The (exponentiated) GP posterior of the person-to-person infection rate $\beta(t)$. The model for the force-of-infection is $\lambda(t) = \beta(t)S(t)I(t)$, where $\beta(t) = \exp(f(t))$, and $f(t)$ is modelled with a GP*

Figure 9.11 (a) shows that the person to person does not appear to be constant over time. In particular, it appears to be pretty low until day 40 and remains fairly constant from day 60 until the end of the epidemic. Since the product $S(t)I(t)$ can be calculated from the data, we also plot the corresponding force of infection $\lambda(t)$. Figure 9.11 (b) also shows some oscillations with a clear pick around day 60 where there is a cluster of infections around that day.

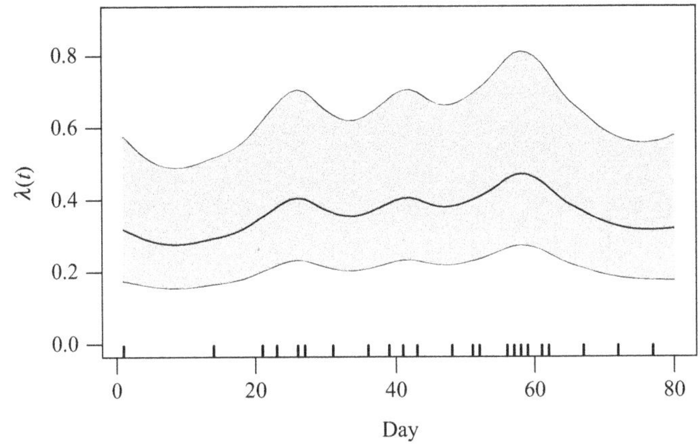

Figure 9.10 *The estimated overall force of infection $\lambda(t)$ for the Abakaliki data when modelled as a log Gaussian Cox process, $\lambda(t) = \exp(f(t))$, with $f(t)$ modelled as a GP. The black line represents the posterior mean, the shaded area represents the 95% credible interval, and the vertical lines represent the infection times*

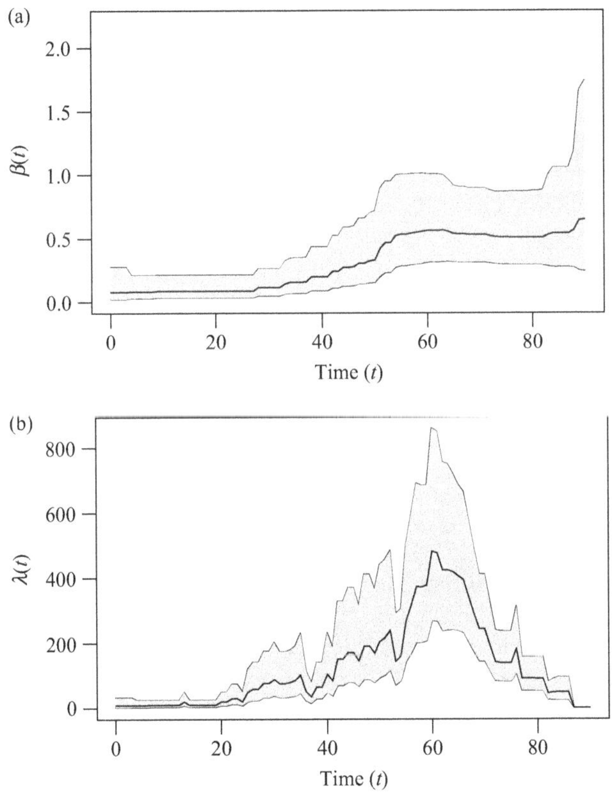

Figure 9.11 *(a) The (exponentiated) GP posterior of the person-to-person infection rate $\beta(t)$ for the Abakaliki data when the overall force-of-infection is $\lambda(t) = \beta(t)S(t)I(t)$, where $\beta(t) = \exp(f(t))$, and $f(t)$ is modelled with a GP. The black line represents the posterior mean, the dashed lines represent 95% credible intervals. (b) The graph at the bottom shows the corresponding overall rate $\lambda(t)$*

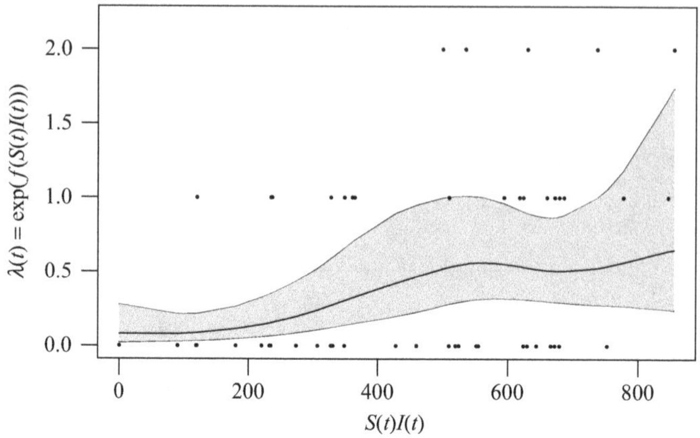

Figure 9.12 Here, the Abakaliki data are modelled as log Gaussian Cox process using $\lambda(t) = \exp\{f(S(t)I(t))\}$, with f modelled using a GP. The posterior mean (black line) and 95% credible intervals (shaded area) of the overall force of infection $\dot{\lambda}()$ are shown along with the observed data

The flexibility of our framework is highlighted when the data are modelled using a log Gaussian Cox process with using $\lambda(t) = \exp\{f(S(t)I(t))\}$. The vast majority of attempts made in the literature to analyse this data assumed a homogeneously mixing mass-action (parametric) model. Figure 9.12 reveals that the assumption of the overall force of infection to increase linearly with the product of $S(t)I(t)$ is questionable.

It is very natural to ask which of the three models best describes the data. Within the proposed framework we are able to compute the marginal likelihood of the data. The (approximate) log marginal likelihoods were -64.52, -58.73, and -63.65 for models M_1, M_2, and M_3, respectively, and indicate that the model that is mostly supported by the data is model M_2.

9.5 Conclusions

We have demonstrated that Bayesian non-parametric inference for epidemic models can be achieved using GP methods. In particular, we have illustrated that the proposed Variational Bayesian framework allows us to fit non-parametric models to large populations. Our work appears worthy of further exploration. An obvious extension to our work would be to develop a framework in which we will assume that the infection times are unknown and would have to be estimated from the observed removal times. The methods that we have developed can be also very naturally extended to other settings, such as epidemic models with non-exponential infection periods and with latent periods, and those with more complex population mixing structures (e.g. households, workplaces).

Acknowledgements

JH was supported by an MRC fellowship and TK by an EPSRC grant (EP/J013528/1).

References

[1] Streftaris G, Gibson G. Bayesian analysis of experimental epidemics of foot-and-mouth disease. *Proc R Soc B Biol Sci* 2004;271(1544):1111.

[2] Chi-Ster I, Ferguson N. Transmission parameters of the 2001 foot and mouth epidemic in great Britain. *PLoS One* 2007;2(6):e502.

[3] Kypraios T. Efficient Bayesian inference for partially observed stochastic epidemics and a new class of semi-parametric time series models. (Ph.D. thesis). Lancaster University; 2007.

[4] McBryde E, Gibson G, Pettitt A, Zhang Y, Zhao B, McElwain D. Bayesian modelling of an epidemic of severe acute respiratory syndrome. *Bull Math Biol* 2006;68(4):889–917.

[5] Forrester M, Pettitt A, Gibson G. Bayesian inference of hospital-acquired infectious diseases and control measures given imperfect surveillance data. *Biostatistics* 2007;8(2):383.

[6] Kypraios T, O'Neill PD, Huang SS, Rifas-Shiman SL, Cooper BS. Assessing the role of undetected colonization and isolation precautions in reducing methicillin-resistant Staphylococcus aureus transmission in intensive care units. *BMC Infect Dis* 2010;10(1):29.

[7] Cauchemez S, Carrat F, Viboud C, Valleron A, Boelle P. A Bayesian MCMC approach to study transmission of influenza: application to household longitudinal data. *Stat Med* 2004;23(22):3469–87.

[8] Cauchemez S, Donnelly C, Reed C, et al. Household transmission of 2009 pandemic influenza a (H1N1) virus in the United States. *N Engl J Med*;361(27):2619–27.

[9] Jewell CP, Kypraios T, Christley RM, Roberts GO. A novel approach to real-time risk prediction for emerging infectious diseases: a case study in avian influenza H5N1. *Prev Vet Med* 2009;91(1):19–28.

[10] Merler S, Ajelli M, Fumanelli L, et al. Spatiotemporal spread of the 2014 outbreak of Ebola virus disease in Liberia and the effectiveness of non-pharmaceutical interventions: a computational modelling analysis. *Lancet Infect Dis* 2015;15(2):204–11.

[11] Hollingsworth T. Controlling infectious disease outbreaks: lessons from mathematical modelling. *J Public Health Policy* 2009;30(3):328–41.

[12] Becker N, Yip P. Analysis of variations in an infection rate. *Aust N Z J Stat* 1989;31(1):42–52.

[13] Huggins RM, Yip PSF, Lau EHY. A note on the estimation of the initial number of susceptible individuals in the general epidemic model. *Stat Prob Lett* 2004;67(4):321–30.

[14] Lau E, Yip P. Estimating the basic reproductive number in the general epidemic model with an unknown initial number of susceptible individuals. *Scand J Stat* 2008;35(4):650–63.
[15] Kenah E. Nonparametric survival analysis of epidemic data. *J R Stat Soc Series B Methodol* 2013;75(2):277–303.
[16] Xu X, Kypraios T, O'Neill PD. Bayesian nonparametric inference for stochastic epidemic models using Gaussian processes. *Biostatistics*; 2016 [to appear], doi: 10.1093/biostatistics/kxw011.
[17] Knock E, Kypraios T. Bayesian non-parametric inference for infectious disease data; 2016. Available from http://arxiv.org/abs/1411.2624.
[18] O'Hagan A, Kingman J. Curve fitting and optimal design for prediction. *J R Stat Soc Ser B Methodol* 1978;40(1):1–42.
[19] Hida T. *Brownian motion*. US, Springer; 1980.
[20] Grewal MS. *Kalman filtering*. Berlin, Springer; 2011.
[21] Kalman RE. A new approach to linear filtering and prediction problems. *J Basic Eng* 1960;82(1):35–45.
[22] Särkkä S. *Bayesian filtering and smoothing*, vol. 3. Cambridge, Cambridge University Press; 2013.
[23] Williams CK, Barber D. Bayesian classification with Gaussian processes. *IEE Trans Pattern Anal Mach Intell*; 1998;20(12):1342–51.
[24] Jylänki P, Vanhatalo J, Vehtari A. Robust Gaussian process regression with a student-t likelihood. *J Mach Learn Res* 2011;12:3227–57.
[25] Rasmussen CE, Williams CK. *Gaussian processes for machine learning*. Cambridge, Massachusetts, MIT Press; 2006.
[26] Lloyd JR, Duvenaud D, Grosse R, Tenenbaum JB, Ghahramani Z. *Automatic construction and natural-language description of nonparametric regression models*; 2014. arXiv preprint arXiv:1402.4304.
[27] Alvarez MA, Luengo D, Lawrence, ND. Latent force models. In: *International conference on artificial intelligence and statistics*. Clearwater Beach, Florida; 2009. p. 9–16.
[28] Blei DM, Kucukelbir A, McAuliffe JD. *Variational inference: a review for statisticians*; 2016. arXiv preprint arXiv:1601.00670.
[29] Beal MJ. *Variational algorithms for approximate Bayesian inference*. London, University of London; 2003.
[30] Bishop CM. *Pattern recognition and machine learning*. Springer, New York; 2006. p. 462–73.
[31] Wainwright MJ, Jordan MI. Graphical models, exponential families, and variational inference. *Found Trends Mach Learn* 2008;1(1–2): 1–305.
[32] Hensman J, Rattray M, Lawrence ND. Fast variational inference in the conjugate exponential family. In: *Advances in neural information processing systems*. Lake Tahoe, Harrahs and Harveys; 2012. p. 2888–96.
[33] Honkela A, Tornio M, Raiko T, Karhunen J. Natural conjugate gradient in variational inference. In: *Neural information processing*. Springer; 2007. p. 305–14.

[34] Hoffman MD, Blei DM, Wang C, Paisley J. Stochastic variational inference. *J Mach Learn Res* 2013;14(1):1303–47.

[35] Gershman S, Hoffman M, Blei D. *Nonparametric variational inference*; 2012. arXiv preprint arXiv:1206.4665.

[36] Rezende DJ, Mohamed S. Variational inference with normalizing flows; 2015. arXiv preprint arXiv:1505.05770.

[37] Kingma DP, Welling M. Auto-encoding variational Bayes; 2013. arXiv preprint arXiv:1312.6114.

[38] Rezende DJ, Mohamed S, Wierstra D. Stochastic backpropagation and approximate inference in deep generative models; 2014. arXiv preprint arXiv:1401.4082.

[39] Kucukelbir A, Ranganath R, Gelman A, Blei D. Automatic variational inference in stan. In: *Advances in neural information processing systems*. Montreal, Canada; 2015. p. 568–76.

[40] Opper M, Archambeau C. The variational Gaussian approximation revisited. *Neural Comput* 2009;21(3):786–92.

[41] Nguyen TV, Bonilla EV. Automated variational inference for Gaussian process models. In: *Advances in neural information processing systems*. Montreal, Canada; 2014. p. 1404–12.

[42] Hensman J, Zwießele M, Lawrence ND. Tilted variational Bayes. In: AISTATS. Iceland; 2014. p. 356–64.

[43] Cox DR. Some statistical methods connected with series of events. *J R Stat Soc Ser B* 1955;17:129–57 [discussion: 157–64].

[44] Møller J, Syversveen AR, Waagepetersen RP. Log Gaussian Cox processes. *Scand J Statist* 1998;25(3):451–482.

[45] Taylor BM, Diggle PJ. Inla or MCMC? A tutorial and comparative evaluation for spatial prediction in log-Gaussian Cox processes. *J Stat Comput Simul* 2014;84(10):2266–84.

[46] Filippone M, Zhong M, Girolami M. A comparative evaluation of stochastic-based inference methods for Gaussian process models. *Mach Learn* 2013;93(1):93–114.

[47] Murray I, Adams RP. Slice sampling covariance hyperparameters of latent gaussian models. In: *Advances in neural information processing systems*. Canada; 2010. p. 1732–40.

[48] Seeger M, Williams C, Lawrence N. Fast forward selection to speed up sparse Gaussian process regression. In: *Artificial intelligence and statistics 9, number EPFL-CONF-161318*. Florida; 2003.

[49] Banerjee S, Carlin BP, Gelfand AE . *Hierarchical modeling and analysis for spatial data*. CRC Press; 2014.

[50] Snelson E, Ghahramani Z. Sparse Gaussian processes using pseudo-inputs. In: *Advances in neural information processing systems*. Vancouver, Canada; 2005. p. 1257–64.

[51] Quinonero-Candela J, Rasmussen CE. A unifying view of sparse approximate Gaussian process regression. *J Mach Learn Res* 2005;6: 1939–59.

[52] Snelson E, Ghahramani Z. Variable noise and dimensionality reduction for sparse Gaussian processes; 2012. arXiv preprint arXiv:1206.6873.

[53] Titsias MK. Variational learning of inducing variables in sparse Gaussian processes. In: International conference on artificial intelligence and statistics. Washington, USA; 2009. p. 567–74.

[54] Hensman J, Fusi N, Lawrence ND. Gaussian processes for big data. In: Conference on uncertainty in artificial intelligence. Bellvue, Washington, USA; 2013. p. 282–90. auai.org.

[55] Hensman, J, Matthews, AGdG, Ghahramani Z. Scalable variational Gaussian process classification. In: *Proceedings of the eighteenth international conference on artificial intelligence and statistics*. California, USA; 2015b.

[56] Matthews AGdG, Hensman J, Turner RE, Ghahramani Z. On sparse variational methods and the Kullback-Leibler divergence between stochastic processes; 2015. arXiv preprint arXiv:1504.07027.

[57] Hensman J, Matthews AGdG, Filippone M, Ghahramani Z. MCMC for variationally sparse Gaussian processes. In: NIPS. Montreal, Canada; 2015a.

[58] Bailey NT. *The mathematical theory of infectious diseases and its applications*. London: Charles Griffin & Company Ltd; 1975.

[59] Becker N. *Analysis of infectious disease data*. vol. 33. Chapman & Hall/CRC; 1989.

[60] Boys RJ, Giles PR. Bayesian inference for stochastic epidemic models with time-inhomogeneous removal rates. *J Math Biol* 2007;55(2):223–47.

[61] O'Neill PD, Roberts GO. Bayesian inference for partially observed stochastic epidemics. *J R Stat Soc Ser A* 1999;162:121–9.

[62] Eichner M, Dietz K. Transmission potential of smallpox: estimates based on detailed data from an outbreak. *Am J Epidemiol* 2003;158(2):110–17.

[63] Mack TM. Smallpox in Europe, 1950–1971. *J Infect Dis* 1972;125(2):161–9.

Chapter 10
Predicting antibiotic resistance from genomic data

Yang Yang, Katherine E. Niehaus and David A. Clifton

Cutting-edge machine learning tools have shown significant promise for infectious disease control using the bacterial genome. In this chapter, an overview of key problems of clinical microbiology surrounding infectious disease management, antibiotic resistance, and clinical susceptibility test to antimicrobial drugs, will be provided, followed by an introduction of genomic data used in genotypic prediction of the phenotype for antimicrobial resistance. This chapter will then provide machine learning models for bacterial resistance prediction using genome, as well as promising tools for exploring the bacterial genomic pattern.

10.1 Antibiotic resistance

While there are many challenges in clinical infectious disease management [1], e.g., identifying the species of an isolates, testing its properties, such as resistance to antibiotics and virulence, and monitoring the emergence and spread of bacterial pathogens, here we will focus our discussion upon antibiotic resistance. The antimicrobial resistance is the resistance of a microorganism to an antimicrobial drug, such as antibiotics, that was originally effective for treatment of infections caused by it. Resistant microorganisms are able to withstand attack by antibiotic, so that standard treatments become ineffective and infections persist, increasing the risk of spread to others.

The evolution of resistant strains is a nature phenomenon that occurs when microorganisms replicate themselves erroneously or when resistant traits are exchanged between them. The use and misuse of antimicrobial drugs accelerates the emergence of drug-resistant strains. Poor infection control practices, inadequate sanitary conditions, and inappropriate food-handling encourage the further spread of antimicrobial resistance. Without effective anti-infective treatment, many standard medical treatments will fail or turn into vary high risk procedures. Infections caused by resistant microorganisms often fail to respond to the standard treatment, resulting in prolonged illness, higher health care expenditures, and a greater risk of death and spreading resistant microorganisms to others.

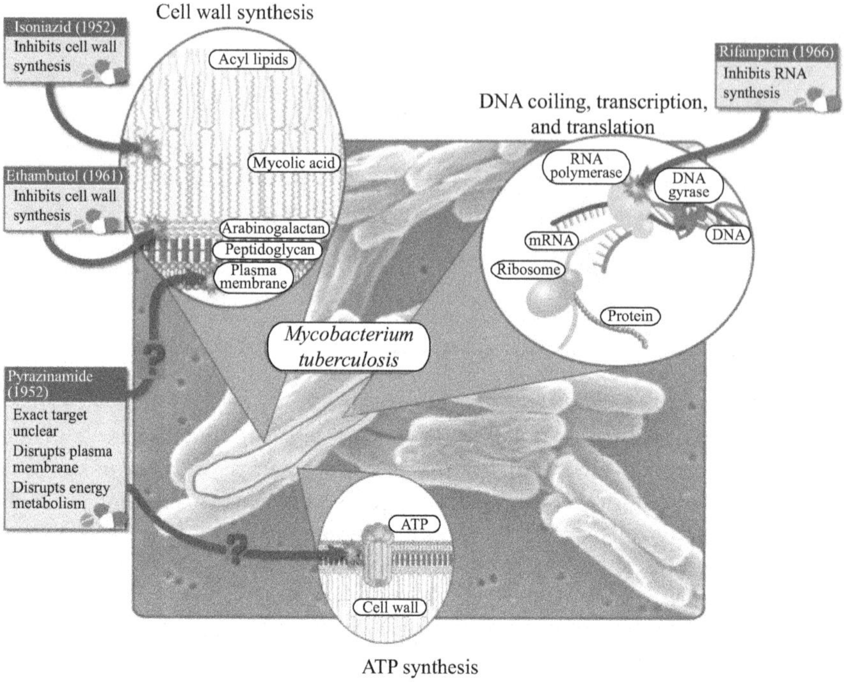

Figure 10.1 First-line TB drugs (Credits: National Institute of Allergies and Infectious Diseases)

This chapter will use the bacterium *Mycobacterium tuberculosis* (MTB) as an example throughout. This is due to the relatively straightforward nature of the MTB genome and the pressing public health concerns worldwide associated with MTB drug resistance. Tuberculosis (TB), caused by the MTB bacterium, infects over one-third of the human population and claims over one million lives each year [1]. While TB caused by a drug-susceptible bacterium is completely curable through antibiotics, drug resistance is increasing worldwide; there was nearly a doubling of diagnosed multi-drug resistant (MDR)-TB cases from 2011 to 2012 [2]. As warned in a 2014 WHO report, "drug-resistant TB threatens global TB control and is a major public health concern in several countries" [3].

Figure 10.1 shows how the most widely used antibiotics for TB, including isoniazid (INH), rifampicin (RIF), ethambutol (EMB), and Pyrazinamide (PZA). These drugs are used in first-line treatment for TB. MDR-TB is defined as being resistant to the most effective first-line antibiotics, which are INH and RIF. MDR now accounts for about 3.6% of all new TB cases and 20.2% of all previously treated cases worldwide. About 10% of these MDR cases are extensively drug-resistant, which is defined as also resistant to two different classes of second-line drugs [3]. Recently, there have been reports in India and Iran of totally drug-resistant MTB, in which the pathogens were not susceptible to *any* of the existing first- or second-line drugs, leaving only experimental treatment options [4].

10.2 Susceptibility test to antibiotics

Determining the drug susceptibility profile, or antibiogram, of a new bacterial isolate is of paramount importance in order to prescribe appropriate drugs. Otherwise, the prescribed drugs will not cure the patient, the patient may develop further resistance, and the patient will go on spreading the (possibly now MDR) infection to others. Current methods for testing susceptibility include phenotypic and genotypic methods.

A schematic representation of the current workflow for processing samples for bacterial pathogens is presented in Figure 10.2, showing high complexity and a typical timescale of a few weeks to a few months. In the case of MTB, phenotypic methods involve growing the MTB isolate in media impregnated with antibiotics. The gold-standard phenotypic method is the "proportion method" on sloped Löwenstein–Jensen (LJ) solid media [5]. This method, performed in specialised reference labs, compares bacterial growth with and without the presence of an antibacterial drug. However, MTB's slow growth-rate means that the LJ proportion method can require up to 2 months to obtain results. The concentration of the drug in the media and the critical proportion of colonies that grow in the antibiotic-impregnated media in order to call the bacteria "resistant" are established based upon clinically defined cut-offs. This produces binary resistant or susceptible labels.

Bacterial drug resistance arises due to mutations in the bacterial genome that enable it to avoid damage caused by the antibiotic. A single nucleotide polymorphism (SNP) is a single-base change in the DNA. Several such resistance-conferring mechanisms are known, and genotypic line-probe assays have been developed to identify the presence of known SNPs in a bacterial sample The "MTBDR*plus*" is a line-probe assay created by Hain (Germany), which tests for the primary mutations associated with resistance to INH and RIF. The Cepheid (USA) "Xpert" system is able to detect resistance to RIF within 2 h. However, these methods only are available for a subset of antibiotics, require further testing to confirm their results, and only probe for the most common resistance-conferring mutations. A much more flexible approach lies in the incorporation of whole genome sequencing (WGS) into the clinical diagnostic pathway [1], which offers the opportunity to identify the presence of any known mutation in a bacterial sequence with a single assay. WGS differs from the genotypic methods presented above in that it reveals all of the SNPs in a given sample using a single test. Currently available sequencing methods require only about 2 days for complete processing (after growing the sample in culture for 7–10 days), with this time requirement only continuing to decrease [6].

However, some resistant bacterial isolates lack an established resistance-conferring mutation, suggesting that unknown mechanisms of resistance remain. Between 10% and 20% of INH-resistant isolates, for instance, lack a mutation in a known resistance gene [7]. Furthermore, other isolates are phenotypically susceptible despite having an established mutation. It is possible that some of this discrepancy may be explained by epistatic interactions (i.e., two or more SNPs may be required to gain drug resistance) or because some of the "established" mutations do not actually cause resistance. These problems motivate further analysis and online predictive systems to provide both improved predictive power for drug resistance and to identify new mechanisms of resistance.

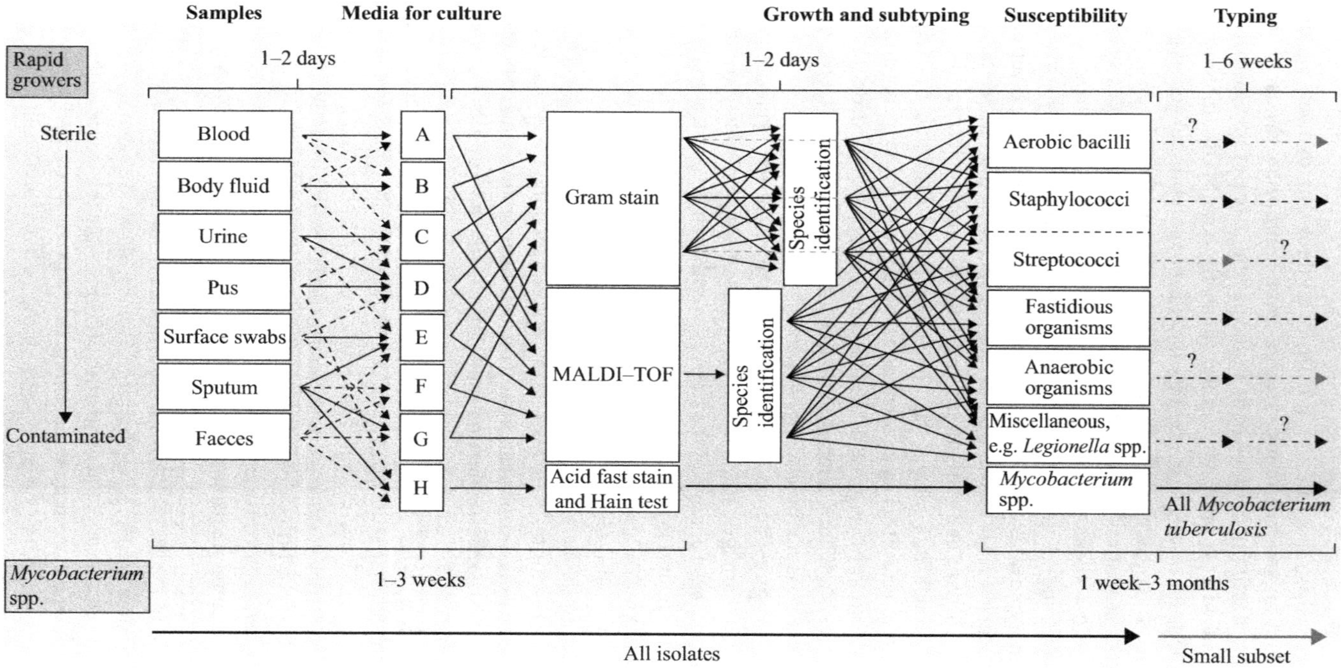

Figure 10.2 Current processing of bacterial pathogens [1]

10.3 Genomic data associated with antibiotic resistance

10.3.1 Overview

Bacterial genetic variation is encoded in two forms: the chromosomal backbone and extrachromosomal plasmids. Both of these are composed of DNA, which consists of long series of nucleotide base pairs: adenine (A), thymine (T), cytosine (C), and guanine (G). Plasmids are small circular rings of DNA that are able to replicate independently from a cell's chromosomal DNA. They often carry drug-resistant and other fitness-enhancing genes. In the process of transcription, portions of DNA are converted into single-stranded RNA. Triplets of RNA bases (codons) are then translated into one of the 20 amino acids, which are building blocks of proteins. The portions of the genome that encode proteins or other functional products are called genes. An SNP is a single-base change in the DNA. SNPs can result in proteins with altered functionality, or, if within a regulatory region, changes in protein production. Our interest here is in relating patterns of SNPs to antibacterial drug resistance.

10.3.2 DNA sequencing

There are several steps to obtain SNP data from a clinical sample. First the DNA must be isolated, next sequenced, then aligned or assembled, and at this point finally SNP is called.

1. *Isolation*
After the collection of human blood or sputum samples, the process for obtaining genetic sequence data begins by culturing the bacteria found in the sample. Bacterial colonies are grown up (often 24 h for most bacteria; about 7 days for MTB), after which DNA is extracted, for instance by using the QuickGene DNA Tissue Kit S (Fujifilm, Japan) or the Nextera DNA sample prep kit [8,9]. This involves the addition of a series of enzymes, together with overnight incubation. The DNA is then randomly fragmented, and adapter sequences are ligated to the fragment ends. This creates multiplexed paired-end DNA libraries, with, for example, an average size of about 200 base pairs [8].

2. *Sequencing*
There are many different sequencing technologies now available. One of the most commonly employed methods is the Illumina HiSeq, which works through sequence-by-synthesis chemistry. DNA is amplified by using solid-phase amplification, which is a clonally amplified template method. DNA binds to random points on the surface of a flow cell (the solid phase), which is covered with a lawn of bound primers. The strands of DNA bind to the primers, a complement DNA strand is formed, and the template strand is washed away. This allows bridge amplification to occur, which is when the single, bound DNA strands flip over to bind to nearby primers. This allows the growth of double-stranded "bridges," which are then denatured to produce a dense cluster of single DNA strands. Amplification produces up to 200 million clusters of DNA strands, each cluster of which may contain thousands of individual strands; the sequence of DNA in each cluster is identical [10,11].

Sequencing then commences with four-colour cyclic reversible termination. Here, labelled reversible terminator nucleotides (deoxynucleoside triphosphate (dNTP)), primers, and DNA polymerase are added to the flow cell. The dNTPs bind to corresponding strands and prevent further lengthening. A laser is used to excite the clusters, which emit fluorescence. Four cameras then capture the emitted colour, which allows the first base in each cluster's sequence to be identified. The dNTP is then cleaved, which allows the cycle to be repeated. The sequence is determined based upon the signal intensity of the emitted colour [10,11]. This process therefore produces thousands of short (e.g., 100–300 base pair), unaligned, overlapping, contiguous "reads" of the DNA sequence, from different locations across the genome.

Sequencing through next-generation platforms promises to be faster and cheaper than current methods. Such platforms are now being commercialised by Pacific Biosciences, Ion Torrent, and Oxford Nanopore, among others [6]. These newer technologies often are able to obtain much longer read lengths than standard methods, which is particularly valuable for untangling the genomic structure for bacteria.

3. *Alignment*

Given these thousands of short reads of the DNA sequence from whole-genome sequencing, they must be aligned or assembled into their coherent whole. The sequence reads can be mapped to bacterial chromosome reference sequences using a tool such as Stampy or Maq. Stampy is a sensitive and fast computational tool that maps short DNA reads to a reference using a hybrid mapping algorithm and a statistical model developed at the Wellcome Trust, Oxford [12]. Extrachromosomal DNA such as plasmids are not included in the reference sequences, so resistance genes contained here will not be assembled. Because chromosomal DNA may only represent 20% of the genome for some bacteria, it is therefore necessary to perform de novo assembly for these bacteria in order to obtain information regarding resistance loci both within plasmids and chromosomal DNA. Tools such as Velvet or Newbler can be used for de novo assembly. Velvet removes errors from short read sequences, identifies repeated regions, and uses graphical models to produce assembled DNA contigs [13].

4. *Calling SNP*

A SNP would be called if any individual is heterozygous or homozygous for a non-reference allele. In the case of MTB, the primary sources of genetic variation include point mutations and indels; extra chromosomal plasmids are not involved. Once aligned to the reference, base calls must be made (for instance, using SAMtools). This is the process of determining the most likely base at each position, given all of the reads that mapped to that position. As a form of quality filtering, bases may be recorded as a "nucleotide null call" (i.e., too much uncertainty to call) if the absolute read depth is too low (e.g., fewer than 10 reads at a given location), if the read at a given position is too mixed (e.g., half of the reads are for guanine, and half are for adenine), or if the mapping quality is not high enough. Analysis on genomic data relies crucially on the accurate calling of SNPs. However, SNP calling for low- or moderate-coverage data entails uncertainty. The uncertainty in SNP calling can be improved and quantified by statistical methods, e.g., calculation of quality scores, recalibration of per-base quality scores, likelihood ratio test or Bayesian procedures and lineage disequilibrium–based methods [14].

10.3.3 Pre-processing

Having assembled a bacterial genome, the next question involves how to capture the relevant information in the form of features. Preparation of the genome feature matrix is a critical pre-processing step for antibiotic resistance prediction.

The pre-processing is commonly consisted three elements: (1) null calls processing; (2) feature translation; and (3) feature reduction.

1. *Null calls processing*
A great number of null calls in the obtained SNPs need to be dealt with properly. According to the quality filtering criteria, the SNPs, whose bases are called "null" since the absolute read depth is too low or mapping quality is not high enough, need to be removed or retested. Other null calls due to the highly mixed reads at a given position can be resulted from more than one population of pathogen in one host and the different mutations in these populations. Such SNPs can be properly interpreted in feature matrix according to the desired feature types in the next step.

2. *Feature translation*
Two simple ways to convert the DNA sequencing data into features are based on binary variable and reading rate. The most common way to interpret the DNA sequencing data is to use binary variables indicating the presence (==1) or absence (=0) of the corresponding SNP in the isolate. In this case, with respect to an SNP with a null call at a given position caused by mixed reads, the base with the maximum read at this position is called for the SNP. If all three bases are the same with the reference of a codon, it is considered to be an SNP; otherwise, it is not an SNP.

Another way to translate the sequencing data is to compute reading rate for one SNP. The reading rate R is defined as

$$R = 1 - r(\mathrm{Ref}_1)r(\mathrm{Ref}_2)r(\mathrm{Ref}_3) \tag{10.1}$$

where Ref_i denotes the read of the reference base over the read of all bases at the ith base site of an SNP. Such rate feature is particularly reasonable for the case when the read at a given position is too mixed.

Figure 10.3 illustrates these two ways of feature matrix construction for the sequencing data. The top table shows an example of data source, where Var stands for the obtained base combination for one SNP. The columns of $\{\mathrm{A}i, \mathrm{C}i, \mathrm{G}i, \mathrm{T}i\}$, $i \in [1, 2, 3]$ provide the reads of four bases at three sites of each SNP. The middle table shows how to represent the SNP with or without the null call in binary case. The bottom table shows how to obtain the reading rate feature.

3. *Feature reduction*
All SNPs found on all genes can be extremely huge, which will result in extremely sparse feature matrix. In the preliminary study, it is encouraged to narrow down to those genes highly suspected to be involved in resistance mechanisms. Taken MTB as

SNP	Ref	Var	A1	C1	G1	T1	A2	C2	G2	T2	A3	C3	G3	T3
1	GAC	AAC	75	0	0	0	76	0	0	0	0	86	0	0
2	CGA	NNA	0	75	25	0	0	20	80	0	40	0	0	0

	SNP1			SNP2		
Ref	G	A	C	C	G	A
Base with max read	A1 (75)	A2 (76)	C3 (86)	C1 (75)	G2 (80)	A3 (40)
Binary feature	1			0		

	SNP1			SNP2		
Ref	G	A	C	C	G	A
Read rate of Ref base	G1 (0/75)	A2 (76/76)	C3 (86/86)	C1 (75/(75+25))	G2 (80/(20+80))	A3 (40/40)
Rate feature	1-G1*A2*C3=1			1-C1*G2*A3=0.4		

Figure 10.3 Feature translation for DNA sequencing data

Table 10.1 A selection of genes suspected to be involved in resistance mechanisms. Starred genes contain specific loci previously documented in the literature as being associated with drug resistance. Chart compiled primarily from References 15, 16

Gene	**Function**	**Relevant drug**
*ahpC**	Oxidative stress	INH
*eis**	Cell surface involvement	Aminoglycosides
*embB**	Cell wall biosynthesis	EMB
*gyrA**	Enzyme for DNA coiling	Fluoroquinolones
inhA	Fatty acid biosynthesis	INH
iniA	Likely transmembrane protein	EMB, INH
*pncA**	Intermediary metabolism	PZA
rmlD	Sugar biosynthesis	EMB
*rpoB**	Transcriptional enzyme	RIF
tlyA	Virulence; methylation	Aminoglycosides

an example, 23 genes are found to be related to antibiotic resistance. All SNPs found within 23 genes suspected to be involved in resistance mechanisms (a representative selection of which are listed in Table 10.1 and their 100 base-pair upstream regions were identified. Upstream regions were included so as to capture SNPs that may potentially be involved in gene regulation. The resulting set of 300 SNPs constituted the feature set for subsequent analysis. The average number of SNPs per isolate was 5.0, ranging between 0 and 23.

Given different purposes, the features can also be limited to: (i) polymorphisms found on genes already thought to be involved in resistance for a given drug; (ii) polymorphisms that were already suspected to confer drug resistance; and (iii) polymorphisms that were not previously suspected to confer drug resistance. Such reduction for features is not compulsive, yet highly recommended, which will benefit efficient validation of new biomarkers by taking advantage of prior knowledge of microbiology.

10.3.4 Direct association

Direct association (DA) method is a simple algorithm to use prior clinical knowledge and essentially represents the best predictive performance that could be obtained based upon those clinical associations already identified in the literature. For an instance, the list of established Hain mutations and a database of MTB mutations is provided in References 15, 16, we assembled a list of mutations that have been previously associated with resistance in clinical and experimental studies. The loci contained in this list of "established" mutations correspond to locations within the starred genes in Table 10.1. A simple "OR" rule is applied: if any of the established mutations was present for a given isolate, the isolate was classified as being resistant to that drug.

10.4 Supervised models

In this section, we assessed several different supervised classification algorithms for the prediction of isolates as being susceptible or resistant to each of the four first-line drugs. This comparison allowed us to understand how well the assumptions of each (e.g., linear combinations of features; independent features) were substantiated in the data. We examined four machine learning models: logistic regression, support vector machine (SVM), random forest (RF), and Bayesian product of marginals. These supervised models are also termed classifiers in this chapter.

We will consider a subset of N isolates to represent a training set of examples $\mathbf{x}_1 \ldots \mathbf{x}_N$ with labels $\ell_1 \ldots \ell_N, \ell \in \{0, 1\}$, with 1 indicating drug resistance for a given drug and 0 indicating susceptibility. Each example $\mathbf{x}_i$ is composed of a vector of D binary features indicating the presence ($x_{ij} = 1$) or absence ($x_{ij} = 0$) of a given SNP.

10.4.1 Logistic regression

Logistic regression (LR) is a linear classification method that optimises a set of weights $\mathbf{w}$ assigned to each input feature to provide the best classification performance using a training dataset. LR can be formulated by considering the sigmoidal hypothesis function:

$$P(\ell_n = 1|\mathbf{x}_n, \mathbf{w}) = h(\mathbf{x}_n) = \frac{1}{1 + \mathrm{e}^{-\mathbf{w}^T \mathbf{x}_n}} \tag{10.2}$$

which is the probability that the given example is of class 1. An example is assigned to class 1 based upon whether the hypothesis function $h(\mathbf{x}_n)$ is greater than or less than a set threshold T. We define a cost function that includes a penalty when the hypothesis is incorrect:

$$f(\mathbf{w}) = -\frac{1}{N}\sum_{n=1}^{N}\left[\ell_n \log(h(\mathbf{x}_n)) + (1-\ell_n)\log(1-h(\mathbf{x}_n))\right] \tag{10.3}$$

Adding an L^2 regularisation term to discourage the weights from overfitting the data by penalising large values in $\mathbf{w}$, the final equation to be minimised is:

$$f(\mathbf{w})_R = f(\mathbf{w}) + \frac{\lambda}{2N}\sum_{i=1}^{D}\mathbf{w}_j^2 \tag{10.4}$$

where λ is an adjustable parameter that governs the degree of regularisation. We also examined LR with the "least absolute shrinkage and selection operator" (LASSO) regularisation method, which imposes the constraint that the L^1 norm $||\mathbf{w}|| = \sum_i |w_i|$ does not exceed some threshold value. From a Bayesian perspective, this is equivalent to putting a zero-mean Laplace prior on the feature weightings, meaning that the prior assumption is that the feature is not important until the training data shows otherwise.

10.4.2 Support vector machine

The SVM is a classification algorithm that attempts to separate two groups by the widest margin possible in some feature space. The hyperplane defining this separation is determined by maximising the distance between it and the closest training points from each class, which are termed the support vectors. Here we will consider a set of labels $\ell_1 \ldots \ell_N$, $\ell \in \{-1, 1\}$, in keeping with the SVM literature.

The formulation of an SVM begins by considering the distance of each training example $\mathbf{x}_i$ from the hyperplane $y(\mathbf{x}_n) = \mathbf{w}^T\mathbf{x}_n + b$, where b is a bias parameter and $\mathbf{w}$ is again a vector of weights. This distance is written as $\frac{|y(\mathbf{x}_n)|}{||\mathbf{w}||}$. This is subject to the constraint that $y_n(\mathbf{w}^T\mathbf{x}_n + b) \geq 1$ because the goal is to classify all examples correctly. The data is not always linearly separable, however, which is taken into account through the introduction of a "slack variable" for every training example, ξ_n, and a cost parameter, C. The slack variable $\xi_n = 0$ if the example datapoint $\mathbf{x}_n$ lies on or within its correct boundary, and $\xi_n = |\ell_n - y(\mathbf{x}_n)|$ otherwise. The parameter C penalises misclassified examples. C is analogous to a regularisation parameter in that lower values of C correspond to more slowly changing decision boundaries (because misclassifications are not penalised heavily), and vice versa. The constraint is therefore $\ell_n y(\mathbf{x}_n) \geq 1 - \xi_n$. As the goal is to maximise the distance between the hyperplane and the closest training example, which requires maximising $||\mathbf{w}||^{-1}$, this is equivalent to minimising $||\mathbf{w}||^2$, where the square is introduced to avoid taking the root in $||\mathbf{w}||$. This therefore requires the minimisation of $f(\mathbf{w}) = C\sum_{n=1}^{N}\xi_n + \frac{1}{2}||\mathbf{w}||^2$, which is referred to as the primal form of the classifier. The primal form can be re-written in terms of the feature vectors themselves in the dual form, which requires maximisation of:

$$f(\alpha) = \sum_{i=1}^{N} \alpha_i - \frac{1}{2} \sum_{j,k=1}^{N} \alpha_j \alpha_k \ell_j \ell_k \mathbf{x}_j^T \mathbf{x}_k, \quad 0 \leq \alpha_i \leq C \quad \text{and} \quad \sum_{i=1}^{N} \alpha_i \ell_i = 0 \qquad (10.5)$$

where α is another vector of weights, with $\mathbf{w} = \sum_{i=1}^{N} \alpha_i \ell_i \mathbf{x}_i$.[1] The dual form allows for the use of the "kernel trick" to project data into a high-dimensional space, in which the two classes may be linearly separable. The kernel trick is a method by which, rather than using the actual vector of features that define each $\mathbf{x}_n$, a kernel function that describes the features of each example in relation to each other is used instead. Through Mercer's theorem, any positive semi-definite kernel function corresponds to a high-dimensional space, for which $\mathrm{k}(\mathbf{x}, \mathbf{x}') = \phi(\mathbf{x})\dot{\phi}(\mathbf{x}')$ and where $\phi(\mathbf{x})$ is some mapping from our original data space to the higher-dimensional space. That is, we can avoid operating in the high-dimensional space because we require only the dot product in 10.5, and our kernel function gives the scalar product in that space. The Gaussian radial basis function kernel is one of the most commonly used kernels because of its straightforward interpretation as a similarity metric between two points:

$$\mathrm{k}(\mathbf{x}, \mathbf{x}') = \exp\left(-\frac{||\mathbf{x} - \mathbf{x}'||^2}{2\sigma^2}\right) \qquad (10.6)$$

10.4.3 Random forest

RFs are ensemble learners, which means that the RF prediction is based upon the votes of a committee of many weak "base learners." The base learner for an RF is a decision tree, each of which is formed from a random subset of the available features and a random subset of the available training set. After all of the trees have been built, the classifier's prediction is based upon majority voting of the trees. For problems involving genomic loci as features, building 40–400 trees and using a random selection of half of the features has been found to be a suitable means of initialising the various parameters [17].

10.4.4 Bayesian naive Bayesian (BNB)

Unlike the classifiers described previously, BNB is a generative model, and it assumes that all features are independent. This assumption rarely holds, but BNB nevertheless often produces good classification performance. With our training examples $\mathbf{X} = \{\mathbf{x}_n\}_{n=1...N}$, π as the prior probability of being in a class, θ_j as the probability that a given feature is "on" (i.e., it has value 1), and again taking $\ell_1 \ldots \ell_N$, $\ell \in \{0, 1\}$, as

[1] In deriving the dual form from the Lagrangian, α is the vector of Lagrange multipliers.

labels, we have $p(x_i, \ell_i) = p(\ell_i|\pi)\prod_j p(x_{ij}|\theta_j)$. Including both classes and taking the logarithm, we obtain

$$\log p(X|\theta) = \sum_c N_c \log \pi_c + \sum_{j=1}^{D} \sum_c \sum_{i:\mathbb{1}(y_i=c)} \log p(x_{ij}|\theta_{jc}) \tag{10.7}$$

with $\mathbb{1}$ as the indicator function and $N_c = \sum_i \mathbb{1}(y_i = c)$; that is, N_c is the number of examples in class c. We could then use a maximum likelihood estimate (which would involve differentiation of the log likelihood, introduction of Lagrange multipliers, and solving for the parameters), but here we will instead obtain full distributions over the model parameters by introducing a set of prior distributions.[2] We will place a $Beta(\beta_0, \beta_1)$ prior over each θ_{jc} and a $Dirichlet(\alpha)$ prior for each π.[3] This then leaves us with

$$p(\theta|X) = p(\pi|X)\prod_{j=1}^{D}\prod_c p(\theta_{jc}|X) \tag{10.8}$$

where $p(\pi|X) = Dirichlet(N_1 + \alpha_1, \ldots N_c + \alpha_c), p(\theta_{jc}|X) = Beta(a, b), a = N_{jc} + \beta_0$, and $b = N_c - N_{jc} + \beta_1$.

The BNB approach provides a probability distribution over the probability that an isolate in class c has the given SNP. After training, predictions are made on new data by calculating the probability of the class label, given the new example and the training data. The class label with the highest probability is the final prediction. This probability is formulated as $p(\ell = c|x, X) \propto p(\ell = c|X)\prod_{j=1}^{D} p(x_j|y = c, X)$. Expanding out, this becomes

$$p(y = c|x, X) \propto \frac{N_c + \alpha_c}{N + \alpha_0}\prod_{j=1}^{D} \bar{\theta}_{jc}^{\mathbb{1}(x_j=1)}(1 - \bar{\theta}_{jc}^{\mathbb{1}(x_j=0)}) \tag{10.9}$$

with $\bar{\theta}_{jc}$ being the mean value of the fitted parameter distribution, equal to $\frac{N_{jc}+\beta_0}{N_c+\beta_0+\beta_1}$.

We used a U-shaped Beta prior, $Beta(0.5, 0.5)$, for every θ_{jc} except for the established SNPs. For these, we used a $Beta(1, 0.25)$ prior for the resistant class, which shifts the prior distribution towards $\theta_{jc} = 1$, and a $Beta(0.25, 1)$ prior for the susceptible class, which shifts the prior distribution towards $\theta_{jc} = 0$, as is illustrated in Figure 10.4. We used a uniform Dirichlet distribution as a prior over each class.

[2]The cumulative distribution function (cdf) is the probability that a given random variable will have a value less than or equal to x, while the probability density function (pdf) is the relative likelihood that a given random variable will take on the value x. The cdf may also be called the "distribution function," while the pdf may also be called the "density." However, the machine learning literature tends to use the word "distribution" to refer to the pdf, as we will in this report.

[3]The Beta distribution provides a distribution over the interval [0, 1]. It is parameterised by $a > 0$ and $b > 0$, which determine the distribution's shape. The Dirichlet distribution is distributed over K random variables and has a single K-dimensional parameter, $\alpha > 0$. The beta distribution is a special case of the Dirichlet distribution, in which $K = 2$.

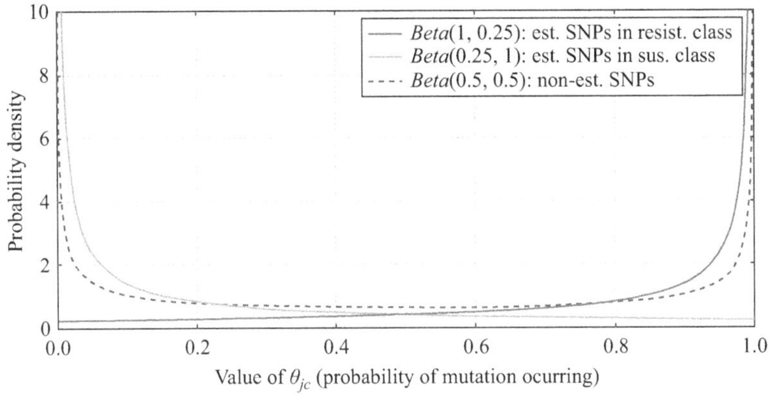

Figure 10.4 Illustration of the prior over the parameters governing features

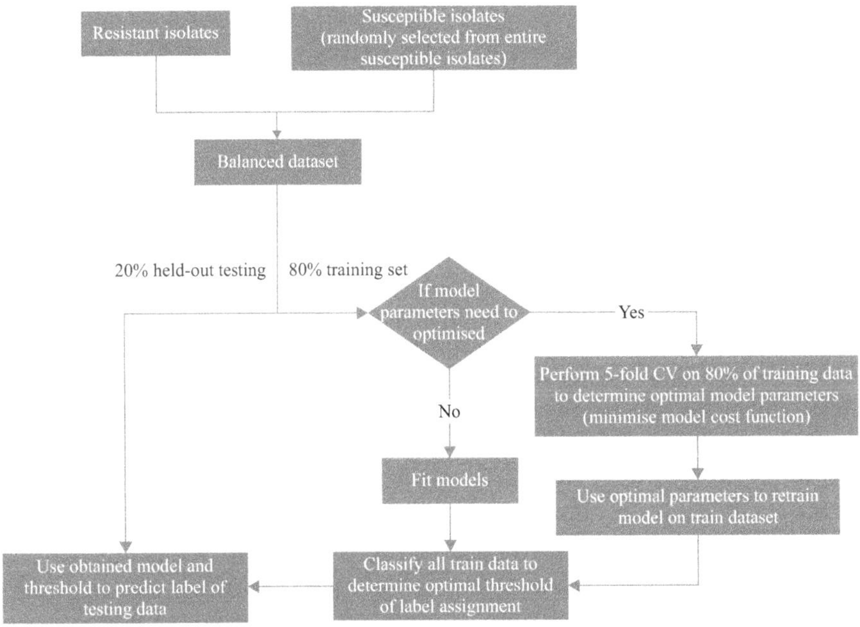

Figure 10.5 Procedure using supervised models for antibiotic resistance prediction

10.4.5 Supervised classification for antibiotic resistance prediction

This part addresses the framework of using supervised models to predict antibiotic resistance, which in essence is supervised classification. Figure 10.5 illustrates the procedure of supervised classification for antibiotic resistance. Validation of supervised classifiers for antibiotic resistance prediction is consisted of three steps: (1) assembling balanced dataset; (2) training the supervised model; (3) testing the model.

1. *Assembling balanced datasets*
Usually, there are many more susceptible isolates than resistant isolates. To avoid bias in the classifier, it is recommended to construct balanced datasets. Taken one data source of MTB as an example, of the 1835 isolates, only 266, 97,47, and 59 isolates were resistant to INH, RIF, EMB, and PZA, respectively. Therefore, to assemble a balanced dataset for training a classifier, a subset of susceptible isolates equal to the number of resistant isolates is randomly selected, for example, for INH analysis, 266 susceptible isolates are selected. In each obtained balanced dataset, the resistant isolates are the same while the susceptible isolates are different. Then, each model can be trained on 80% of this balanced dataset and tested on the held-out 20%.

2. *Training a classifier*
The parameters of these supervised models, e.g., width of SVM kernel, soft margin of SVM, and the regularisation parameter of LR, should be determined based on internal fivefold cross-validation on 80% of training data. These optimised parameters will then be used train a final model using all the training data, meanwhile, the decision threshold is determined by maximising the classification performance.

3. *Testing a classifier*
The final obtained model after the training stage is used for prediction on the "held-out" 20% data in the test set. This process can be repeated for many times with each time random samplings from the pool of susceptibility examples. Ultimately, the mean and standard deviation of the accuracy, sensitivity, and specificity can be subsequently calculated across all iterations, allowing an assessment of the variation in the process due to the stochastic selection of the training and testing data. These results also provide a fair comparison among all available models as well as the DA method.

10.5 Unsupervised models

Unsupervised learning is used to cluster objects when they are given without associating labels, which is promising as an exploratory tool for discovering hidden structures of the dataset, and especially useful to examine whether there are new, undetected groups of similar samples within the dataset. It has played a crucial role in the analysis of gene expression data. The nature basis for organising gene expression data is to group together genes with similar patterns of expression. Ongoing antibiotics resistance analysis using unsupervised learning is limited and challenged, mainly because the mechanism of antibiotics resistance of the pathogen still needs to be well understood.

Unsupervised learning is promising given the uncertainty of phenotype test. Sometime, phenotypic testing has proved to be unreliable in some well-described situations. For example, the susceptibility tests are subject to many assumptions about the degree of susceptibility based on the minimum inhibitory concentration

(MIC), and they require the selection of a "breakpoint" for each antibiotic: an MIC level above which the isolate is deemed to be resistant to therapy. These breakpoints are chosen on the basis of diverse but imperfect factors. There is considerable debate on how to set the breakpoints, and these are not always agreed across countries and organisations. The effect of susceptibility testing on the clinical response to infection is difficult to study, given the multiple factors that influence patient outcome, so that the sensitivity and specificity for determining resistance or susceptibility of phenotypic tests are often poorly measured.

Unsupervised clustering methods that are potentially usable for analysing genomic data in infectious disease management will be focused in the section. Typical clustering is consisted of discriminative and generative models. K-means clustering, as non-probabilistic model, is a representative of discriminative models. Generative model in an unsupervised fashion is often termed latent variable model which assumes the data is generated by unseen variables. The variables to be discovered can be latent feature, latent cause or latent class. We will introduce two typical unsupervised models: mixture model and latent feature model.

In this section, we will consider a subset of N isolates to represent a training set of examples $\mathbf{X} = \{\mathbf{x}_1 \ldots \mathbf{x}_N\}$ only without phenotypic labels. Both the binary and percentage representation of genomic data are considered. For example, each example $\mathbf{x}_i$ can be composed of a vector of D binary features indicating the presence ($x_{ij} = 1$) or absence ($x_{ij} = 0$) of a given SNP j, or, a vector of percentage features indicating the probability of being a mutation for the given SNP.

10.5.1 Mixture model

Instead of assigning hard label to examples, mixture models tend to associate an example with the probability of mixture components responsible for generating the example. A mixture model, also termed latent class model, assumes each example in a component c_i with probability

$$p(c_i = k|\pi) = \pi_k \tag{10.10}$$

which is a multinomial and π_k is prior or mixing weights of the kth component. In the mixture model, the probability of the assignment satisfies $\sum_{k=1}^{K} \pi_k = 1$. The assignment is the latent variable to be estimated. To model the probability of the data with the latent variable is to marginalise likelihood with the probability of being in a class,

$$p(\mathbf{X}) = \prod_{i=1}^{N} \sum_{k=1}^{K} p(\mathbf{x}_i|c_i = k, \boldsymbol{\theta}) p(c_i|\pi) \tag{10.11}$$

where for each component k, $p(\mathbf{x}_i|c_i = k, \boldsymbol{\theta})$ is component-conditional probability (density) function. $\boldsymbol{\theta}$ is the parameters of the mixture components. This can be seen as a generative model that first selects the kth component with probability $p(c_i = k)$ and then generates $\mathbf{x}_i$ in accordance with $p(\mathbf{x}_i|c_i = k, \boldsymbol{\theta})$. Note that (10.11) assumes an upper bound on the number of mixture components, since it only allows assignments of objects up to K clusters.

For such a mixture model, the maximise likelihood estimation (MLE) cannot be solved since the derivative of the log likelihood of the model with summation in the log cannot be computed explicitly. Expectation maximisation (EM) is often preferred for finding MLE estimates of mixture models because of its simplicity. In the E-step, the current model values are used to evaluate the posterior of the latent variable $p(\mathbf{C}|\mathbf{X};\boldsymbol{\theta}^{old})$, termed responsibility. Then, in the M-step, the model parameters is re-estimated using the current responsibility, the objective function of this step is,

$$\boldsymbol{\theta}^{new} = \arg\min_{\boldsymbol{\theta}} \sum_{\mathbf{c}} p(\mathbf{C}|\mathbf{X};\boldsymbol{\theta}^{old}) \ln p(\mathbf{C},\mathbf{X}|\boldsymbol{\theta}) \tag{10.12}$$

which is to maximise the expectation of the $\ln p(\mathbf{C},\mathbf{X}|\boldsymbol{\theta})$ with respect to $\mathbf{C}$ drawn according to the distribution given by $p(\mathbf{C}|\mathbf{X};\boldsymbol{\theta}^{old})$. The EM procedure is similar to the iterative update in the K-means. The update iterates as: (1) assign every data point to pre-defined cluster with probability; (2) update cluster using the assigned data points.

Any conditional density to model each cluster in each cluster. In particular, the use of the Bernoulli mixture model (BMM) is discussed below. BMM is used to model the probability distribution of binary data. A Bernoulli model is a particular case of (10.11), where each component k has D-dimensional Bernoulli probability function governed by its own vector of parameters or prototype $\mu_k = (\mu_{k,1}, \ldots, \mu_{k,D})^T \in [0,1]^D$,

$$p(\mathbf{x}_i|\mu_k) = \prod_{d=1}^{D} \mu_{k,d}^{\mathbf{x}_i}(1-\mu_{k,d})^{1-\mathbf{x}_i} \tag{10.13}$$

The parameters of mixture component in BMM is $\boldsymbol{\theta} = \{\pi_k, \mu_k\}$. Note that (10.13) is just the product of independent, unidimensional Bernoulli probability functions. Therefore, for a fixed k, it cannot capture any kind of dependencies or correlations between individual SNP. Unlike a single product of Bernoulli, the mixture distribution can capture correlations between variables.

Using mixture models for antibiotic resistance, prediction is based on the assumption that the population of resistant isolates with respect to one specific antibiotic usually includes MDR isolates and isolates that are resistant to other drugs. The mixture model for modelling data given the label is called class-conditioned mixture model or mixture discriminant analysis, which is to model the conditional density of each class. To model the genomic data, given the phenotype using class-conditioned mixture model is to train mixture model with respect to the resistant and susceptible isolates, respectively.

$$p(\mathbf{x}|\ell) = \sum_{i=1}^{K} p(c_i|\ell)p(\mathbf{x}|\ell, c_i) \tag{10.14}$$

Then, the optimal Bayes decision rule is to assign each example $\mathbf{x}$ to a class $\ell^*(\mathbf{x})$ giving maximum a posteriori probability or, equivalently,

$$\ell^*(\mathbf{x}) = \underset{\ell}{\text{argmax}} \quad \log p(\ell) + \log p(\mathbf{x}|\ell) \tag{10.15}$$

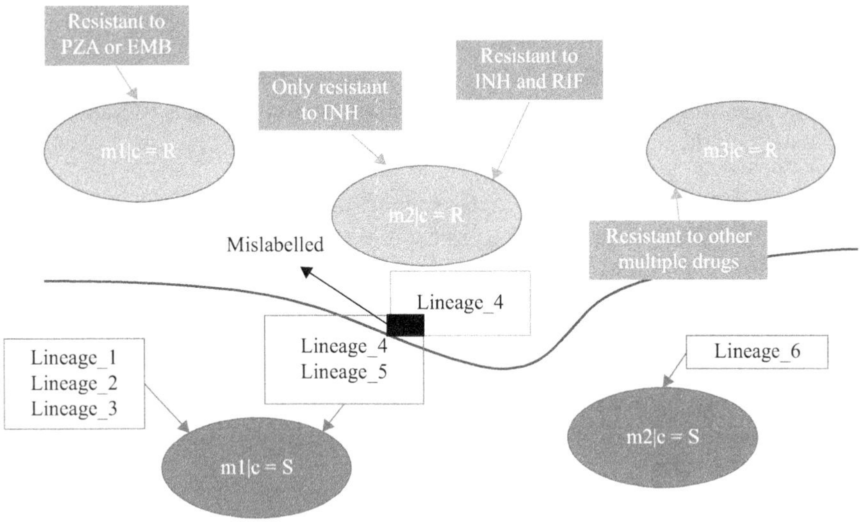

Figure 10.6 Illustration of mixture modelling on genomic data for antibiotic resistance prediction. Top three grey ellipses with notation of "c = R" represent clusters in resistance class. Black solid line in the middle represents boundary between resistant and susceptible classes. Bottom two grey ellipses with notation of "c = S" represent clusters in susceptible class. Grey rectangles represent resistant profile for anti-TB drugs. Outlined rectangles associated with an ellipse represent lineage profile for this cluster

Figure 10.6 illustrates the class-conditioned mixture model in antibiotic resistance prediction given the class labels in terms of INH. It shows that there are multiple mixture components in both classes, which either relate to the subgroup of isolates with different phenotype profile for all tested antibiotic drugs or relate to different lineages of isolates. According to the established model, one can also inference the pattern of the mixture component that is most likely responsible for every isolate. The misclassified isolates could either be mislabelled or be resistant to other drugs except for INH. Noted that black area means that isolates of lineage 4 labelled by resistant class have same pattern with that lineage in susceptible class, which could be mislabelled.

10.5.2 Bayesian mixture model

In real practice, we don't really believe there is a "true" number of clusters, which motives the application of non-parametric Bayesian mixture models, or infinite mixture model. Such model assumes that the data comes from a mixture of an infinite number of distributions, which means to specify the probability of **X** in terms of infinitely many classes.

The Bayesian approach offers an appealing strategy, which is to allow an "infinite" (i.e., unbounded) number of mixture components. A merit of infinite mixture model is as the dataset gets larger and more heterogeneous, the number of components grows automatically. One scheme to develop infinite mixture models is to apply prior distribution on the mixing weight and to take limit of analytic marginal distribution as the number of class approaches infinity.

Specifically, in Bayesian approaches to mixture modelling, mixing weights π is assumed to follow a prior distribution $p(\pi)$, with a standard choice being a symmetric Dirichlet distribution. The Dirichlet distribution on multinomials over K classes has parameters $\alpha_1, \alpha_2, \dots \alpha_K$, and is conjugate to the multinomial. In a symmetric Dirichlet distribution, all α_k are equal, which take $\alpha_k = \frac{\alpha}{K}$ for all k. The probability model of the Dirichilet-multinomial model is

$$\begin{aligned} \pi \,|\alpha &\sim \text{Dirichilet}\left(\tfrac{\alpha}{K}, \dots, \tfrac{\alpha}{K}\right) \\ c_i|\pi &\sim \text{Discrete}(\pi) \end{aligned} \tag{10.16}$$

where Discrete(π) is the multiple-outcome analogue of a Bernoulli event. The marginal probability of an assignment vector $\mathbf{c}$, integrating over all values of π is,

$$p(\mathbf{c}) = \frac{\prod_{k=1}^{K} \Gamma(m_k + \frac{\alpha}{K})}{\Gamma(\frac{\alpha}{K})^K} \frac{\Gamma(\alpha)}{\Gamma(N+\alpha)} \tag{10.17}$$

where $m_k = \sum_{i=1}^{N} \delta(c_i = k)$ is the number of objects assigned to class k. Considering two assignment vectors that result in the same division of objects correspond to the same partition, we denote $[\mathbf{c}]$ as an equivalence class of assignment vectors. The probability of each equivalence class assignments is

$$p([\mathbf{c}]) = \sum_{\mathbf{c} \in [\mathbf{c}]} p(\mathbf{c}) = \frac{K!}{K_0!} \left(\frac{\alpha}{K}\right)^{K_+} \left(\prod_{k=1}^{K_+} \prod_{j=1}^{m_k - 1} \left(j + \frac{\alpha}{K}\right) \right) \frac{\Gamma(\alpha)}{\Gamma(N+\alpha)} \tag{10.18}$$

where K_+ is the number of classes for which $m_k > 0$, K_0 is the number of classes for which $m_k > 0$, so $K = K_0 + K_+$. Rearrange the first two terms, we can compute the limit of the probability of a partition as $K \to \infty$, which is

$$\begin{aligned} &\lim_{K\to\infty} \alpha^{K_+} \cdot \frac{K!}{K_0! K^{K_+}} \cdot \left(\prod_{k=1}^{K_+} \prod_{j=1}^{m_k - 1} \left(j + \frac{\alpha}{K}\right) \right) \cdot \frac{\Gamma(\alpha)}{\Gamma(N+\alpha)} \\ &= \alpha^{K_+} \cdot 1 \cdot \left(\prod_{k=1}^{K_+} (m_k - 1)! \right) \cdot \frac{\Gamma(\alpha)}{\Gamma(N+\alpha)} \end{aligned} \tag{10.19}$$

A simple process that produces the same distribution over partitions specified above is Chinese restaurant process (CRP). Figure 10.7 illustrates the generative process for CRP, where each observed example is assigned to one table (cluster) and the number of tables is unbounded.

Inference in an infinite mixture model is only slightly more complicated than inference in a mixture model with a finite, fixed number of classes. The standard

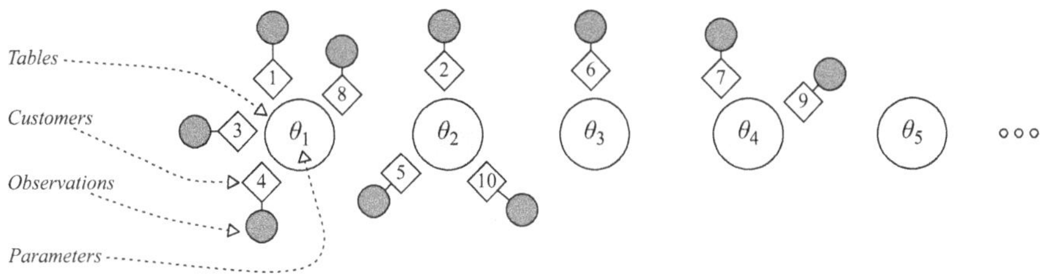

Figure 10.7 Generative process of CRP [18]. The shaded circles indicate observed examples, and the large circles represent tables (clusters) and associated parameters, respectively

algorithm used for inference in infinite mixture models is Gibbs sampling. Interested readers please refer to Reference 19.

The introduction of Bayesian mixture model shows that infinite statistical models can be defined by specifying priors over infinite combinatorial objects, which can be derived by taking the limit of priors for finite models. Although the large hypothesis spaces are implied, the inference in these models can remain possible. Infinite mixture models are still fundamentally limited in their representation of objects, assuming that assume each example can only belong to a single class.

10.5.3 Latent feature model

Unlike mixture model, latent feature model assumes the multiple latent features are responsible for generating each object. In another word, it assumes that each object belongs to multi-classes simultaneously. Latent feature models are known for dimension reduction. Typical latent feature models include factor analysis, principal component analysis, cooperative vector quantisation, etc.

In a latent feature model, each object is represented by latent feature values $\mathbf{f}_i$, and the properties $\mathbf{x}_i$ are generated from a distribution determined by those latent feature values. Latent feature model is to represent objects in terms of latent features values $\mathbf{F} = [\mathbf{f}_1^T \mathbf{f}_2^T \ldots \mathbf{f}_N^T]$ for all N objects. Similar to latent class model, latent feature model is defined as

$$p(\mathbf{X}) = \sum_{\mathbf{F}} p(\mathbf{X}|\mathbf{F})p(\mathbf{F}) \tag{10.20}$$

Then, break matrix $\mathbf{F}$ into two components as, $\mathbf{F} = \mathbf{Z} \otimes \mathbf{V}$,where $\mathbf{Z}$ defines which features are processed by each object, $\mathbf{V}$ stores value of each feature for each object, $\otimes$ denotes elementary product and $\mathbf{Z}$ contains the information about the latent feature.

As using Bayesian approach to obtain the infinite mixture model, define a prior for infinite latent feature models is to define a distribution over infinite binary matrices $\mathbf{Z}$. The prior is defined as

$$\begin{aligned} \pi_k|\alpha &\sim Beta\left(\tfrac{\alpha}{k}, 1\right) \\ z_{ik}|\pi_k &\sim Ber(\pi_k) \end{aligned} \tag{10.21}$$

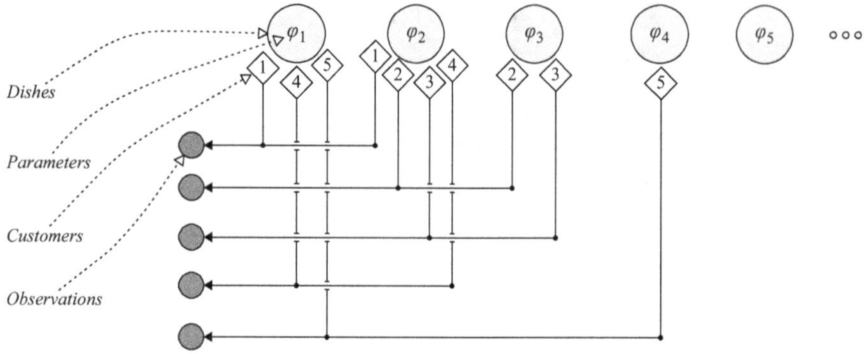

Figure 10.8 Generative process of IBP [18]. The shaded circles indicate observed examples, and the large circles represent dishes (factor) and associated parameters, respectively

The probability mode of the data is derived as marginal probability as,

$$p(\mathbf{Z}) = \prod_{k=1}^{K} \int \sum_{i=1}^{N} p(z_{ik}|\pi_k)p(\pi_k)d\pi_k \tag{10.22}$$

Similar to the infinite mixture model, consider the limit of analytic marginal distribution as the number of latent features approaches infinity.

$$\lim_{K\to\infty} p(\mathbf{z}) = \frac{\alpha_+^K}{\prod_{h=0}^{2^N-1} K_h} \cdot 1 \cdot \exp\{-\alpha H_N\} \cdot \prod_{k=1}^{K} \frac{(N-m_k)(m_k-1)}{N} \tag{10.23}$$

This distribution over partitions provides a prior over class assignments matrices for an infinite feature model. The equivalent stochastic process to obtain the same distribution is termed Indian buffet process (IBP). Interested readers can refer to Reference 19 for sampling from the distribution defined by IBP. Figure 10.8 illustrates the generative process for IBP, where each observed example possesses multiple dishes (features) and the number of dishes is unbounded. Also noted that in the latent feature model, the obtained features are shared by all observations.

Combining this prior with Gaussian likelihood, the linear Gaussian latent feature model is given by,

$$p(\alpha, \sigma_A, \sigma_X, \mathbf{Z}, \mathbf{A}, \mathbf{X}) = p(\alpha)p(\sigma_X)p(\sigma_A)p(\mathbf{Z}|\alpha)p(\mathbf{A}|\sigma_A)p(\mathbf{X}|\sigma_X, \mathbf{A}, \mathbf{Z}) \tag{10.24}$$

where $\mathbf{Z} \sim IBP(\alpha)$, $\mathbf{A} \sim N(0, \sigma_A^2\mathbf{I})$, $\mathbf{x_i} \sim N(\mathbf{z_i}\mathbf{A}, \Sigma_X)$, $\Sigma_X = \sigma_X^2\mathbf{I}$. Figure 10.9 shows the graphical model of the linear Gaussian latent feature model.

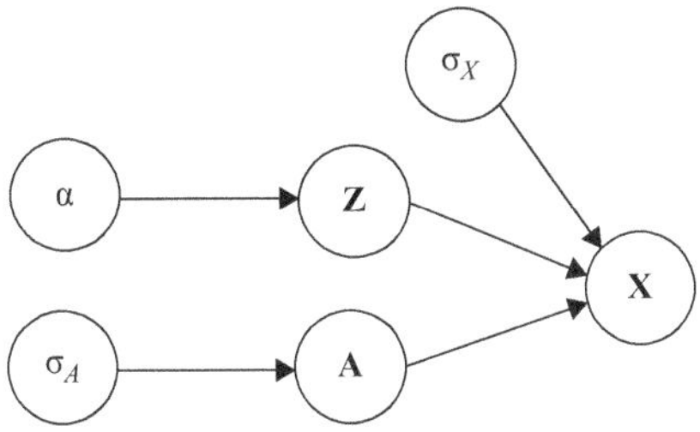

Figure 10.9 Graphical model of the linear Gaussian latent feature model [19]

The distribution of **X** given **Z**, σ_X and σ_A is

$$p(\mathbf{X}|\mathbf{Z},\sigma_X,\sigma_A) = \frac{1}{(2\pi)^{(ND/2)}\sigma_X^{(N-K)D}\sigma_A^{KD}|\mathbf{Z}^T\mathbf{Z}+\frac{\sigma_X^2}{\sigma_A^2}\mathbf{I}|^{d/2}}$$
$$\exp\left\{-\frac{1}{2\sigma_X^2}\mathrm{tr}\left(\mathbf{X}^T\left(\mathbf{I}-\mathbf{Z}\left(\mathbf{Z}^T\mathbf{Z}+\frac{\sigma_X^2}{\sigma_A^2}\mathbf{I}\right)^{-1}\mathbf{Z}^T\right)\mathbf{X}\right)\right\} \tag{10.25}$$

The assignment **Z** can be inferred as

$$P(z_{ik}|\mathbf{X},\mathbf{Z}_{-(i,k)},\sigma_X,\sigma_A) \propto p(\mathbf{X}|\mathbf{Z},\sigma_A,\sigma_X)P(z_{ik}|z_{-i,k}) \tag{10.26}$$

The latent features can be computed as posterior mean as,

$$E(\mathbf{A}|\mathbf{Z},\mathbf{X}) = \left(\mathbf{Z}^T\mathbf{Z}+\frac{\sigma_X^2}{\sigma_A^2\mathbf{I}}\right)^{-1}\mathbf{Z}^T\mathbf{X} \tag{10.27}$$

The dependencies among the variables in this model are shown in Figure 10.9. The inference of other hyper-parameters relies on Monte Carol Markov Chain (MCMC). Within each iteration of MCMC, the IBP is sampled with straightforward Gibbs sampling. The inference based on MCMC for Bayesian latent feature models is time consuming especially for genomic data of infectious disease pathogen. Variational inference can be an alternative option to fulfil the task of antibiotics resistance prediction. The underlying assumption of the latent feature model matches the hidden structure of the genomic data, which implies great potential of this type of models for modelling genomic data for antibiotic resistance prediction and infectious disease management.

10.6 Summary

In the infectious disease management, accurate antibiotic resistance prediction using genomic data of pathogen will shorten the treatment significantly. Both supervised and unsupervised machine learning in this task have shown valuable merits to date.

Developing more robust machine learning methods is desired, given the following reasons:

1. When evaluating the predictive performance of a machine learning system, it is necessary to keep in mind that the analysis operates upon statistical associations across the input features. Improved prediction can be due to the discovery of new resistance-conferring mutations, epistatic interactions between mutations that together cause resistance, phylogenetic associations, or the fact that isolates are commonly resistant to multiple drugs.
2. Machine learning can be used in many of the steps of clinical infectious disease management and resistance prediction. Considering increasingly more coming sequencing data and limited phenotype labels, the merits of semi-supervised and unbounded latent variable model is promising for infectious disease management and resistance prediction in the future.
3. To make full use of genomic data, unbalanced case needs to be considered. Unbalance data is one of the key concerns in machine learning community, which highly affects the performance of one classifier. In classification, machine learning algorithms will suffer a performance bias when datasets are unbalanced. Increasing the accuracy of minority class can result in lower accuracy on majority class. To overcome the bias, various solutions are available, that is, multiobjective optimisation [20], over- and under-sampling [21], adaptive evaluation measurement [22], etc.
4. A human error is always possible in lab based susceptible test and an error in the phenotype could have big effects on the decision phase, particularly if the size of the learning example is small. It is therefore very important to provide supervised classifiers robust enough to deal with data with uncertain labels.
5. Cross-resistance phenomena, also termed resistance co-occurrence, have been frequently found in MTB, e.g., MTB that are resistant to PZA are more likely to be resistant to INH as well. Machine learning techniques should take cross-resistance information explicitly into account to improve classification and prediction of drug resistance.

In addition, any promising mutations must be validated through additional experimental analysis before being deemed as causative. For instance, it is very easy to find highly predictive mutations of MTB for PZA drug resistance simply because MTB that are resistant to PZA are more likely to be resistant to INH as well. This can lead to the incorrect conclusion that INH-causative mutations are mechanistically involved in PZA drug resistance. This does not necessarily limit the benefit of the learned association (indeed, this is an intuition that doctors have developed as well when designing a drug regimen for patients), but it does mean that a predictive system should be continually updated to adapt to a changing bacterial population.

Acknowledgements

Y.Y. gratefully acknowledges the support of K.C. Wong Fellowship. K.E.N. acknowledges funding from the Rhodes Trust and the RCUK Digital Economy Programme grant number EP/G036861/1 (Centre for Doctoral Training in Healthcare Innovation).

References

[1] X. Didelot, R. Bowden, D. J. Wilson, T. E. Peto, and D. W. Crook, "Transforming clinical microbiology with bacterial genome sequencing," *Nature Reviews Genetics*, vol. 13, no. 9, pp. 601–612, 2012.

[2] World Health Organization, *Tuberculosis: Fact Sheet*, 2013. [Online]. Available: http://www.who.int/mediacentre/factsheets/fs104/en/index.html.

[3] World Health Organization, *Antimicrobial Resistance: Global Report on Surveillance 2014*, 2014. [Online]. Available: http://www.who.int/drugresistance/documents/surveillancereport/en/.

[4] Z. F. Udwadia, R. A. Amale, K. K. Ajbani, and C. Rodrigues, "Totally drug-resistant tuberculosis in India," *Clinical Infectious Diseases*, vol. 54, no. 4, pp. 579–581, 2012.

[5] C. C. Boehme, S. Saacks, and R. J. O'Brien, "The changing landscape of diagnostic services for tuberculosis," *Seminars in Respiratory and Critical Care Medicine*, vol. 34, no. 1, pp. 17–31, 2013.

[6] C. U. Köser, M. J. Ellington, E. J. Cartwright, *et al.*, "Routine use of microbial whole genome sequencing in diagnostic and public health microbiology," *PLoS Pathogens*, vol. 8, no. 8, p. e1002824, 2012.

[7] M. H. Hazbón, M. Brimacombe, M. B. del Valle, *et al.*, "Population genetics study of isoniazid resistance mutations and evolution of multidrug-resistant *Mycobacterium tuberculosis*," *Antimicrobial Agents and Chemotherapy*, vol. 50, no. 8, pp. 2640–2649, 2006.

[8] N. Stoesser, *et al.*, "Predicting antimicrobial susceptibilities for *Escherichia coli* and *Klebsiella pneumoniae* isolates using whole genomic sequence data," *Journal of Antimicrobial Chemotherapy*, vol. 68, no. 10, pp. 2234–2244, 2013.

[9] C. U. Köser, M. T. Holden, M. J. Ellington, *et al.*, "Rapid whole-genome sequencing for investigation of a neonatal MRSA outbreak," *New England Journal of Medicine*, vol. 366, no. 24, pp. 2267–2275, 2012.

[10] M. L. Metzker, "Sequencing technologies: the next generation," *Nature Reviews Genetics*, vol. 11, no. 1, pp. 31–46, 2009.

[11] E. R. Mardis, "The impact of next-generation sequencing technology on genetics," *Trends in Genetics*, vol. 24, no. 3, pp. 133–141, 2008.

[12] G. Lunter and M. Goodson, "Stampy: a statistical algorithm for sensitive and fast mapping of Illumina sequence reads," *Genome Research*, vol. 21, no. 6, pp. 936–939, 2011.

[13] D. R. Zerbino and E. Birney, "Velvet: algorithms for de novo short read assembly using de Bruijn graphs," *Genome Research*, vol. 18, no. 5, pp. 821–829, 2008.

[14] R. Nielsen, J. S. Paul, A. Albrechtsen, and Y. S. Song, "Genotype and snp calling from next-generation sequencing data," *Nature Reviews Genetics*, vol. 12, no. 6, pp. 443–451, 2011.

[15] A. Sandgren, M. Strong, P. Muthukrishnan, B. K. Weiner, G. M. Church, and M. B. Murray, "Tuberculosis drug resistance mutation database," *PLoS Medicine*, vol. 6, no. 2, p. e1000002, 2009.

[16] J. M. Lew, A. Kapopoulou, L. M. Jones, and S. T. Cole, "Tuberculist–10 years after," *Tuberculosis*, vol. 91, no. 1, pp. 1–7, 2011.

[17] B. A. Goldstein, A. E. Hubbard, A. Cutler, and L. F. Barcellos, "An application of random forests to a genome-wide association dataset: methodological considerations & new findings," *BMC Genetics*, vol. 11, no. 1, p. 49, 2010.

[18] S. J. Gershman and D. M. Blei, "A tutorial on Bayesian nonparametric models," *Journal of Mathematical Psychology*, vol. 56, no. 1, pp. 1–12, 2012.

[19] T. L. Griffiths and Z. Ghahramani, "The Indian buffet process: an introduction and review," *The Journal of Machine Learning Research*, vol. 12, pp. 1185–1224, 2011.

[20] U. Bhowan, M. Johnston, M. Zhang, and X. Yao, "Evolving diverse ensembles using genetic programming for classification with unbalanced data," *Evolutionary Computation, IEEE Transactions on*, vol. 17, no. 3, pp. 368–386, 2013.

[21] T. M. Padmaja, N. Dhulipalla, P. R. Krishna, R. S. Bapi, and A. Laha, "An unbalanced data classification model using hybrid sampling technique for fraud detection," in *Pattern Recognition and Machine Intelligence*. Springer-Verlag Berlin, Heidelberg, 2007, pp. 341–348.

[22] C.-Y. Yu, L.-C. Chou, and D. T. Chang, "Predicting protein-protein interactions in unbalanced data using the primary structure of proteins," *BMC Bioinformatics*, vol. 11, no. 1, p. 167, 2010.

Chapter 11
Machine learning for chronic disease

Katherine E. Niehaus and David A. Clifton

11.1 Introduction

Chronic disease is a hugely growing healthcare burden, with patients experiencing symptoms and requiring therapy throughout life. Studies in the USA have found that, with direct healthcare costs combined with lost productivity, the total economic cost of diabetes, heart disease, and hypertension was over 300 billion dollars annually from 2008 to 2010 [1]. Within this chapter, much of our motivation will be from the application area of inflammatory bowel disease (IBD), a chronic disease characterised by severe gastrointestinal inflammation. Approximately 620,000 patients in the UK have IBD, with estimates of healthcare costs per patient ranging from £631 to £3,000 per year [2]. IBD incidence is growing throughout the world, making efforts to better understand the underlying disease pathophysiology all the more important [3].

Within chronic disease, there are a variety of clinical areas in which machine-learning approaches can provide clinical value. Here, we will start with an overview of the types of data that may be encountered in the setting of chronic disease. We will then explain how extreme value theory (EVT) can be applied to better quantify severity and risk in chronic disease, and we will finally introduce a variety of methods for examining underlying patient subgroups within heterogeneous diseases.

11.2 Data

Within the realm of chronic disease, a wide range of data types may be available. We will focus here on the types of data that may be available in large retrospective analyses, as these are the settings in which machine-learning specialists most commonly find themselves. These typically fall into two categories: clinical data obtained from the electronic health record (EHR) and genomic data. EHRs have been developed for the purposes of aiding physicians in clinical practice, but their nature as a repository of patient information, accumulated during the routine care of patients, also makes them an attractive source of data for research. With legislation in the USA and elsewhere incentivising the implementation of EHR systems, there has been a

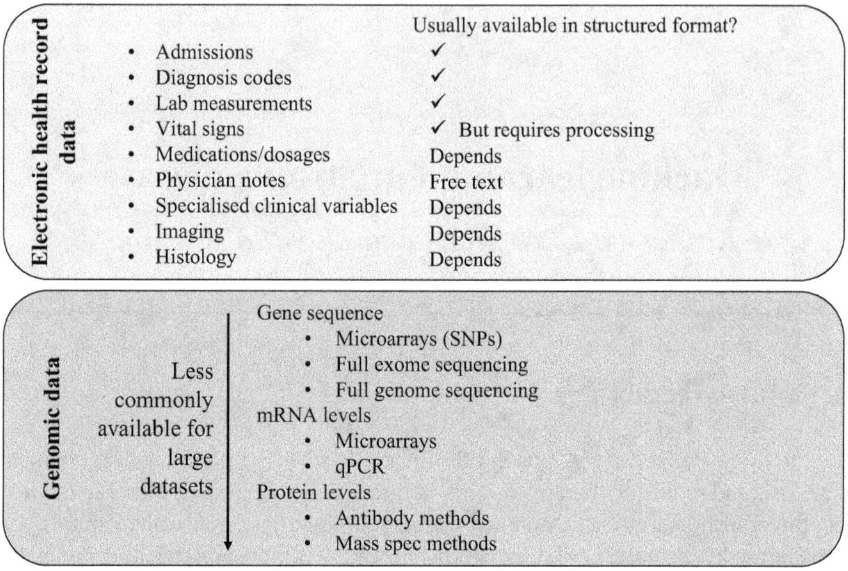

Figure 11.1 Data types commonly available for the analysis of chronic diseases

significant growth in the EHR uptake, and as a result, much of patient information collected in hospitals is now accessible in electronic formats. Simultaneously, the declining cost of genome sequencing has allowed for the possibility of creating large biobanks of linked clinical and genomic data sources. These databases are built upon the hypothesis that human genetic information (i.e., genotype) can help us to predict or augment our understanding of a patient's phenotype. While genome-wide association studies have illustrated that the links between genotype and phenotype are more complex than originally thought, there is still great potential for research to uncover how genomic factors are involved in different types of disease [4]. Exemplifying this purpose, a number of large EHR/biobank databases have been initiated, including the Electronic Medical Records and Genomics (eMERGE) network, the Kaiser Permanente Research Program on Genes, Environment, and Health (RPGEH), the "i2b2" service created by the National Center for Biomedical Computing in the USA, the China Kadoorie Biobank, and the UK Biobank [5–7].

We will now delve further into the types of information commonly encountered in EHR and genomic studies. Figure 11.1 provides a summary of the different data types that may be available.

11.2.1 EHR data

EHRs contain a number of different data types. These generally include diagnosis codes (e.g., International Classification of Diseases – ICD10); procedural codes (e.g., the USA uses Current Procedural Terminology – CPT); laboratory results; data such as vital-sign summary values; and free text. While some information, such as laboratory data, is generally stored in a structured form, other information can be much more difficult to ascertain. Specific characteristics of the data are often unique to individual EHRs (and even between different specialties within the same hospital), making data extraction methods difficult to standardise across systems. For instance, drug prescription and dosage may be included in structured formats in some EHRs, while this information may only be included in free text in others.

Because EHR data are collected for clinical care, patient records are often partially missing, incorrect, systematically misleading, and contradictory. The process of extracting meaningful EHR data that reflects true patient physiology (this is often referred to in the literature as "phenotyping" the patient) is not a simple task. Hripcsak and Albers outline several of the associated challenges [8]. As various authors have identified, within the scope of machine-learning analysis, a pertinent drawback of EHR data is that the labels required for supervised learning may be confounded by the fact that care is being provided [9,10].

Particularly in chronic disease applications, measurements taken repeatedly over time are relevant for analysis. In terms of structured data, such measurements can include blood measures of various metabolites ("labs"), ICD10 codes, or specialised relevant clinical variables that are collected for particular diseases. Modelling these metrics directly can provide insight into a patient's physiological progression over time, as well as relevant comorbidities. For instance, there have been recent developments on using ICD10 codes and specialised clinical variables to model subtypes of disease progression [11–14]. The type of data that is most relevant will depend, of course, upon the disease of interest and the availability within the record.

Free text in the medical notes also provides a potentially rich source of information regarding patient progression. However, the frequent misspellings, abundance of abbreviations, and multiple meanings of many medical terms means that advanced natural language processing (NLP) is often required to glean meaningful textual information beyond what is already present in the rest of the record.

Often particular diseases will involve specialised variables that may not be routinely collected in the EHR. For instance, in IBD, the specific locations of inflammation are particularly relevant to how physicians manage and treat the disease. Such information can be obtained through NLP of the free text, or, if such approaches have proved too difficult, manual extraction from the notes may be required. This is particularly the case for hospital systems where not all aspects of the patient record are available in electronic formats. Information contained in imaging studies such as MRIs or endoscopy images may also be relevant for analysis.

11.2.2 Genomic data

The declining cost of human genome sequencing means that genomic information has the potential to inform routine clinical practice. Human genetic variation is encoded in our DNA, which is composed of a long series of nucleotide base pairs (adenine, thymine, cytosine, and guanine). In the process of transcription, portions of DNA are converted into single-stranded RNA. Triplets of RNA bases (codons) are then translated into one of the 20 amino acids, which are the building blocks of proteins. The portions of the genome that encode proteins or other functional products are called genes. Only about 3% of the 3 billion nucleotide bases in the human genome constitute genes. Understanding the role of the rest of the genome is still a work in progress, but it is well-established that parts are involved in regulating gene expression (i.e., protein production). Heritable (and non-heritable) gene expression regulation can also be accomplished through changes to the macro-structure of the DNA through chemical alterations such as methylation. Such changes are termed "epigenetic" because they result in changes in gene expression without altering the underlying DNA sequence.

Human genomic variation can occur through many mechanisms. A single nucleotide polymorphism (SNP) is a single-base change in the DNA. SNPs can result in proteins with altered functionality, or, if within a regulatory region, changes in protein production. Across populations, there may be a few different common variants of a gene, termed alleles. Insertions and deletions of nucleotide bases (indels) and copy-number variants (CNVs) are also sources of inter-human variation. CNVs are large portions of the genome that have been deleted or duplicated; they constitute approximately 12% of human DNA [15]. Most multicellular organisms, including humans, have two copies of each chromosome. If the alleles on both chromosomes are the same, the allele is said to be homozygous; if the alleles differ, then it is said to be heterozygous.

Patient genetic information may be obtained in a variety of ways. Microarrays (also known as DNA chips) are perhaps the most common source of data in large databanks of phenotypic and genetic information. Microarrays are small chips that contain thousands of DNA probes attached to their surface. When a fluorescently labelled sample is introduced, any pieces of DNA that are complementary to the attached DNA probes will bind to the probe, indicating which sequences were present in the sample. Specialised microarrays can be created for specific purposes; for instance, the Immunochip is a microarray that has been designed to provide coverage of SNPs suspected to be involved in inflammatory diseases (e.g., IBD and rheumatoid arthritis).

Microarrays can be very cost-effective for wide coverage of common SNPs, but they do not provide information about every mutation in a patient's genome. Alternatively, whole-genome sequencing methods can be used to obtain the full genome sequence, which identifies SNPs and indels throughout the genome; CNVs are still sometimes difficult to identify. Illumina (USA), the current market leader in sequencing platforms, announced the sale of the first machines capable of the long-heralded "$1,000" human genome in early 2014.[1] Some newer sequencing companies are offering longer read lengths, allowing for perhaps easier interpretation of CNVs. Full exome sequencing is another sequencing alternative, in which all protein-coding regions of a patient's genome are sequenced (as mentioned, the exome represents only about 1–3% of the human genome).

[1]This $1,000 genome is practically only achievable for large-scale research labs: Illumina only sells the machines in batches of 10 for $10 million.

While sequencing data can provide information about a patient's genetic background, it does not answer which proteins are actually being produced in particular cells in the body at any given time (due to the advanced regulatory mechanisms involved). For this, mRNA levels or protein levels must be obtained. mRNA can be measured through microarrays (again, most useful for known and common gene transcripts), real-time quantitative polymerase chain reaction (allows for very specific exact measurements of the amount of mRNA in a sample), or RNAseq (which relies upon next-generation sequencing to assess RNA levels). Proteins levels can be assessed through antibody-based methods or mass spectrometry. mRNA and protein levels are less commonly available for large patient populations with EHR data, but they are increasingly being used (particularly in more targeted studies) to examine how gene expression levels influence disease phenotype.

There are a wide variety of additional data types that may also be relevant for a particular question. For instance, the microbiome, which consists of all microorganisms in the body, has been shown to be particularly relevant for IBD pathogenesis. The "exposome", the record of environmental exposures a given patient has been exposed to, is also important for unravelling the pathogenesis of many diseases [3]. Of course, a detailed record of such information is not available in nearly any setting, but thinking about how environmental exposures can influence disease progression can guide which information may be useful to collect.

A key aspect of any study of patient disease progression and modelling is a deep understanding of the data collected. It is important to ascertain, for instance, how a hospital's local practices may influence how one should interpret specific variables. The application of diagnosis codes is notoriously inconsistent, with coding practices varying by institution. Lab machinery may change over time, which means that reference ranges and the maximum/minimum possible values may shift. Interpreting such clinical data will likely require close consultation with physicians or nurses who are experienced with the hospital practices.

11.3 EVT applied to longitudinal data

Often when monitoring patients over long periods of time, as is the case for chronic disease, it is desirable to understand how recent trends in measured data points compare to a patient's previous levels and to those of the patient population. However, it is often only deviations beyond a certain range (i.e., "normal") that are of interest. For instance, for a patient with IBD, a physician may want to understand how concerning the results of a high C-reactive protein or lymphocyte level may be; the physician may be unconcerned if the value is within the normal patient range. For applications in which this is the case, it is desirable to focus specifically on modelling the extremes of the distribution of data points.

EVT is a branch of statistics that seeks to model the behaviour of the tails of distributions. Here, we will provide an introduction to the basic models and explain how they may be applied in healthcare settings. For more details, References 16 and

17 provide good introductions to EVT, each containing additional references for a more mathematical treatment of the models.

11.3.1 Classical EVT

There are two primary formulations for classical EVT models: a block maxima approach and a peaks-over-threshold approach. We start with a sequence of independently and identically distributed (IID) random variables, $X_1, \ldots, X_n \sim F$, collected at time points $1 \ldots n$. See Figure 11.2 for a visual overview of these models. The block maxima approach attempts to model the maximum of these random variables obtained within a given time frame: $M_n = \max(X_1, \ldots, X_n)$. The probability of M_n being less than some value z_m is therefore $F(z_m)^n$. However, since we do not know F, and since estimates of F^n will vary greatly depending upon the estimate of F, we instead focus on modelling the extremes themselves. In the limit of infinite data $(n \to \infty)$, M_n will approach a dirac delta function on the maximum possible value of F. To avoid this, we re-normalise M_n as $M_n^* = \frac{M_n - \mu}{\sigma}$ for two constants, the scale: $\sigma > 0$ and the location: μ.

It can then be shown that, regardless of the distribution of F, in the limit as $n \to \infty$, the distribution of M_n^* approaches the generalised extreme value (GEV) distribution [16]. The GEV cumulative distribution function (CDF) is as follows:

$$P(M_n^* \leq z) \to G(x) = \exp\left(-\left[1 + \xi\left(\frac{x-\mu}{\sigma}\right)\right]^{-1/\xi}\right) \tag{11.1}$$

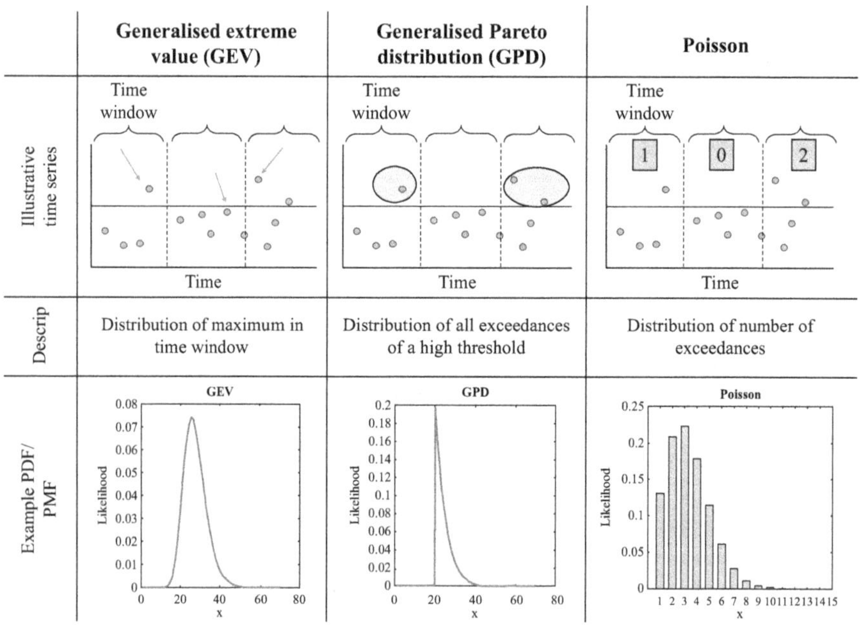

Figure 11.2 Illustration of EVT distributions

where ξ is termed the shape parameter. $G(x)$ is defined for $1 + \frac{\xi(x-\mu)}{\sigma} > 0$. When $\xi = 0$, the limit is taken to obtain $G(x) = \exp\left(-\exp\left(-\frac{x-\mu}{\sigma}\right)\right)$. The values of ξ correspond to three special cases of the GEV: when $\xi > 0$, the distribution is called the Frechet type; when $\xi < 0$, the distribution is called the Weibull; and when $\xi = 0$, the distribution is called the Gumbel.[2] In sum, this tells us that the maximum value of a set of IID variables collected over a period of time will follow a GEV distribution. We can fit the parameters for the GEV using training data from multiple periods of time with maximum likelihood or Bayesian methods, if desired.

As mentioned, an alternative perspective is to model points exceeding a set, high threshold. This allows us to use more of the data, rather than simply the maximum values within each time window. Here, we are interested in a slightly different question: the probability of seeing a point above the threshold, u. Formally, we are interested in $P(X > u + y \mid X > u)$. We can obtain this by building upon our findings for the GEV above. Because $F(x)$ is a CDF, it tends towards one with large values of x. Therefore, the Taylor expansion of $\log F(x) \approx F(x) - 1$ with large x. Using this fact to rewrite our formulation of the GEV above, we can obtain [16]:

$$P(X > u + y \mid X > u) \approx H(y) = 1 - \left(1 + \frac{\xi y}{\sigma_p}\right)^{-1/\xi} \quad (11.2)$$

$$\sigma_p = \sigma + \xi(u - \mu) \quad (11.3)$$

$H(y)$ is the form of a family of distributions called the generalised Pareto distribution (GPD). As is evident, the GPD and GEV models are closely related; the parameter ξ is shared between the two models; and σ_p is a function of σ and μ. It makes intuitive sense that the distribution governing the probability of high values above a set threshold will be related to the maximum value observed within a given time window.

These two models form the cornerstone of classical EVT. As has been emphasised, these rely upon the assumption of IID data. In the case of a stationary time series, however, there are temporal dependencies in the data. Fortunately, it turns out that, given a time dependency that decreases with increasing time distance, the GEV model is still an appropriate model for block maxima. The parameters governing a series of IID datapoints versus those governing a stationary time series are different, but since the parameters are being fit anyway, this is not of practical importance. In the case of the exceedances-over-threshold model, the GPD model is no longer as appropriate because exceedances will tend to occur in clusters. For instance, a high value is more likely to be followed by a high value. Traditionally, the common way to manage this issue has been to "decluster" the data. This involves using a (typically rule-based) approach to identify clusters of exceedances, and to keep only the maximum value in the cluster. The resulting exceedances should still follow the GPD.

In the case of non-stationary data, it is also possible to model trends parametrically. For instance, if there is clear information that the values in a time series are

[2]These distributions are often presented with slight reparameterisations in different references and textbooks.

increasing over time, the location parameter can be modelled as having a linear trend, for example in a simple case as $\mu(t) = a_0 + a_1 t$. Or, if the occurence of extreme points is related to a covariate, this can also be directly modelled in the same way (time is really a special case of a covariate). Of course, more complex trends will require more sophisticated modelling techniques. We will come back to non-parametric methods for modelling non-stationary time series in Section 11.3.5.

11.3.2 EVT from a point process perspective

We will now take a slightly different approach, which is that of modelling a time series as a point process. We will define a set $\mathscr{M}$ (e.g., a defined period of time), upon which there is some stochastic process that generates events. The point process approach is also valid for higher dimensional space, though we will focus on the two-dimensional case (value vs. time) here. The expected number of points in any subset of the time series is termed the intensity measure of the process: $\Lambda = \mathrm{E}\{N(M)\}$, for every $M \subset \mathscr{M}$. The prototypical example of a point process is the Poisson process (PP), in which we model a homogeneous point process with the number of points according to the Poisson: $P(N(M) = n) = \frac{\lambda^n}{n!}e^{-\lambda}$, where λ is the Poisson parameter. We can also make λ a function of time to allow for a non-homogeneous PP. The general form for the likelihood of the PP is $L(\theta) = \exp(-\Lambda(\mathscr{M}))\prod_{i=1}^{n}\lambda(x_i)$, with $\Lambda(\mathscr{M}) = \int_{\mathscr{M}}\lambda(x)dx$.

We take this approach because it turns out that the block maxima and points-over-threshold models (the GEV and GPD models just presented, respectively) are special cases of the point process approach. This makes the PP model often more useful when modelling in practice because all parameters of both models can be fit simultaneously. Given a sequence of IID random variables, the points that appear above a high threshold u converge to a non-homogeneous PP as the number of points, $n \to \infty$ [16]. The intensity measure for a region $[t_1, t_2]$ can be derived to obtain

$$\Lambda = (t_2 - t_1)\left[1 + \xi\left(\frac{u-\mu}{\sigma}\right)\right]^{-1/\xi} \tag{11.4}$$

The PP likelihood with this intensity measure is then:

$$L \propto \exp\left(-n_y\left[1 + \xi\left(\frac{u-\mu}{\sigma}\right)\right]^{\frac{-1}{\xi}}\right)\prod_{i=1}^{N(A)}\sigma^{-1}\left[1 + \xi\frac{(x_i-\mu)}{\sigma}\right]^{\frac{-1}{\xi}-1} \tag{11.5}$$

where n_y is a scaling parameter (the number of years of data) and $N(A)$ is the number of points exceeding the threshold. The parameters for the PP model for EVT can then be determined via maximum likelihood. Of course, Bayesian methods can also be used if a prior is specified over the model parameters, but we will not go into detail for those here.

The PP approach is therefore very powerful because simply by fitting this single model, we obtain the parameters for the GEV, GPD, and Poisson: μ, σ, ξ, σ_p, λ. We can then use the corresponding models to answer questions about the likelihood of observing a given value as the maximum in a time window, etc.

11.3.3 Practicalities

A few practical questions remain. For instance, how should the threshold be chosen? How should the model fit be evaluated?

In choosing a threshold, this is a trade-off between model bias and variance. A too-low threshold will lead to bias in the model because the assumption of a high threshold, which was needed to derive the limiting approximation, will be violated. A too-high threshold will mean that there is very little data with which to estimate the model, leading to large variance in parameter estimation. One approach is to use a mean residual life plot. In such a plot, the threshold u is varied and the GPD parameters are fit to the training data, D, for each u. A separate plot is then created for each u: m_e, the mean of all excesses above a threshold w, where $u < w < \max(D)$, is plotted against w. While in practice this line will be rather jagged, it should roughly follow a linear trajectory with a slope equal to $\frac{\xi}{1-\xi}$. This comes from the fact that for a set of points $Y = X - u$, $\mathrm{E}(Y - w|y > w) = \frac{\sigma+\xi w}{1-\xi}$. Confidence bands can also be included using Monte Carlo sampling (see Reference 17 for more details).

Another approach for choosing the threshold is to again vary the threshold and assess how the parameters change. If the GPD is an appropriate model, the parameters chosen should be valid for any subset of the data above the high threshold. Therefore, the threshold can be chosen as the point at which the fitted model parameters begin to stabilise.

In some cases, a "high" threshold has already been established through clinical experience. Lab measurements, for instance, typically are accompanied by a reference range. Though this cutoff may need to be adjusted if a particular patient population has consistently elevated or low measurements, it can often serve as a first-estimate threshold. Alternatively, physiological factors may be informative for determining a threshold. For example, IBD patients often have persistently elevated CRP measurements above the "normal" reference maximum of 8 mg/L. However, clinical experience has shown that measurements of up to 40 mg/L are associated with viral infection, and measurements greater than this associated with either bacterial infection or systemic inflammation. Therefore, a cutoff of 40 may prove to be reasonable, depending upon the question at hand.

In regards to model fit, of course standard approaches of using training and validation sets can be used to maximise the log-likelihood. It is also instructive to view the actual density in comparison to a histogram of the underlying data to qualitatively evaluate the model fit. In addition, the overall applicability of the model can be assessed via a quantile plot (Q–Q plot). In a Q–Q plot, the quantiles of the empirical distribution of the data are plotted versus the quantiles of the theoretical distribution (as obtained by the fitted model parameters). In a well-fitting model, the Q–Q plot should yield a line on the unit diagonal. As a note, if a covariate is built into the model (as was presented in the case of a non-stationary time series), the quantiles must be adjusted to take the changing distribution into account. Basically, the modelled variable must be standardised based upon the included covariates (see Reference 16, Chapter 6, for more details). A Q–Q plot can also be used to assess whether points are outliers. Points may appear to be outliers when plotted simply as a histogram, but a Q–Q plot can indicate whether the point is actually in-line with the fitted model.

Particularly in healthcare applications, it may be that all of the measurements are only positive-valued. In this case, it may be necessary to take the natural log transform of the data before fitting the model so as to ensure that the resulting probability distributions only have support over positive values.

In some cases, it is not actually the exceedances of a threshold that are of interest, but the shortfalls. In this case, the same machinery can be used, but the data can simply be transformed so as to make it mirror an extreme distribution. For instance, if examining a set of data D_l where points below a low threshold u_l are of interest, the data can be transformed as $D_T = -D_l + c$ where c is a constant to ensure that all of the resulting data is again in the positive domain (if, for instance, the log transform is taken as described above).

11.3.4 Application of EVT models to healthcare

As presented, the EVT approach is well-suited for problems in which the points of interest are those that are positioned in the extremes. EVT has indeed been applied for many years to applications in environmental and financial applications. Recently, the theory has been extended to model extreme functions, with motivating applications from hospital monitoring of vital signs [18]. Within chronic disease, this theoretical approach has not been widely adopted. However, it is an appropriate model: particularly when examining measurements of blood metabolites for patients over long periods of time, it is often the deviations from normality that are of interest. To capture this information in a probabilistic sense, we can fit the EVT model to training data and use this model to describe and evaluate new patients.

We now present an example of simulated patient data to represent a lab series over time, to illustrate the points from this section of the chapter. For this illustration, we have simply taken a time series as samples from a constant-mean linear function over time, with Gaussian noise. While idealised, this patient time series is representative of the behaviour of many patient blood measurements over time. In Figure 11.3, we show a sample time series, with a histogram of the entire set of simulated data to show the full distribution.

We then use maximum likelihood to fit the μ, σ, ξ, and λ parameters using (11.5). We then find σ_p using (11.3). The effect of varying the threshold is shown in Figure 11.4. As is evident, the μ, σ, and ξ parameters are quite constant as the threshold is varied, showing that any threshold greater than one results in a valid GPD model. As would be expected, as the threshold is increased, the λ parameter will decrease, because there will be fewer exceedances in a given time window.

In Figure 11.5, we show the model fit with $u = 1$. We present superpositions of the empirical histograms with the model probability density functions or probability mass function (in the case of the Poisson), as well as Q–Q plots. As would be expected from such an idealised dataset, the model provides a very good fit to the data.

This model can then be used to ask various questions about a newly seen patient dataset. For example, one could calculate the probability of the number of exceedances

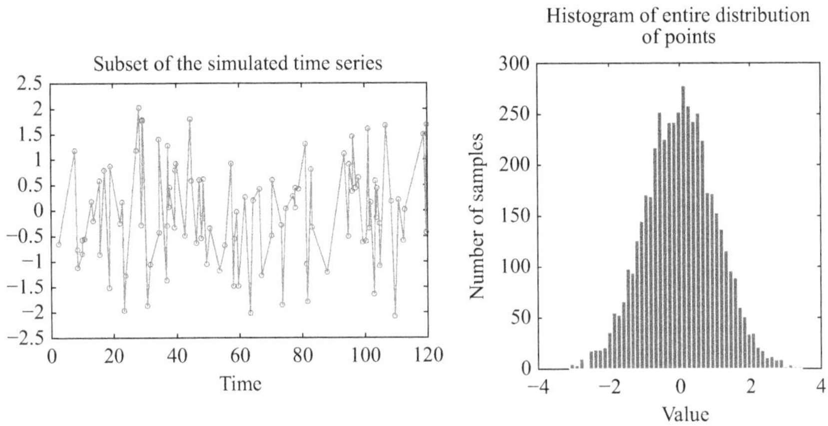

Figure 11.3 Example subset of a simulated time series, and the distribution of the entire set of simulated data

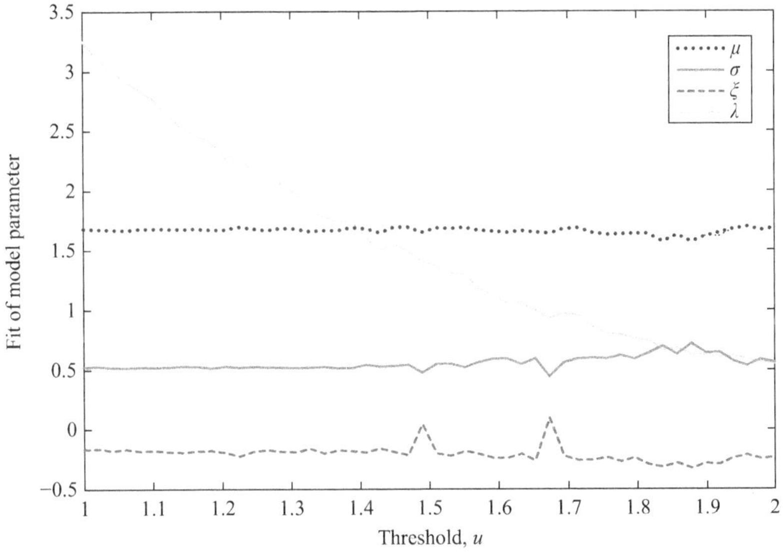

Figure 11.4 Illustration of the effect of varying the cutoff threshold on the values of the fit parameters

seen within a given window of time, or the probability of seeing a given high value. Given enough data, this can be done in a patient-specific manner to make personalised estimates of severity at a given time point. Alternatively, to compare patients across time and cohorts, "severity" scores over time can be created that combine different aspects of these EVT models. For instance, a simple model that makes

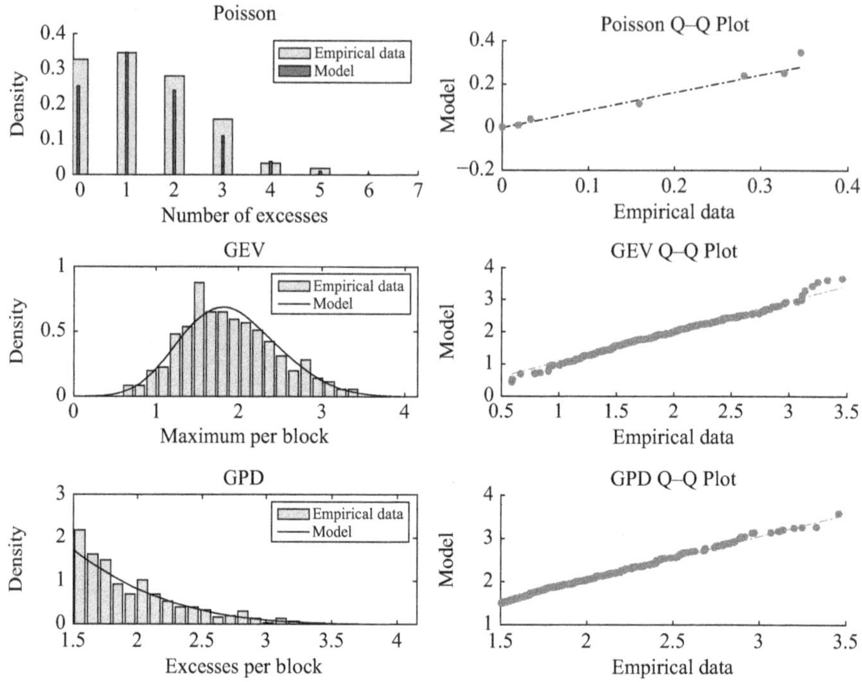

Figure 11.5 Model fit for simulated data extremes

an assumption of independence among the GPD, GEV, and Poisson can be used to combine information across these three characteristics [19].

Of course, in a healthcare application, it is important to validate that the extreme values actually correspond to periods of patient deterioration. This can be done by linking lab measurements with hospital admissions or other metrics of severity. For instance, in IBD, extremely high measurements of CRP are indicative of a relapse event. High CRP measurements in the record typically co-occur with multiple hospital admissions and/or surgery. Thus, probability densities over extreme CRP lab measurements are useful indicators of a patient's physiological state.

Of particular note, measurements are often repeated as a patient is monitored in-hospital, which will invalidate the assumption of the IID nature of the data for a PP. As was mentioned, one approach for dealing with this is to de-cluster the exceedances, so that only the highest value in a cluster of exceedances is retained. More advanced methods are described in the following section.

11.3.5 Advanced topics

As described above, it is possible to directly parameterise changing dynamics over time in an inhomogeneous PP. However, an alternative approach is to allow the complexity of the data itself to determine the model using non-parametric models. For instance, the intensity function can be modelled as a Gaussian process (GP) to provide a smooth function of events over time. Such a model is called a Gaussian Cox process (GCP) or a doubly stochastic PP. The initial presentation of full inference on this model with minimal approximations is from Reference 20. Their model, the sigmoidal GCP, models the intensity function as a GP squashed through a logistic function and scaled by a set maximum intensity. Their inference scheme was through MCMC. There have been further developments on this model recently, with a new variational Bayes scheme for inference [21] as well as an approach for modelling multiple-dependent GCPs [22]. In the latter approach, multiple latent underlying functions are modelled, as well as the parameters for the individual GCPs; the model was fit with multiple types of MCMC, in a similar fashion to the Adams model [20].

11.3.6 Conclusions on EVT

EVT provides a useful way to assess and model "beyond-normal" patient measurements. This is particularly relevant for chronic disease applications, where there may not be readily available data-driven metrics through which to monitor patient severity over time. Such scoring metrics also can be used as input into clustering methods to better elucidate the underlying subtypes of a disease, which often points towards distinct biological mechanisms and involved genetic factors. We now shift towards this question.

11.4 Patient clustering

Many diseases have very heterogeneous trajectories. IBD is one such disease; patients vary greatly in their age of onset, the severity of their initial presentation, the frequency of relapse, the response to medication and surgery, etc. There are many other diseases (e.g., autism, asthma, heart disease) for which this heterogeneity is similar. Indeed, it is likely that within many broad disease categories, there are distinct subtypes [23–27]. Disease subtypes may be related to underlying genetics or to environmental factors that influence changes in gene expression patterns. Better understanding these subtypes will allow for both improved scientific understanding of disease physiology as well as progress towards "precision medicine" by enabling the delivery of personalised treatments.

Unsupervised machine-learning techniques provide a powerful way to probe the types of data now available to identify subgroups of patients. In this section, we will introduce various methodologies that can be used for patient clustering, using EHR and genetic data. Of course, this only represents a subset of possible clustering methods that may be used, and the most appropriate methods will depend on the specific question and the nature of the data. We will provide examples of how the overviewed methods have been extended for specific questions related to disease subtyping.

11.4.1 Clustering overview

There are a number of ways in which one can begin to assess groups of patients with similar characteristics. Of course, in this context any patient must first be represented by a set of features, which may include continuous, binary, categorical, or one of many other data types (as presented in Section 11.2). The input into a clustering model can either be the raw features (i.e., an $N \times D$ matrix, where N is the number of patients and D is the number of features) or a distance matrix specifying the distance between each patient in terms of some specified metric (i.e., a $D \times D$ matrix).

A very common first approach for clustering patient data is hierarchical clustering. Hierarchical clustering involves the iterative joining (or separating, if using divisive clustering) of the "most similar" groups of patients. Distance between data points of course must be defined; some example metrics are shown in Table 11.1. There are additionally a number of ways in which the clusters can be co-joined. In many real-world applications, Ward's criterion, which minimises the covariance within clusters, often results in distinctive cluster identification when other methods (e.g. average linkage, maximum linkage) do not.

Clustering methods for time-series data, such as is available for many chronic disease and critical care medical applications, is often more challenging than clustering of static data because the distance metric between two time-series is less well-defined. Relevant distance metric options include Euclidean distance, Pearson's correlation factor, and dynamic time warping methods [28].

However, hierarchical clustering is heuristic in nature. Another approach is to model the underlying data, rather than defining a distance metric. This has the benefit that new patients can be assigned a probability of belonging to any of the clusters, and the clusters are defined by a generative model. The parameters can therefore be used as identifying descriptions for the given cluster. Particularly within a Bayesian framework, generative mixture models also can very easily handle missing data through marginalisation. The common starting point for such modelling is the Gaussian mixture model (GMM), though depending on one's data types, Bernoulli or categorical mixture models (which follow the same framework) may be appropriate. We will not go into the derivations of mixture modelling here; References 29 and 30 provide excellent introductions to this material. Mixture modelling essentially makes the

Table 11.1 Commonly used distance metrics

Metric	**Type of data**	**Distance formula**
Euclidean	Continuous	$(x_1 - x_2)^2$
City block	Continuous	$\lvert x_1 - x_2 \rvert$
Correlation coefficient	Time series	$\sum_{d=1}^{D} x_{1,d} x_{2,d}$
Hamming	Categorical	$\sum_{d=1}^{D} \mathbf{1}(x_{1,d} \neq x_{2,d})$

For two data points, x_1, x_2, with feature dimension D.

assumption that the underlying data can be separated into discrete latent variables, defined by the number of clusters, K, and a set of parameters to describe the underlying parametric cluster distributions. In a GMM, for instance, these parameters would be the mean μ_k and covariance Σ_k for every cluster.

A challenge, not particular to modelling of chronic disease patients, but certainly encountered in this application, is the high-dimensional nature of the data involved. For instance, suppose we have $D = 500$ continuous clinical measurements available for a set of patients, and we wish to model these patients with a Gaussian mixture model. This means that 628, 754 parameters would need to be fit in order to model $K = 5$ clusters with full covariance functions. While feasible with large numbers of patients, access to patients is often challenging in medical applications; the model becomes impossible to fit if less than 500 patients are available (as will be covered shortly, modifications have been developed to handle this situation). This high-dimensional situation is particularly common when incorporating genetic data. For instance, a full microarray will contain $> 100,000$ SNPs. If the included SNPs are not filtered prior to modelling their distribution across patients, the use of the basic generative clustering models necessitates impossibly large patient sample sizes.

One approach for managing a large number of variables is to regularise the model, for instance by applying L1 (ridge) or L0 (lasso) penalties. Another approach to dealing with the situation of a large number of variables is to assume that the "true" number of variables is much smaller, and that the dimensionality of the problem can be greatly reduced. This is essentially assuming that there is a continuous latent space upon which the data can be projected (in contrast to the discrete latent space of mixture models). These models, latent factor models, attempt to find a low-dimensional representation, L, of some D-dimensional data, X onto a subspace of dimension M. So $L = SX + \varepsilon$, where S is termed the loading matrix (of size M by N), and ε is some Gaussian noise; we will say $W = S^{-1}$. In other words, it is a matrix factorisation of one matrix (X) into two low-rank matrices (W and L). Principal component analysis (PCA), independent component analysis (ICA), and canonical correlation analysis are all special cases of latent factor models.

PCA attempts to find an orthogonal projection of some input data that maximises the variance of the projected data. We can derive PCA in a probabilistic way from our framework above ($X = WL + \varepsilon$), if we assume that the latent variables are normally distributed with isotropic covariance: $L \sim N(\mu, \mathbf{I})$, and that the noise is also Gaussian: $\varepsilon \sim N(\mathbf{0}, \sigma^2\mathbf{I})$. This means that $X|L \sim N(WL, \sigma^2\mathbf{I})$. When maximum likelihood is used to estimate the parameters of this model, this yields the PCA result. The full probabilistic formulation is sometimes termed probabilistic PCA (pPCA). When the model is relaxed and the latent variables are no longer assumed to have a Gaussian distribution, this is equivalent to ICA.

As the above outline derivation suggests, all of these clustering models can be approached from first principles from a Bayesian graphical modelling framework, with priors specifying the required constraints. In linear regression, for example, L1 regularisation is equivalent to placing Gaussian priors over the weight vector. To induce sparsity in the loading matrix S, spike-and-slab and automatic relevance detection (ARD) priors have been proposed. Spike-and-slab priors place large probability mass at zero, with uniform low probability mass elsewhere [31]; ARD priors consist of hyperparameters governing each weight vector (e.g., a Gaussian prior over each weight vector), such that when the values of the hyperparameters approach infinity, a given weight parameter is dropped from the model. Engelhardt and Stephens explain how mixture models can also be formulated as latent factor models, with modelling choices such as Bayesian priors acting as constraints on the matrix factorisation [32]. Reference 33 explains how various model-based mixture methods build upon each other and are related.

When this perspective is taken, it becomes more apparent how to combine design principles to develop a modelling approach specific to the problem at hand. For instance, models have been developed that combine aspects of both latent continuous and discrete variables. These can be viewed as mixtures of pPCA decompositions, so that within each mixture component, there is a different PCA decomposition.

11.4.2 Modelling choices applicable to chronic disease applications

There are many examples of how models may be developed for a particular question in identifying patient subgroups; we present a few examples here. Schulam et al. use a latent variable approach combined with a generative GP model of time series to capture consistent progression trajectories in patients with scleroderma [13]. Scleroderma is a connective tissue disease in which patients may experience different subsets of symptoms to varying degrees. The authors modelled specialised clinical variables and also employed additional covariates to help explain some of the patient variability.

Ross and Dy developed a non-parametric model for clustering chronic obstructive pulmonary disorder (COPD) patient time-series data [34]. They used a Dirichlet mixture of GPs, performing inference using variational methods. They also allowed for domain knowledge through the inclusion of "must-link" and "cannot-link" constraints. Ross et al. further extended this method to allow for certain features to be important only in certain groups and to allow individuals to belong to multiple groups [35]. They formulated this as a dual beta process over GPs, again performing variational inference to determine the most probable clusters in their application of COPD patient subtypes. They related these subgroups to the presence of several genetic mutations known to be associated with certain forms of COPD.

Kirk et al. used a Dirichlet-multinomial allocation mixture model (a finite approximation to a Dirichlet Process mixture model) to integrate multiple datasets [36]. The underlying idea is that the clustering within one dataset informs the clustering in other datasets, which the authors refer to as "correlated clustering." The study used GP models (for time-series gene expression data) combined with multinomial models (for discrete gene expression data), with comparable performance to other clustering methods, but with the advantage of being able to incorporate more than two distinct data types. Kirk et al. applied this method to identify genes with similar behaviour across yeast datasets, but such a method could also conceivably be used to identify clusters of patients with similar disease trajectories.

Zhao et al. developed a Bayesian group factor analysis model, which is an extension of factor models to the case of multiple observation matrices [37]. Their goal is to capture the covariance structure of a low-rank approximation to their original data X. They therefore place a sparsity-inducing prior on the loading matrix S: the three parameter Beta prior. This model is applicable to the problem of finding gene subsets that are co-regulated.

11.4.3 Clustering extensions

While some data is best formulated as a matrix, sometimes it makes more sense as a tensor. Just as matrices can be decomposed, tensors can also be decomposed in various ways. Kolda and Bader provide a review of the general techniques, the most notable of which include Parafac and Tucker decompositions [38]. Parafac decomposition is a generalisation of singular value decomposition (SVD) to higher dimensions, while Tucker decomposition is essentially a higher-dimensional form of PCA. Parafac can be formulated as a special case of Tucker decomposition. In Parafac, a tensor is decomposed into a sum of first-order tensors that describe each dimension of the tensor; in Tucker, a tensor is decomposed into a core, compressed tensor, which is multipled by additional matrices that describe each tensor mode.

Tensor-based methods are particularly appropriate when examining data collected across repeated experiments or consistent time points, such as often encountered with gene expression experiments. For instance, if 300 patients have the same 100 mRNA levels measured across 10 different experiments where various pathways are stimulated, this data naturally makes sense as a $300 \times 100 \times 10$ tensor. A decomposition may reveal which mRNAs are consistently involved across patients in certain types of experimental scenarios. While gene expression data is currently less commonly available in large biobank repositories, this is likely to change in the future.

11.4.4 Practical considerations in unsupervised clustering

An important aspect of clustering is determining the stability of the identified clusters. For instance, just as evaluation of a supervised machine-learning model's performance will involve cross-validation to estimate the model performance across different subsets of the data, an unsupervised clustering across an entire dataset is vulnerable to the idiosyncrasies of the given dataset. To better assess the generality of the identified clusters, it is recommended that the dataset is resampled multiple times to repeatedly evaluate clustering structure.

Of course, since there is usually no known "true" clustering when attempting to identify patient phenotypes, the identified clusters must be compared in some way across sampling iterations. This is not a trivial task, as the cluster label will change with different iterations of the algorithm, and the composition of assigned patients to each cluster will vary (unless the clusters are extremely well defined). If a non-parametric clustering model is being used, then the number of clusters may also vary across iterations. There are many metrics that can be used to compare the similarity of clusters that are generated from the same underlying dataset, some of which are presented in Table 11.2. Each cluster in one iteration of a subsampling can be compared with each cluster in another iteration using one of these metrics to "match" clusters across iterations. The overall consistency across subsamplings can

Table 11.2 Commonly used cluster comparison metrics

Metric	Formula	Intuition
Purity	$\frac{\sum_i (\sum_{j=1}^{K} N_{ij})(\max_j p_{ij})}{N}$	Consistency of group assignments
Rand index (RI)	$\frac{TP+TN}{TP+FP+FN+TN}$	Proportion of "correct" clustering decisions
Mutual information (MI)	$\sum_{i=1}^{R} \sum_{j=1}^{C} P(i,j) \log \frac{P(i,j)}{P_A(i)P_B(j)}$	Overlap between two clusters
Jaccard index (JI)	$\frac{TP}{TP+FP+FN}$	Number shared in both groups divided by total number across both groups

Purity: N_{ij} is the number of class i in class j; $p_{ij} = N_{ij}/(\sum_{j=1}^{K} N_{ij})$; K is the number of classes.
RI, JI: TP = true positive; TN = true negative; FP = false positive; FN = false negative.
MI: R, C = number of clusters in two partitions of the dataset, A and B, respectively.
$P(i, j)$ = probability of patient being in class A_i and B_j; $P_A(i)$ = probability of being in class A_i.
$P_B(i)$ = probability of being in class B_i.

then be compared. While some of these indices, such as the Rand index, rely on a "true" label, a single instance I_0 of the subsampling procedure can be identified as the "true" label, and other clusterings can be compared to I_0 to assess consistency.

Some of these metrics have been further developed to account for chance in cluster similarity. It is particularly important to take chance similarities into account when the number of clusters within the dataset is large. The adjusted Rand index is formulated as $ARI = \frac{RI - I_{exp}}{I_{max} - I_{exp}}$, where RI is the Rand index as above, I_{exp} is the expected index, and I_{max} is the maximum index. The adjusted mutual information follows the same formulation. Assuming two clusterings of a dataset, A and B, the ARI written out fully is

$$ARI = \frac{\sum_{i,j} \binom{n_{ij}}{2} - \frac{\left[\sum_i \binom{a_i}{2} \sum_j \binom{b_j}{s}\right]}{\binom{n}{2}}}{0.5\left[\sum_i \binom{a_i}{2} + \sum_j \binom{b_j}{2}\right] - \frac{\left[\sum_i \binom{a_i}{2} \sum_j \binom{b_j}{s}\right]}{\binom{n}{2}}} \tag{11.6}$$

where n_{ij} is the number of patients contained in both cluster A_i and B_j, a_i is the total number of patients in cluster A_i, and b_i is the total number of patients in cluster B_i.

Figure 11.6 illustrates a comparison of different clustering outcomes, ranging from random class assignments (panel a) to perfect agreement (panel b). As is evident, some metrics require first the matching up of corresponding groups. For instance, the JI is only able to match groups with the same label, yielding a low score even in the case of perfect agreement.

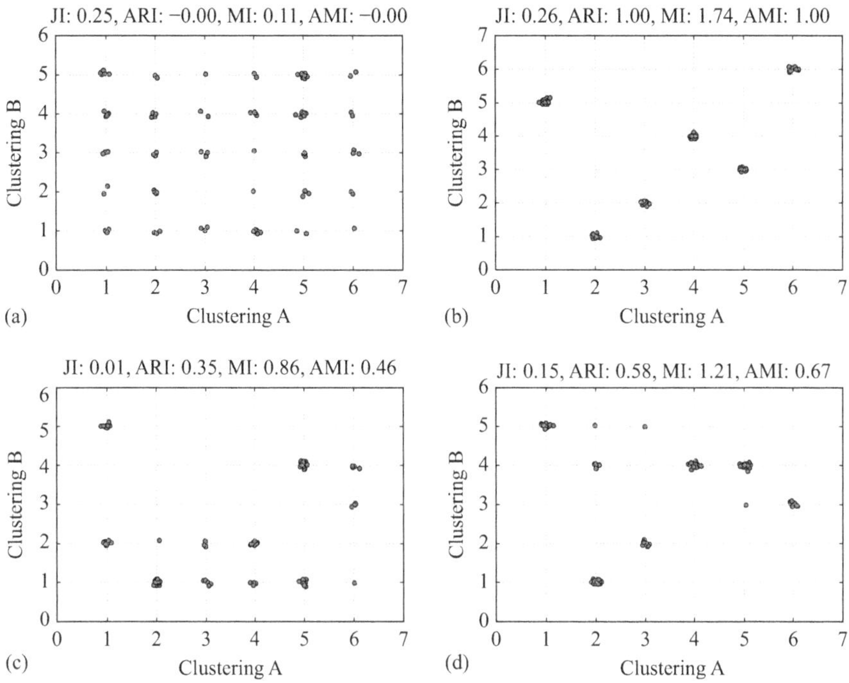

Figure 11.6 *Comparison of various cluster evaluation metrics. (a) Random clustering, (b) perfect agreement between clusters, and (c) and (d) situations between these two extremes. JI = Jaccard index, ARI = adjusted Rand index, MI = mutual information, AMI = adjusted mutual information*

11.4.5 Clustering conclusions

The utility of any identified clusters will depend upon the specific question and whether the featured form of the patient data can answer this question. For instance, a clustering of IBD patients based on various clinical variables may reveal consistent subtypes. However, these groups may not correspond with drug response to infliximab (a last line medication) because the question presented was to find the underlying structure of the input dataset. If patient response to infliximab is determined by some factor not present or captured in the input dataset, then the resulting clusters cannot be expected to be useful for understanding infliximab response. However, since they represent the general structure of the data they might point towards specific sub-populations within the spectrum of IBD symptomology.

If training for a specific outcome is of interest, and it is believed that there is latent structure in the data, then unsupervised approaches can also be used within two-step algorithms, to generate features as input for secondary supervised analyses.

This is particularly appropriate when it is unclear which aspects of the data may be discriminatory (e.g., within a complex physiologic time series), but it is suspected that underlying structure in the data does exist and correlates to the desired outcome predictor variable. This approach is taken, for example, by Reference 39.

11.5 Conclusion

Here, we have presented illustrations of how techniques from machine learning can be used specifically for the purposes of modelling chronic disease. EVT provides a method by which to assess patient severity by providing a principled framework for defining how "abnormal" an extreme measurement may be. This is particularly beneficial for chronic disease applications in which fluctuations of measurements within the normal range are not relevant for treatment, but in which deviations outside of this range become important. We have also explained how clustering techniques can be used to probe the underlying structure of large disease phenotypic cohorts to uncover latent sub-phenotypes. Given the growing evidence that many chronic diseases are in fact composed of patient with similar but distinct underlying disease mechanisms, these methods are particularly important in the application area of chronic disease. The high-dimensional nature of genetic data, combined with the variety of data types commonly encountered in patient databases, motivates the use of specialised clustering techniques, as discussed. The growing availability of data and the increasing research focus on novel machine-learning approaches suggests that the modelling of chronic disease will continue to yield beneficial findings for patients and doctors.

References

[1] A. Chatterjee, S. Kubendran, J. King, and R. DeVol, "Checkup time: chronic disease and wellness in America," *Milken Institute*, 2014.

[2] I. S. Group, "IBD standards: standards for the healthcare of people who have inflammatory bowel disease (IBD), 2013 update," 2013.

[3] A. N. Ananthakrishnan, "Epidemiology and risk factors for IBD," *Nature Reviews Gastroenterology & Hepatology*, 2015.

[4] P. B. Jensen, L. J. Jensen, and S. Brunak, "Mining electronic health records: towards better research applications and clinical care," *Nature Reviews Genetics*, vol. 13, no. 6, pp. 395–405, 2012.

[5] O. Gottesman, H. Kuivaniemi, G. Tromp, *et al.*, "The electronic medical records and genomics (eMERGE) network: past, present, and future," *Genetics in Medicine*, vol. 15, no. 10, pp. 761–771, 2013.

[6] D. Gotz, F. Wang, and A. Perer, "A methodology for interactive mining and visual analysis of clinical event patterns using electronic health record data," *Journal of Biomedical Informatics*, vol. 48, pp. 148–159, 2014.

[7] eMERGE, *PheKB: Phenotype KnowledgeBase*. [Online]. Available: http://phenotype.mc.vanderbilt.edu/, 2012.

[8] G. Hripcsak and D. J. Albers, "Next-generation phenotyping of electronic health records," *Journal of the American Medical Informatics Association*, vol. 20, no. 1, pp. 117–121, 2013.

[9] C. Paxton, A. Niculescu-Mizil, and S. Saria, "Developing predictive models using electronic medical records: challenges and pitfalls," in *AMIA Annual Symposium Proceedings*, vol. 2013. American Medical Informatics Association, 2013, p. 1109.

[10] L. Tarassenko, D. A. Clifton, M. R. Pinsky, M. T. Hravnak, J. R. Woods, and P. J. Watkinson, "Centile-based early warning scores derived from statistical distributions of vital signs," *Resuscitation*, vol. 82, no. 8, pp. 1013–1018, 2011.

[11] F. Doshi-Velez, Y. Ge, and I. Kohane, "Comorbidity clusters in autism spectrum disorders: an electronic health record time-series analysis," *Pediatrics*, vol. 133, no. 1, pp. e54–e63, 2014.

[12] B. Kim, J. A. Shah, and F. Doshi-Velez, "Mind the gap: a generative approach to interpretable feature selection and extraction," in *Advances in Neural Information Processing Systems*, 2015, pp. 2251–2259.

[13] P. Schulam, F. Wigley, and S. Saria, "Clustering longitudinal clinical marker trajectories from electronic health data: applications to phenotyping and endotype discovery," in *Twenty-Ninth AAAI Conference on Artificial Intelligence*, 2015.

[14] P. Schulam and S. Saria, "A framework for individualizing predictions of disease trajectories by exploiting multi-resolution structure," in *Advances in Neural Information Processing Systems*, 2015, pp. 748–756.

[15] P. Stankiewicz and J. R. Lupski, "Structural variation in the human genome and its role in disease," *Annual Review of Medicine*, vol. 61, pp. 437–455, 2010.

[16] S. Coles, J. Bawa, L. Trenner, and P. Dorazio, *An Introduction to Statistical Modeling of Extreme Values*. vol. 208, Springer, 2001.

[17] R. Smith, "Extreme value statistics in meteorology and the environment," *Environmental Statistics*, vol. 8, pp. 300–357, 2001.

[18] D. A. Clifton, L. Clifton, S. Hugueny, D. Wong, and L. Tarassenko, "An extreme function theory for novelty detection," *Selected Topics in Signal Processing, IEEE Journal of*, vol. 7, no. 1, pp. 28–37, 2013.

[19] K. E. Niehaus, H. H. Uhlig, and D. A. Clifton, "Phenotypic characterisation of Crohn's disease severity," in *Engineering in Medicine and Biology Society (EMBC), 2015 37th Annual International Conference of the IEEE*. IEEE, 2015, pp. 7023–7026.

[20] R. P. Adams, I. Murray, and D. J. MacKay, "Tractable nonparametric bayesian inference in Poisson processes with gaussian process intensities," in *Proceedings of the 26th Annual International Conference on Machine Learning*. ACM, 2009, pp. 9–16.

[21] C. Lloyd, T. Gunter, M. A. Osborne, and S. J. Roberts, "Variational inference for Gaussian process modulated Poisson processes," *International Conference on Machine Learning*, 2015.

[22] T. Gunter, C. Lloyd, M. A. Osborne, and S. J. Roberts, "Efficient Bayesian nonparametric modelling of structured point processes," *arXiv preprint arXiv:1407.6949*, 2014.

[23] I. S. Kohane, "Deeper, longer phenotyping to accelerate the discovery of the genetic architectures of diseases," *Genome Biology*, vol. 15, no. 5, p. 115, 2014.

[24] M. W. State and N. Šestan, "The emerging biology of autism spectrum disorders," *Science (New York, NY)*, vol. 337, no. 6100, p. 1301, 2012.

[25] J. Lötvall, C. A. Akdis, L. B. Bacharier, *et al.*, "Asthma endotypes: a new approach to classification of disease entities within the asthma syndrome," *Journal of Allergy and Clinical Immunology*, vol. 127, no. 2, pp. 355–360, 2011.

[26] G. W. De Keulenaer and D. L. Brutsaert, "The heart failure spectrum time for a phenotype-oriented approach," *Circulation*, vol. 119, no. 24, pp. 3044–3046, 2009.

[27] J. Loscalzo, I. Kohane, and A.-L. Barabasi, "Human disease classification in the postgenomic era: a complex systems approach to human pathobiology," *Molecular Systems Biology*, vol. 3, no. 1, 2007.

[28] T. Warren Liao, "Clustering of time series data: a survey," *Pattern Recognition*, vol. 38, no. 11, pp. 1857–1874, 2005.

[29] C. M. Bishop, *Pattern Recognition and Machine Learning (Information Science and Statistics)*. Secaucus, NJ, USA: Springer-Verlag New York, Inc., 2006.

[30] K. P. Murphy, *Machine Learning: A Probabilistic Perspective*. MIT Press, 2012.

[31] T. J. Mitchell and J. J. Beauchamp, "Bayesian variable selection in linear regression," *Journal of the American Statistical Association*, vol. 83, no. 404, pp. 1023–1032, 1988.

[32] B. E. Engelhardt and M. Stephens, "Analysis of population structure: a unifying framework and novel methods based on sparse factor analysis," *PLoS Genet*, vol. 6, no. 9, p. e1001117, 2010.

[33] C. Bouveyron and C. Brunet-Saumard, "Model-based clustering of high-dimensional data: a review," *Computational Statistics & Data Analysis*, vol. 71, pp. 52–78, 2014.

[34] J. Ross and J. Dy, "Nonparametric mixture of gaussian processes with constraints," in *Proceedings of the 30th International Conference on Machine Learning (ICML-13)*, 2013, pp. 1346–1354.

[35] J. C. Ross, P. J. Castaldi, M. H. Cho, and J. G. Dy, "Dual beta process priors for latent cluster discovery in chronic obstructive pulmonary disease," in *Proceedings of the 20th ACM SIGKDD International Conference on Knowledge Discovery and Data Mining*. ACM, 2014, pp. 155–162.

[36] P. Kirk, J. E. Griffin, R. S. Savage, Z. Ghahramani, and D. L. Wild, "Bayesian correlated clustering to integrate multiple datasets," *Bioinformatics*, vol. 28, no. 24, pp. 3290–3297, 2012.

[37] S. Zhao, C. Gao, S. Mukherjee, and B. E. Engelhardt, "Bayesian group latent factor analysis with structured sparse priors," *arXiv preprint arXiv:1411.2698*, 2014.

[38] T. G. Kolda and B. W. Bader, "Tensor decompositions and applications," *SIAM Review*, vol. 51, no. 3, pp. 455–500, 2009.

[39] B. M. Marlin, D. C. Kale, R. G. Khemani, and R. C. Wetzel, "Unsupervised pattern discovery in electronic health care data using probabilistic clustering models," in *Proceedings of the 2nd ACM SIGHIT International Health Informatics Symposium*. ACM, 2012, pp. 389–398.

Chapter 12
Big data and optimisation of treatment strategies

Shamim Nemati and Mohammad M. Ghassemi

12.1 Introduction

Deviations from established treatment protocols in a complex clinical environment, such as the intensive care unit (ICU), are both common and often necessary. While some of these deviations are errors, which can result in harmful outcomes [1,2], others are innovative adjustments made by clinicians to adapt treatments to individual patients. Clinicians often refer clinical context, patient preference, provider bias, prior training and experience, local medical practice, and lack of (or conflicting) randomised clinical trials (RCTs)-based evidence as some of the driving factors behind variability in clinical practice. For instance, the decision to administer intravenous fluids or vasoactive agents, and the volume or dose chosen largely depends on local practice patterns, and unsystematic process-related factors at the time of the hypotensive event [3]. While this can be potentially dangerous from a patient safety viewpoint, it provides a unique opportunity for learning optimal treatment policies from clinical databases. A major assumption we make in this chapter is that given a large patient cohort (or the so-called clinical "big data"), the inherent variability in the patient care allows for adequately exploring the space of possible patient phenotypes and corresponding clinical actions to arrive at optimal treatment strategies (or *policies*).

Medication dosing is one example where deviations from the policy and error are common [4,5]. For many drugs, these errors are harmless; however, misdoing medications with sensitive therapeutic windows, such as Heparin (an anticoagulant drug), can place patients at unnecessary risk [6]. Too much Heparin and the patient can bleed to death. Too little, and a blood clot may cause a stroke [7]. In practice, patients who are over- or under-dosed can experience issues which may unnecessarily extend their hospital length of stay, or require additional follow-up interventions, driving up costs, and reducing hospital productivity. The same holds true for warfarin (an oral anticoagulant used to prevent heart attacks and strokes) which is currently being used by 20 million patients in the United States alone, and requires frequent office visits for blood tests and dose management. Adjustment of such medications can be challenging not only due to their narrow therapeutic window and variation in individual responses but also due to patient factors, physician factors, or regional practice variations and sub-optimal patient management may also occur. Systematic reviews have estimated that less than 50% of patients receive oral anticoagulation therapy on a routine basis and that patients are in the therapeutic range only 64% of the time [8].

In this chapter, we look at how machine-learning techniques for classification, prediction, and sequential decision-making (such as *reinforcement learning*) can be used to learn actionable policies for medication dosing from the clinical big data. The former two belong to the class of single-stage decision-making methods, while the latter tackles the problem of multistage decision-making [9]. The need for sequential decision-making algorithms arises in clinical practice due to the fact that treatments often consist of a sequence of clinical actions without any immediate feedback, which makes it difficult to assign credit or blame to every single action, when considering the final patient outcome. To illustrate this point, we provide an example of dosing of Heparin in ICU patients from a large-scale retrospective clinical database to demonstrate the utility of data-driven techniques to both minimise dosing error and the total amount of time patients spend outside of their therapeutic windows.

Translating statistical relationships to treatment policies however is a non-trivial task. Algorithms must have the ability to begin with simple population-level assumptions, based on sparse data available at admission, and gradually evolve into increasingly patient-specific estimates as the length of stay, and individual data density increases. Such online methods have been explored for a variety of phenomenon, especially mortality prediction. The factors that may influence a patient's mortality (genomic, molecular or cellular, lifestyle and social factors being among them) are so immense however that only with the advent of clinical big data [10], we may begin to adequately sample the space of possible factors (or feature), in order to achieve clinically acceptable levels of predictive generalisability. Even for drugs with limited serious misdosing risks, dosing adjustments should still, in principal, be designed such that the number of trials to reach the state intended by the physician is minimal. That is, an ideal data-driven approach should empower clinicians to accomplish their goals more quickly and effectively, not dictate those goals themselves.

12.2 Heparin dosing as an illustrative example

Figure 12.1 shows a typical Heparin dosing trial. A trial begins by intravenous administration of first dosage of Heparin based on patient's weight. Within 4–6 h a laboratory test is performed to determine the activated partial thromboplastin time (aPTT), which is an indicator of time it takes for blood to form clot, and a decision is made to increase or decrease the Heparin dosage. Our goal is to devise an optimal dosing strategy that not only takes into account a patient's aPTT level but also his/her evolving clinical phenotype, by incorporating commonly recorded time series of clinical measurements within the patient's electronic medical record (EMR).

The example shown in Figure 12.1 was selected from the publicly available multiparameter intelligent monitoring in intensive care (MIMIC) database [11]. MIMIC contains structured and unstructured clinical data from over 30,000 critical care

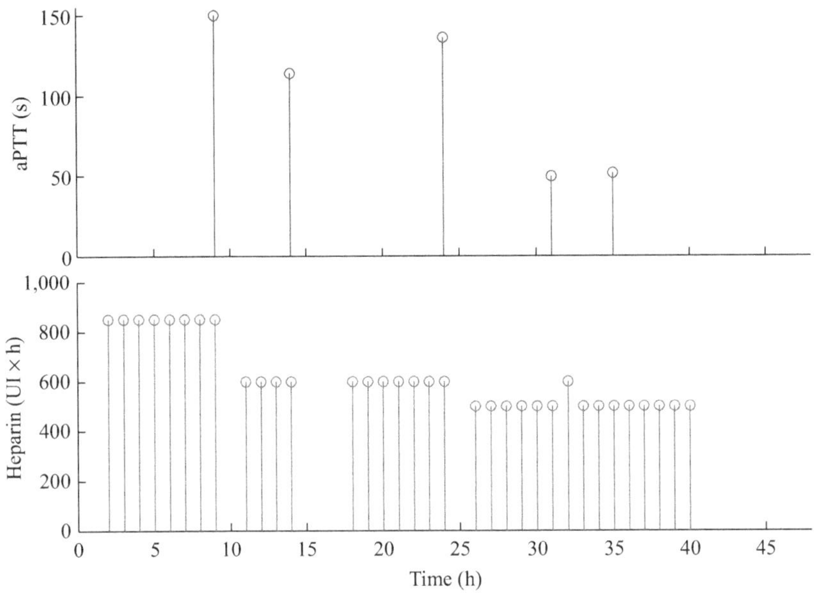

Figure 12.1 An example of Heparin dosing. Each trial starts with an initial dosing of Heparin (bottom plot) followed by sequential adjustments over the next 24–48 h upon availability of new test results (aPTT; top plot) and according to a hospital dosing protocol/policy. An aPTT of 60–100 s is often considered therapeutic. If the aPTT value is too high, clinicians may (over) react by turning the drip off, resulting in zero Heparin levels

patients at the Beth Israel Deaconess Medical Center in Boston, Massachusetts from 2001 to 2008. We extracted 4,470 patients from MIMIC which received a Heparin intravenous infusion at some point during their ICU stay (randomly assigned to 80% training and 20% testing sets). Our extracted features included Heparin dose level and aPTT measurements over the last 4 h, comprehensive laboratory measurements (such as vital signs, white blood count, haematocrit) updated hourly or otherwise interpolated using sample-and-hold, and all known static confounders of Heparin dosing (such as age, gender, ethnicity, existence of pulmonary embolism) according to the previous work by Ghassemi *et al.* [12].

For all patients we extracted the first 48 h of asynchronous continuous measures from MIMIC, starting from the time of Heparin initiation. These measures included: arterial carbon dioxide (CO_2) level, heart rate (HR), aPTT, Heparin dose, albumin, systolic and diastolic arterial blood pressure (SBP and DBP), bilirubin, creatinine, Glasgow Coma Score (GCS), haematocrit, haemoglobin, international normalised ratio (INR) of prothrombin, blood pH, platelet count, prothrombin time, respiration rate, oxygen saturation of arterial blood (SaO2), daily Sequential Organ

Failure Assessment (SOFA) scores, temperature, troponin, urea, and white blood cell (WBC) count. Additionally, we collected the following binary indicators: ethnicity (white/non-white), ICU service type (surgical/medical), gender, transfer from another hospital, pulmonary embolism, and obesity. We also extracted the following continuous static features: age and weight. From these measures, aPTT was selected as the outcome of interest. We excluded all patients which were transferred from another institution as we had no way of accessing their medication history.

For prediction and classification purposes (as described below), we evenly sampled the data into 8-h bins, while for the sequential decision-making we utilised 1-h bins (multiple measurements within the same time bin were replaced by their median value). To account for missing values, we utilised sample-and-hold interpolation which we consider the most practical form of interpolation at the bedside, given the non-random (and generally unknown) nature of the missing data in most clinical settings. A subset of the extracted features was selected for inclusion in our model by discarding those which were missing more than 10% of their data. This threshold was chosen based on the number of missing data-points observed in the weight-normalised Heparin dose (which was also 10%). We performed a two-sample t-test to test the null hypothesis that the distribution of features in our final cohort was representative of the population which received Heparin, which could not be rejected at $p = 0.05$ significance level. This shows that our extracted cohort is, for the most part, representative of the population available in MIMIC.

12.2.1 Medication dosing as a classification problem

Let x and y represent all available clinical data for a patient (i.e., features) and the target medication dose level we are trying to optimize, respectively. Generally, x and y are time series; henceforth we use the superscript n to index a time bin, and the subscript i to index the ith patient. Moreover, we use the notation $1{:}n$ to denote a time-range. When dosing medications, patients may be thought of as taking on one of three therapeutic states $S = \textit{Therapeutic, Sub-therapeutic, Supra-therapeutic}$. According to the guidelines at the Beth Israel Deaconess Medical Center, the continuous aPTT ranges which define these states are:

$$S(aPTT) = \begin{cases} \textit{Supra-therapeutic} & aPTT > u \\ \textit{Therapeutic} & l \leq aPTT \leq u \\ \textit{Sub-therapeutic} & aPTT < l \end{cases}$$

where u and l describe the upper and lower bounds of the therapeutic state, respectively. In the categorical approach, our goal is to estimate the probability of patient i being in state s at time n using a combination of data from the population training set, x_p and y_p, and the available individual measurements $x_i^{1:n-1}, y_i^{1:n-1}$:

$$p(S_i^n = s | x_p, y_p, x_i^{1:n-1}, y_i^{1:n-1}, \theta_i^n) \tag{12.1}$$

where θ_i^n describes the parameters of our chosen model, and is determined by minimising the sum of squared error (SSE) cost function. In Ghassemi *et al.* [12], a simple method to estimate the optimal setting of a patient's initial dose was described.

This form can be extended to estimate the probability of supra- and sub-therapeutic aPTT at each stage as:

$$p(S_i^n = supra) = \frac{1}{1 + e^{-(\beta_{i,o}^n d_i^n + \kappa_{i,o}^n)}} \tag{12.2}$$

$$p(S_i^n = sub) = \frac{1}{1 + e^{-(\beta_{i,u}^n d_i^n + \kappa_{i,u}^n)}} \tag{12.3}$$

where β models the effects of dose d on the state probability and κ models the effects of the other selected features on the state probability estimate ($\beta_{i,o}^n, \beta_{i,u}^n, \kappa_{i,o}^n, \kappa_{i,u}^n \in \theta_i^n$ and $d \in x_i^n$). It follows from (12.2) and (12.3) that the probability of a therapeutic dose may be estimated as:

$$p(S_i^n = therapeutic) = 1 - [p(S_i^n = supra) + p(S_i^n = sub)] \tag{12.4}$$

The optimal Heparin dose at each interval (n) then corresponds to the dose value which jointly minimises the probability of overshoot and undershoot modelled by supra- and sub-therapeutic sigmoidals. Given the monotonic natures of the functions, this joint minimum will always occur where the curves intersect:

$$d_i^n = \frac{\kappa_{i,u}^n - \kappa_{i,o}^n}{\beta_{i,o}^n - \beta_{i,u}^n} \tag{12.5}$$

This form allows a clinician to, at each aPTT draw, prescribe an increasingly individualised dose, with an optimal probability of yielding a therapeutic state.

We estimate the optimal model parameters at each stage (θ_i^n), through a slight modification to the cost function of the supra- and sub-therapeutic logistic generalized linear models, which include weighted population and patient specific residuals:

$$SSE_i^n = \sum_{n'=1}^{M} (r_p^{n'})^2 + \sum_{n'=1}^{n-1} (\phi(n') r_i^{n'})^2 \tag{12.6}$$

$$SSE_i^n = SSE_p + \sum_{n'=1}^{n-1} (\phi(n')(y_i^{n'} - \hat{y}_i^{n'})^2 \tag{12.7}$$

where M denotes the size of the population data, and the population and individual residuals are denoted by $r_p^{n'}$ and $r_i^{n'}$, respectively. The function $\phi(\cdot)$ describes the weight of the individual residuals as a function of dosing stage. In our case, the function was chosen to be of a sigmoidal form:

$$\phi(n) = \frac{\alpha}{N(1 + e^{-(\gamma_0 + \gamma_1 n)})} \tag{12.8}$$

where the α and γ parameters control the shape and magnitude of the weighting function ($\alpha, \gamma \in \theta$). The optimal parameter values in (12.6) and (12.7), $\arg\min_{\theta_i^n} SSE_i^n$ can then be selected using any of the standard global optimisation techniques including scatter search, genetic algorithm, or Bayesian optimisation [13]. In our case, simple scatter search was deployed.

To ensure the integrity of our results, we employed leave-one-out cross-validation (LOOCV). For each fold, patients falling into the training set simulate a known "population" at the hospital, while the testing data simulates an individual patient with sequentially available incoming data streams. Given the retrospective nature of our dataset, comparing the performance of our model against clinicians will require us to make certain assumptions about clinical intent at the time of each aPTT draw. Our task is thus to develop a fair measure of error. If we assume that clinicians are aiming to bring all patients to the therapeutic state, each time they adjust the dose (i.e., we assume that clinicians do not intend to over- or underdose the patients), then we can define error as the proportion of non-therapeutic subjects at each state, which resulted from the dose. We compared the area under the curve (AUC) measure of the $p(S)$ for each of the three states, in addition to the overall state classification performance of our model, versus the performance of the clinician for comparison. Once again, as we do not know the clinician's true intent, we assume that clinicians were attempting to dose Heparin to bring patients to the therapeutic state.

We acknowledge that there may be circumstances where the above assumption is invalid. It is possible, particularly for patients at risk for bleeding [14], that clinicians may intentionally underdose Heparin to mitigate the probability of an adverse reaction. It follows that we may be unfairly penalising the clinician's performance by misjudging what their actual intentions were when providing the dose. To account for this, we performed a subgroup analysis in which we excluded any patient whose final aPTT state after dose adjustment was sub-therapeutic. By excluding these patients, we can be more certain of the validity in our assumption, that is, a clinician's goal at each dose adjustment was to bring the patient into the therapeutic state. This in turn allows us to more robustly compare our model against the clinicians.

Figure 12.2 illustrates the number of subjects receiving multiple sequential aPTT draws, partitioned by therapeutic state. The figure highlights that misdoing remains consistently problematic even after multiple aPTT draws (and consequent opportunities for dose adjustment). Importantly, over 80% of our sample stopped receiving aPTT draws after their fifth draw and a mere 5% of the original 3,883 patient sample had a sixth aPTT draw.

In Figure 12.3, we show the magnitude of aPTT estimation error made by clinicians at each aPTT and compare it to the population and individualised model estimates. We observed a statistically significant decrease in model error using the individualised approach, when compared to the clinician (assuming a clinician goal of aPTT = 80), and the population-level model which does not explicitly account for individual error. We observed a statistically significant decrease in the error ($p < 0.05$ according to a two-sample t-test) for the individualised model when compared to the population model for the third, through the sixth aPTT draw (Table 12.1). In Figure 12.4, we show the same analysis after excluding patients whose final therapeutic state was sub-therapeutic. In this case, we observe a statistically significant decrease in dosing error from the third, through the fifth aPTT draws for the individual model when compared to the population or clinician performance.

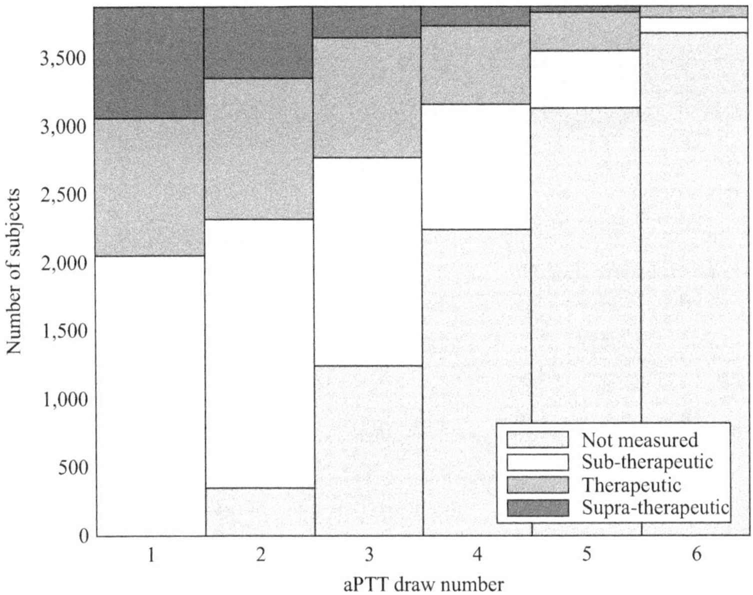

Figure 12.2 The aPTT state distribution of the patient cohort after various aPTT draws

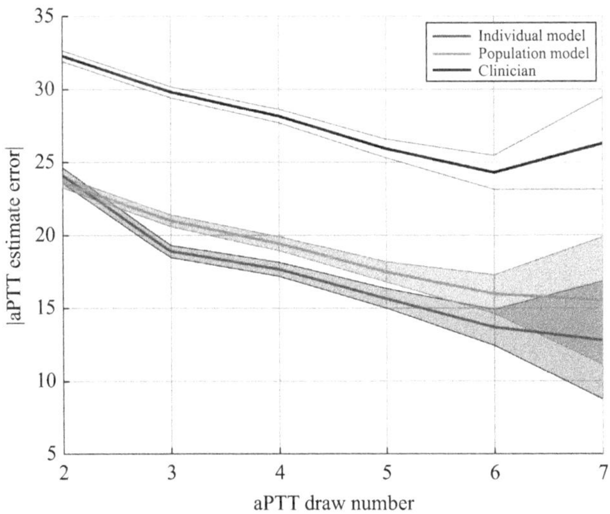

Figure 12.3 The magnitude of aPTT estimation error at successive draws for the individual (bottom) and population (middle) models compared to the clinician (top). The first draw is reported in the main text. The shaded areas around each line segment represent the standard error of each estimate. p-value < 0.05 for aPTT draw numbers less than 8. p-value < 0.05 for aPTT draws less than 6 and greater than 2 between the population and individual model according to the Wilcox rank sum test

Table 12.1 Population model for continuous aPTT

	Estimate	SE	*t*-Statistic	*p*-Value
Intercept	−7.45	28.68	−0.26	0.80
Age	0.19	0.03	5.99	0.00
Dose (units/kg)	1.92	0.11	17.05	0.00
Gender (male)	−5.90	0.95	−6.21	0.00
ICU type (surgical)	−7.85	0.99	−7.93	0.00
Ethnicity (white)	−3.65	0.99	−3.68	0.00
Transfer	−4.15	0.96	−4.31	0.00
End-stage renal disease (ESRD)	3.71	2.70	1.37	0.17
Treatment of pulmonary embolism	6.52	1.59	4.11	0.00
CO_2	−0.22	0.10	−2.23	0.03
HR	0.01	0.03	0.26	0.79
Creatinine	−0.11	0.41	−0.28	0.78
GCS	0.14	0.13	1.03	0.30
Haematocrit	0.64	0.28	2.24	0.02
Haemoglobin	−1.15	0.81	−1.41	0.16
INR	6.13	1.22	5.03	0.00
Platelet	−0.02	0.00	−5.43	0.00
prothrombin time	0.97	0.21	4.68	0.00
Peripheral capillary oxygen saturation	0.47	0.18	2.54	0.01
Temperature	−0.27	0.21	−1.31	0.19
Urea	0.07	0.03	2.52	0.01
WBC	0.13	0.08	1.60	0.11

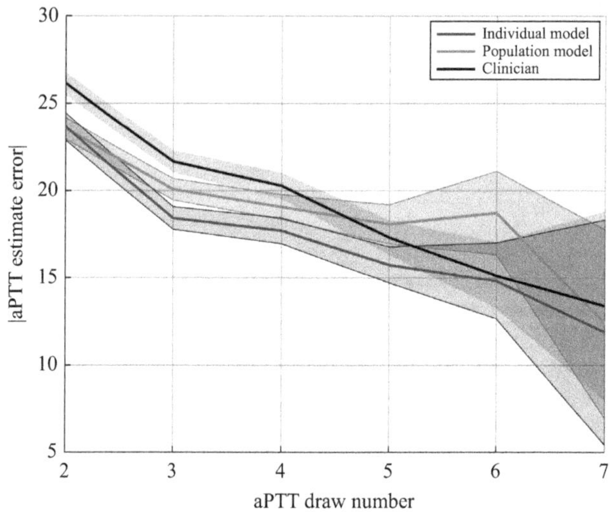

Figure 12.4 The magnitude of aPTT estimate error at successive draws for the individual (bottom) and population (middle) models compared to the clinician (top) excluding those patients with a final aPTT draw which was sub-therapeutic. The first draw is reported in the main text. The shaded areas around each line segment represent the standard error of each estimate. p-value < 0.05 for aPTT draw numbers less than 6. p-value < 0.05 for aPTT draws less than 6 and greater than 2 between the population and individual model according to the Wilcox rank sum test

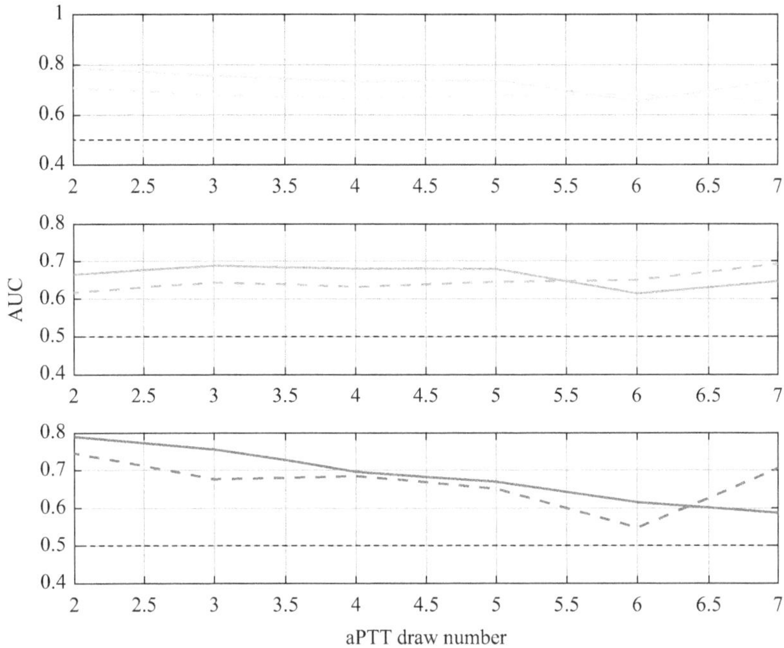

Figure 12.5 A comparison of the population and individual model AUCs for each state, at each stage in the dosing process. The individual model is represented as a solid line while the population model is represented as a dashed line. The top, middle, and bottom plots represent sub-therapeutic, therapeutic, and supra-therapeutic AUC, respectively

In Figure 12.5, we illustrate the AUC of our categorical approach for the prediction of sub-therapeutic, supra-therapeutic, and therapeutic aPTT states. For all three states, we see an improvement in the performance of the individualised method when compared to the population-based approach up until the fifth aPTT draw. The performance of the individualised model at the sixth and seventh draws, where the cohort sizes are much smaller, is less reliable. The average improvement across AUC draws is 0.07%, 0.044%, and 0.038% for the sub-therapeutic, therapeutic, and supra-therapeutic classification AUCs, respectively (Table 12.2). The same performance plot, excluding patients whose final state was sub-therapeutic, is shown in Figure 12.6. Here we observe even stronger performance for our model, with increased AUC of 0.081%, 0.075%, and 0.038% for the sub-therapeutic, therapeutic, and supra-therapeutic classifications, respectively. The average improvement in AUC above the performance of the clinician was 0.178% for the individual model and 0.135% for the population-level model. For the subgroup of patients whose final state was not sub-therapeutic, we observed an average increase in AUC of 0.058% for the population-level model versus 0.13% for the individualised model.

Table 12.2 The average p-values for each of our features in the overshoot and undershoot cases

	Overshoot *p*-values	Undershoot *p*-values
Intercept	0.0821	0.0449
Age	0.0225	0.0173
Dose/weight	0.0004	0.0000
Gender (male)	0.0088	0.0422
ICU service type	0.0056	0.0044
Ethnicity	0.0550	0.1359
Transfer flag	0.0259	0.1143
End-stage renal disease	0.2494	0.3553
Pulmonary embolism	0.0852	0.0023
CO_2	0.1382	0.0789
Heart rate	0.0840	0.1145
Creatinine	0.4454	0.3550
GCS	0.1138	0.0945
Haematocrit	0.0442	0.0326
Haemoglobin	0.0869	0.0544
INR	0.0211	0.3134
Platelet	0.0183	0.0421
Prothrombin time	0.1009	0.0073
Peripheral capillary oxygen saturation	0.1043	0.2670
Temperature	0.1156	0.2785
Urea	0.0662	0.0517
WBC	0.0698	0.2979

In Figures 12.7 and 12.8, we compare the classification performance of our approach against the clinician both with, and without the sub-therapeutic cohort. In both cases, we observe a significant improvement in the classification performance of the individualised model when compared to the population-based model. Importantly, Figure 12.8 shows that the population model underperforms the clinician by the fourth dose adjustment while the individualised model consistently outperforms the clinician.

12.2.2 Medication dosing as a prediction problem

At the population level, we assume a linear relationship between continuous aPTT ($\hat{y}_p$) and our feature set (X, which includes Heparin dose):

$$\hat{y}_p = X\beta - \varepsilon \tag{12.9}$$

In this model, ε models the effects of all covariates not explicitly accounted for by other model parameters (β). Given the random effects imposed by the error term, the value of the parameters that minimise the SSE cost function will estimate the

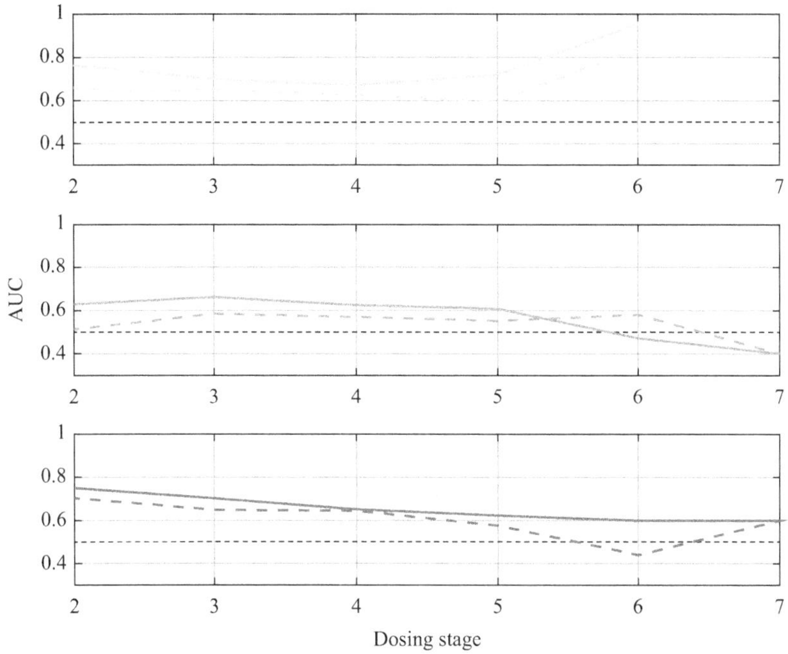

Figure 12.6 A Comparison of the population and individual model AUCs for each state, at each stage in the dosing process, excluding patients whose final aPTT state was sub-therapeutic. The individual model is represented as a solid line while the population model is represented as a dashed line. The top, middle, and bottom plots represents sub-therapeutic, therapeutic, and supra-therapeutic AUC, respectively

mean of the outcome $\hat{y}_p$ for the training population. One simple way to adapt this population-level estimate to an individual estimate is to simply identify the error of the population-based estimate $\hat{y}_p$ for each individual. Such a model would be of the following form:

$$\hat{y}_i = \hat{y}_p + \hat{\varepsilon}_i \tag{12.10}$$

where $\hat{y}_i$ describes the aPTT estimate for the individual, i, as a function of the population estimate, after correcting for the estimated individual error ε_i. The estimate of the individual error, however, can only be inferred as individual patient data becomes available, which demands a model of the following form:

$$\hat{y}_i^n = \begin{cases} \hat{y}_p, & \text{if } n = 1 \\ \hat{y}_p + \hat{\varepsilon}_i^n, & \text{if } n > 1 \end{cases}$$

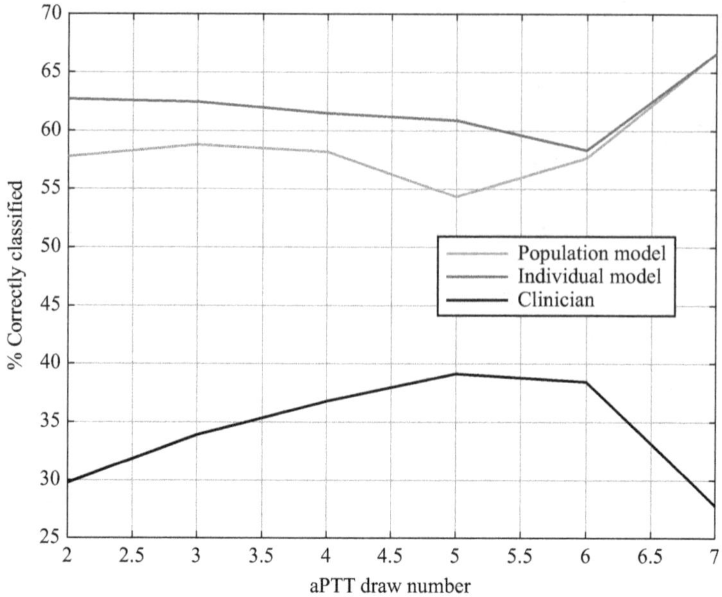

Figure 12.7 A comparison of the classification performance of the population model, the individual model, and clinician at each of the dose adjustment stages

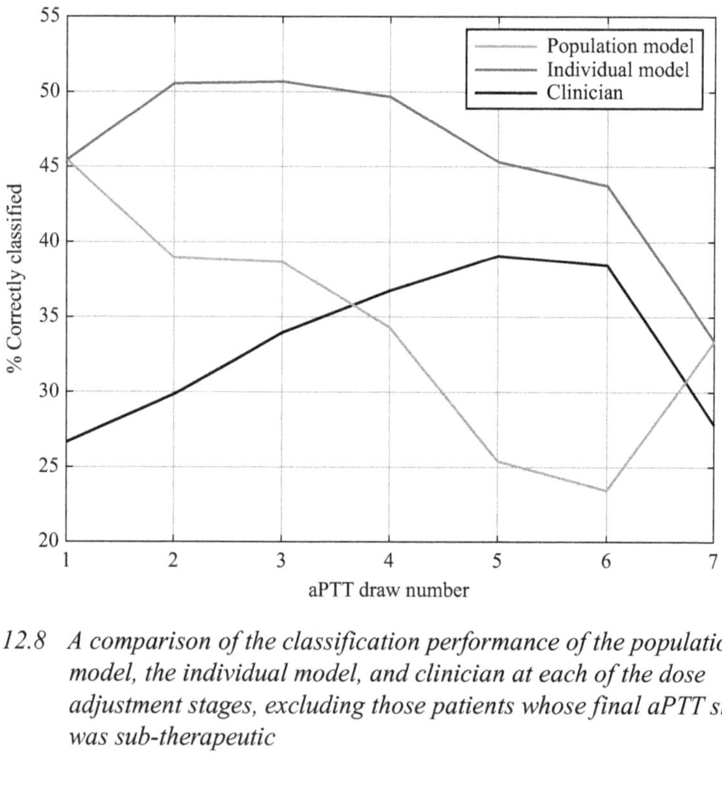

Figure 12.8 A comparison of the classification performance of the population model, the individual model, and clinician at each of the dose adjustment stages, excluding those patients whose final aPTT state was sub-therapeutic

where $\hat{y}_i^n$ describes the estimated relationship between our features and the aPTT, given the error estimate generated using all data available up till discrete time n and $n \in [1 : N]$, while N is the total number of dose adjustments. Assuming that the variance of the individual error is significantly smaller than the variance of the population error, then a simple form of the error estimate is the average difference between the measured and estimated aPTT values:

$$\hat{\varepsilon}_i^n = \sum_{n'=1}^{n-1} \frac{y_i^{n'} - \hat{y}_i^{n'}}{n-1} \tag{12.11}$$

which is in fact the maximum likelihood estimate of the error. With this error estimate, we can specify a model which grows increasingly capable of estimating patient-specific aPTT as more measurements are made increasingly available.

12.2.3 Medication dosing as a sequential decision-making problem

Reinforcement learning (RL) is a mathematical framework for learning optimal policies for taking actions in an environment so as to maximise some notion of cumulative reward [15]. Our medication dosing problem can be mapped into an RL framework (see Figure 12.9) by assigning a positive award to every aPTT measurements that falls

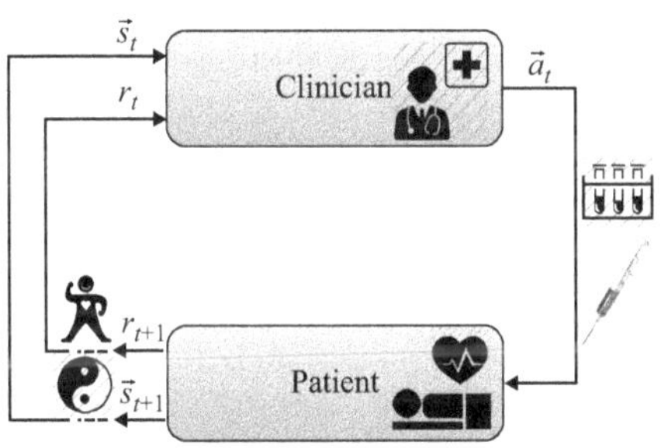

Figure 12.9 A conceptual framework for the closed-loop patient–clinician interaction in a typical ICU setting. At any given time t, the clinician observes the patient state s_t as well as the risk associated with the state, r_t. In its simplest form, a patient's state may be a vector of patient's vital signs (HR, BP, respiration, etc.), or more generally, an abstract vector representing position of the patient within a multidimensional space of deterioration and recovery. In general, state estimation requires integration of multiple sources of data (socio-demographic, genetics, imaging, laboratory tests, and vital signs), to provide an evolving view of a patient's trajectory towards physiological deterioration or recovery. The upper block represents the clinical decision-making process, that is, observing the patient's state and risk and taking an appropriate action a_t, such as administration or adjustment of a medication or ordering of a lab test

within a clinically pre-defined therapeutic range. The objective of the RL agent is to learn a dosing policy that maximises the overall fraction of time a given patient stays within his/her therapeutic aPTT range. Here by *policy* we mean a set of rules that recommends a set of actions given the patient "state", where a patient's *state* aggregates everything we like to know about the patient at a given point in time. Since the actual state of the patient is not observed, the agent has to infer both the state of the patient and an optimal policy from sample trajectories of its interaction with the environment. Therefore, in the case of Heparin dosing, the agent is confronted by the problem of learning latent factors (or states) in routinely collected clinical time series that are directly optimised to assist in sequential adjustment of Heparin dosage.

Moreover, often consequences of medical interventions are not immediately available (this known as the problem of *delayed rewards*). In the extreme case, the learning agent may only receive a single reward upon the completion of a long sequence of actions (e.g., hospital discharge after a long ICU stay). In such scenarios, not only there is no explicit teacher signal (immediate reward) to indicate a correct action at each time step, the agent is confronted with a credit assignment problem upon the completion of the tasks, i.e., must determine credit and blame to each of the states and actions that resulted in the final outcome of the sequence. Moreover, the effect of interventions for a given patient can be non-deterministic, and attempting to predict the effects of a series of treatments over time only adds to this uncertainty. The RL literature is intimately connected to the work on Markov decision processes (MDPs), as a way of performing probabilistic inference over time given non-deterministic action effects. Partially observable Markov decision processes (POMDPs) extend MDPs by maintaining internal belief states about patient state, response to interventions, etc. This is essential for dealing with real-world clinical issues of noisy observations and missing data. Here we cast the medication dosing problem into a POMDP framework and provide approximate solutions through an RL method known as *Q*-learning. Within the RL framework, a reward ($r(s_t, a_t)$; typically a scalar) is a measure of the immediate utility of an action in given state. Agent's objective is to maximise the expected long-term reward by following a policy $\pi : S \rightarrow A$, where S denotes the state space, and A denotes the set of possible actions. The *value function* for a policy is defined as the expected discounted long-term reward under that policy: $V^{\pi}(s_t) = E[\sum_{t=0}^{\infty} \gamma^t r(s_t, \pi(s_t))]$, where γ is the *discount* factor and assumes values between zeros and one. Following a dynamic programming (DP) approach, the expected reward under the optimal policy V^* starting from time t is given by: $V^*(s_t) = \max_{a' \in A} [r(s_t, a') + \gamma \sum_{s' \in S} P(s'|s_t, a')V^*(s')]$. The first term inside the bracket is the immediate reward associated with the state s_t and action a', and the second term is the discounted long-term reward the agent can expect by following its policy thereafter. Following a similar DP approach, the optimal policy is given by: $\pi^*(s_t) = \arg\max_{a' \in A} [r(s_t, a') + \gamma \sum_{s' \in S} P(s'|s_t, a')V^*(s')]$. A simple and powerful approach to solving this DP problem is Watkins's method of *Q-learning*, which works by learning an action-value function that ultimately gives the expected utility of taking a given action in a given state and following the optimal policy thereafter. The Q-function for a state-action pair is defined as [16]:

$$Q(s_t, a_t) = \max_{\pi} \mathbf{E}[r_t + \gamma r_{t+1} + \gamma^2 r_{t+2} + \cdots | s_t = s, a_t = a, \pi] \tag{12.12}$$

where r_t is a shorthand notation for $r(s_t, a_t)$. Within the *fitted Q-learning* framework [17], the Q-function is represented by a neural network, and so β represents all the network weights. We can rewrite a parametrised version of (12.12) using DP:

$$Q^*(s_t, a_t; \beta) = r(s_t, a_t) + \gamma \sum_{s' \in S} P(s'|s_t, a_t) \max_{a' \in A} Q^*(s', a'; \beta) \tag{12.13}$$

The first term in the right-hand side of the equation is the immediate reward of taking action a_t in state s_t, and the second term is the discounted long-term reward the agent can expect by taking the best action thereafter. Given the optional Q-function, the optimal value and policy functions are given by $V^*(s_t; \beta) = \max_{a' \in A} Q^*(s_t, a'; \beta)$ and $\pi^*(s_t; \beta) = \arg\max_{a' \in A} Q^*(s_t, a'; \beta)$, respectively. The Q-learning algorithm updates the parametric Q-function (or the Q-network [18]) by minimising the following cost function:

$$L(\beta_{i+1}) = \frac{1}{2|N_i|} \sum_{n \in N_i} \sum_{t=1}^{T^{(n)}} [Y(n, t; \beta_i) - Q(s_t, a_t; \beta_{i+1})]^2 \tag{12.14}$$

where $Y(n, t; \beta_i) = r(s_t, a_t) + \gamma \sum_{s' \in S} P(s'|s_t, a_t) \max_{a' \in A} Q(s', a'; \beta_i)$ is the expected value of the state-action pair under the current Q-function (parametrised by β_i) at time t and for example n within the current training batch. Note that, we have replaced $Q^*(.,.;\beta)$ by its best current estimate $Q(.,.;\beta_t)$; this is a form of bootstrapping. Gradient of this cost function with respect to the weights β_{i+1} is given by:

$$\frac{\partial L(\beta_{i+1})}{\partial \beta_{i+1}} = -\frac{1}{|N_i|} \sum_{n \in N_i} \sum_{t=1}^{T^{(n)}} [Y(n, t; w_i) - Q(s_t, a_t; \beta_{i+1})] \frac{\partial Q(s_t, a_t; \beta_{i+1})}{\partial \beta_{i+1}} \tag{12.15}$$

The above gradient can be directly plugged into an optimisation routine[1] to optimise β [19]. When optimising over a large patient cohort, we found that a stochastic optimisation approach – using mini-batches with a few iterations per batch and a momentum term – yielded improved generalisation performance with significant speed up.

We used the range of values of Heparin over six quantile intervals to define a discrete set of actions (see Figure 12.10, top panel). Next, we defined the therapeutic range of Heparin as an aPTT between 60 and 100 s [12], and constructed a reward function according to the curve $r_t = \frac{2}{1+e^{-(aPTT_t-60)}} - \frac{2}{1+e^{-(aPTT_t-100)}} - 1$ when there was an aPTT measurement, and zero elsewhere. This reward function assigns a reward of one when a patient's aPTT value was within the therapeutic window and rapidly

[1] For instance, see the *minFunc* optimisation package: http://www.di.ens.fr/ mschmidt/Software/minFunc.html

drops to -1 outside of these window (it is straight forward to define more complex reward functions that take into account a patient's risk for bleeding or stroke).

The results presented in Figure 12.10(b) show that end-to-end training of the discriminative Hidden Markov model and Q-network yielded a dosing policy superior to the hospital protocol. In fact, while the expected reward over all dosing trajectories in our cohort is negative, patients whose administered Heparin trajectory most closely followed the RL agent's policy could on average expect a positive reward (i.e., spending the majority of their time within the therapeutic range).

12.3 Discussion

The results presented in this chapter illustrate that a data-driven approach to Heparin dosing on average performs better than the state of the heart in clinical practice. Nevertheless, there is plenty of room for improvement in the Heparin dosing paradigm. Whether the suboptimal Heparin dosing we observe are from intentional actions on the part of the clinician, mistakes, or simply due to a lack of adherence to hospital guidelines was beyond our ability to investigate with the dataset. Indeed, there are clear advantages and disadvantages, in the use of retrospective data to inform clinical practice. One major advantage of retrospective analysis is its low cost, high volume, and easy scalability. More importantly, retrospective data often provides diverse representations of the critically ill, including members of the population which might be too ill to include in a clinical trials. Hence, there are some areas of research that, in the interest of ethics, can only be carried out retrospectively. Retrospective data is not without its problems however. The rational for treatment decisions are often unknown, and some features which may be important for understanding outcomes may be missing, possibly not at random.

Given the complexity of sequential decision-making in a clinical setting, the example presented here should be taken as illustrative. In fact, the validity of the results hinges on an assumption that the clinicians were dosing patients with an intention to achieve the therapeutic aPTT outlined by the institution. We acknowledge that this could be untrue in some cases. Patients with a high propensity for bleeding [14], for instance, are known to receive more conservative doses of Heparin. To address this, we performed a subgroup analysis, where we observed an even stronger indication of our approach's predictive power. As we see when inspecting Figure 12.8, the clinician's ability to classify remaining patients grows increasingly adept over dose adjustments while the population-based model eventually exhibits a predictive performance lower than the clinicians. The individualised approach we proposed, however, consistently outperformed both the clinician and the individual model.

As illustrated in this chapter, the era of big data and digital medicine contains a simple but enticing promise: with better bookkeeping in the hospital and rigorous retrospective analysis, we can better replicate what works, and avoid what does not [20,21]. The knowledge already generated from passive monitoring is immense, with countless papers describing improved procedures for treatment, prognostication, and false alarm detection. While several of these approaches are quick to identify

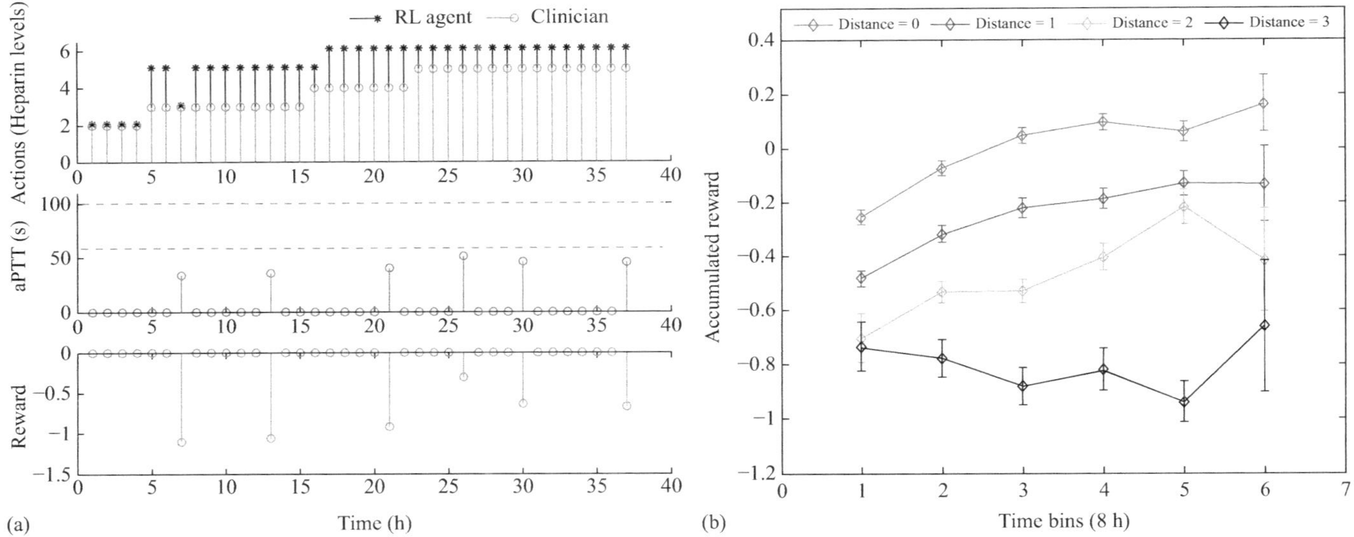

Figure 12.10 *An example of medication dosing, viewed as a reinforcement learning problem. Panel (a): each trial starts with an initial dosing of Heparin (stemmed open circles) followed by sequential adjustments over the next 24–48 h upon availability of new test results (aPTT; middle plot) and according to a hospital dosing protocol/policy (π_H). The prescribed actions by the trained RL agent (π_{RL}) are superimposed (stemmed asterisks). Panel (b): The x-axis shows the absolute difference between the actual policy followed on a given patient and the policy of the reinforcement learning agent, and the y-axis is the total reward received during the trial. Each patient is presented by an open circle, for the training (left) and testing (right) folds. The red lines represent means and standard errors over 10 quantiles (0.05–0.95) of $|\pi_H - \pi_{RL}|$, indicating a downward trend in accumulated reward with deviation from the RL agent's policy. (b) Quantifying dosing performance (accumulated reward) as a function of time, and distance from RL policy (colour-coded)*

relationships between features and outcomes, most stop short of identifying how this knowledge can practically inform clinician's decisions at the bedside and assist patients with managing their evolving state of health. Members of the medical community are aware of this translational gap, and there have been increasing calls to advance "precision medicine" through personalisation of patient care. Nevertheless, application of machine learning to medicine is still at its infancy, and we believe that advances in sequential decision-making will play an important role in the future of precision medicine and achieving a learning health care system [22].

References

[1] Kohn LT, Corrigan JM, Donaldson MS (eds.). To err is human: building a safer health system. National Academies Press; 2000 Apr 1.

[2] James JT. A new, evidence-based estimate of patient harms associated with hospital care. *J Patient Safety* 2013;9(3):122–28.

[3] Kastrup M, Markewitz A, Spies C, Carl M, Erb J, Grosse J, et al. Current practice of hemodynamic monitoring and vasopressor and inotropic therapy in post-operative cardiac surgery patients in Germany: results from a postal survey. *Acta Anaesth Scand* 2007;51(3):347–58.

[4] Wahr JA, Shore AD, Harris LH, Rogers P, Panesar S, Matthew L, *et al.* Comparison of intensive care unit medication errors reported to the United States' MedMarx and the United Kingdom's National Reporting and Learning System: a cross-sectional study. *Am J Med Qual* 2014;29(1):61–9. doi: 10.1177/1062860613482964.

[5] Alban S. Adverse effects of heparin. In: *Heparin – a century of progress*. Lever R, Mulloy B, Page CP. (eds.). Berlin: Springer; 2012. vol. 207.

[6] Raschke RA, Gollihare B, Peirce JC. The effectiveness of implementing the weight-based heparin nomogram as a practice guideline. *Arch Inter Med* 1996;156(15):1645.

[7] Landefeld CS, Cook EF, Flatley M, Weisberg M, Goldman L. Identification and preliminary validation of predictors of major bleeding in hospitalized patients starting anticoagulant therapy. *Am J Med* 1987;82(4):703–13.

[8] Health Quality Ontario. Point-of-care international normalized ratio (INR) monitoring devices for patients on long-term oral anticoagulation therapy: an evidence-based analysis. *Ont Health Technol Assess Ser.* 2009;9(12):1.

[9] Chakraborty B, Murphy SA. Dynamic treatment regimes. *Annu Rev Stat Appl* 2014;1:447.

[10] Celi L, Mark R, Stone D, Montgomerey R. "Big data" in the intensive care unit: closing the data loop. *Am J Resp Crit Care Med* 2013;187(11):1157–60.

[11] Saeed M, Villarroel M, Reisner AT, Clifford G, Lehman L-W, Moody G, et al. Multiparameter intelligent monitoring in intensive care II (MIMIC-II): a public-access intensive care unit database. *Crit Care Med* 2011;39(5):952.

[12] Ghassemi MM, Richter SE, Eche IM, Chen TW, Danziger J, Celi LA. A data-driven approach to optimized medication dosing: a focus on heparin. *Intens Care Med* 2014;40(9):1332–39.

[13] Ghassemi M, Lehman L-W, Snoek J, Nemati S. Global optimization approaches for parameter tuning in biomedical signal processing: a focus on multi-scale entropy. In: Computing in cardiology conference (CinC), 2014. Piscataway (NJ): IEEE; 2014. p. 993–96.

[14] Levine M, Hirsh J, Kelton J. Heparin-induced bleeding. In: *Heparin: chemical and biological properties clinical applications*. Land DA, Lindahl U (eds.), London: Edward Arnold; 1989. p. 517–32.

[15] Sutton RS, Barto AG. *Reinforcement learning: an introduction*, vol. 1. Cambridge (MA): MIT Press; 1998.

[16] Watkins CJ, Dayan P. *Q*-learning. *Mach Learn* 1992;8(3–4):279–92.

[17] Riedmiller M. Neural fitted *q* iteration – first experiences with a data efficient neural reinforcement learning method. In: Proceedings 16th European Conference on Machine Learning (ECML-05), volume 3720 of Lecture Notes in Computer Science; 2005. Porto, Portugal, p. 317–28.

[18] Mnih V, Kavukcuoglu K, Silver D, Rusu AA, Veness J, Bellemare MG, et al. Human-level control through deep reinforcement learning. *Nature* 2015;518(7540):529–33.

[19] Schmidt M. minFunc: unconstrained differentiable multivariate optimization in MATLAB; 2012. Available from http://www.cs.ubc.ca/~schmidtm/Software/minFunc.html

[20] King J, Patel V, Furukawa M. Physician adoption of electronic health record technology to meet meaningful use objectives: 2009–2012: ONC Data Brief No. 7; Dec 2012. Available from http://www.healthit.gov/sites/default/files/onc-data-brief-7-december-2012.pdf.

[21] Kellermann AL, Jones SS. What it will take to achieve the as-yet-unfulfilled promises of health information technology. *Health Affair* 2013;32(1):63–8.

[22] Friedman CP, Wong AK, Blumenthal D. Achieving a nationwide learning health system. *Sci Transl Med* 2010;2(57):1–3.

Chapter 13

Decision support systems for home monitoring applications: Classification of activities of daily living and epileptic seizures

Stijn Luca, Lode Vuegen,*,† Hugo Van hamme,* Peter Karsmakers* and Bart Vanrumste*,†*

13.1 Introduction and overview

Home monitoring systems (HMSs) are an application of ambient intelligence that, by making use of ICT, enable home environments to become sensitive, adaptive, and responsive to the presence of people [1]. The aim of HMSs is to support the lives of people at home with respect to care and well-being and to postpone the transfer to a nursing home for people who need care. In recent years, the research to develop these services has known a rapid growth, partially due to the increasing pressure induced by the ageing population on our healthcare system.

Related to HMSs are *telemonitoring systems*, which are defined as the use of telecommunication technologies to transmit data on patients' health status from home to a healthcare centre [2]. Consider, for example remote monitoring systems where the data of blood pressure monitors are transmitted to an external monitoring centre or emergency nurse call systems facilitating the ability to call for assistance with the push of a button. In contrast to HMSs however, telemonitoring systems do not consider the inclusion of easy-to-use technology (e.g. automated data acquisition by sensors integrated in an item of clothing) and are not adjusted to patient-specific needs, nor is there any possibility for automatic adaptation when these needs are evolving.

Generally a HMS can be assigned to one of the following three different types. A first set of systems provide early diagnosis such as fall prevention methods or early diagnoses of mild-cognitive decline. A second set of systems allow patients to return sooner to their homes after a hospital admittance. Consider, for example systems that allow patients to do their rehabilitation exercises at home. A third and last set of systems are those that allow elderly people to postpone their transfer to a nursing home

*Department of Electrical Engineering, KU Leuven, Kasteelpark Arenberg 10, B-3001 Leuven, Belgium
†iMinds Future Health Department – STADIUS, KU Leuven, Kasteelpark Arenberg 10, B-3001 Leuven, Belgium

such as fall detection systems and systems that detect epileptic seizures. An essential aspect in all these systems is that real-life data is collected to build these systems. This gives more guarantees that the developed systems can be applied in practice, although this is an expensive task since (i) annotation of data leads to substantial costs; (ii) the data is often highly unbalanced due to the relevance of rare events such as falls or epileptic convulsions, requiring a lot of data to be collected; and (iii) data is often patient-specific inducing the need of training models on different patients [3].

HMSs consist of two main components: (i) sensor technology and (ii) machine learning techniques. In this chapter the use of machine learning techniques is illustrated on data acquired by the sensors of a HMS to perform two main tasks: *activity recognition* and *novelty detection*.

The goal of activity recognition is to identify common normal activities (e.g. 'make coffee' or 'brush teeth') as they occur based on data collected by sensors. Machine learning techniques that are used to model and recognize activities include decision trees, naïve Bayes classification, Bayesian networks, instance-based learning, support vector machines (SVMs), and ensembles of classifiers that are mostly trained in a *supervised* setting where fully annotated data is needed [1].

Novelty detection aims to identify abnormal events (e.g. 'fall with elderly' or 'epileptic seizures') that typically occur rarely but may indicate a crisis or an abrupt change related to health. Approaches to novelty detection include frequentist, Bayesian and information theoretic approaches, one-class support vector machines (OCSVM), and neural networks [4]. Also the use of extreme value theory (EVT) is shown to be suitable for novelty detection [5].

The remainder of this chapter is structured as follows. In section 13.2 a tutorial on SVMs and GMMs is given. The use of these models is illustrated in a HMS where audio data is acquired to classify activities of daily living. Section 13.3 treats OCSVMs and EVT as approaches to novelty detection. The techniques are applied on an epileptic seizure detection problem. The chapter ends with some concluding remarks.

13.2 Supervised classification

In this section the classification problem is discussed in which the class $\mathscr{K}_c$ $(1 \leq c \leq C)$ is estimated to which an input vector $\mathbf{x} \in \mathbb{R}^d$ belongs, for example the classification of handwritten digits based on pixel data. In a supervised setting this estimation is based on a training set of data containing observations whose class membership is known:

$$\mathscr{D} = \{(\mathbf{x}_i, t_i) \mid 1 \leq i \leq n\}$$

where $\mathbf{x}_i$ denotes input vectors or data points in input space $\mathbb{R}^d$ and t_i denotes scalar outputs or targets presenting class membership in $\{1, \ldots, C\}$.

One might divide supervised classification methods into three main categories: (i) *generative models*[1] that approach the classification problem by estimating a joint distribution $p(\mathbf{x}, t)$ on as well inputs $\mathbf{x}$ as outputs t, (ii) *discriminative models* that

[1]Generative models owe their name to the fact that they can be used to generate synthetic data points.

only provide a model for the conditioned probabilities $p(t|\mathbf{x})$, and (iii) *discriminant functions* $f(\mathbf{x})$ that map each input $\mathbf{x}$ directly onto a class label. This section focuses on two widely known examples of models belonging to categories (i) and (iii), respectively. In particular in the following sections GMMs are used in a generative setting of classification and (2-class) SVMs are discussed as an example of a discriminant function approach where $f(\mathbf{x})$ maps each instance to one of two class labels. A typical example of a model belonging to category (ii) is given by a logistic regression model that estimates the probability of a class given an input by using a logistic function [6].

13.2.1 Gaussian mixture models for classification

In this section GMMs are introduced as a generative approach to the classification problem.

The likelihood of a GMM. The density function $p(\mathbf{x})$ of a GMM on $\mathbb{R}^d$ is given by a weighted sum of m multivariate Gaussian densities:

$$p(\mathbf{x}) = \sum_{j=1}^{m} w_j \mathcal{N}(\mathbf{x}, \boldsymbol{\mu}_i j, \boldsymbol{\Sigma}_j)$$

where $w_1, \ldots w_m$ are *mixture weights* that satisfy the constraint $\sum_{j=1}^{m} w_j = 1$ and $\mathcal{N}(\mathbf{x}, \boldsymbol{\mu}_j \boldsymbol{\Sigma}_j)$ $(1 \leq j \leq m)$ are the density functions of d-dimensional multivariate Gaussian distributions given by:

$$\mathcal{N}(\mathbf{x}, \boldsymbol{\mu}_j, \boldsymbol{\Sigma}_j) = \frac{1}{(2\pi)^{d/2}|\boldsymbol{\Sigma}_j|^{1/2}} \exp\left(-\frac{1}{2}(\mathbf{x} - \boldsymbol{\mu}_j)^T \boldsymbol{\Sigma}_j^{-1}(\mathbf{x} - \boldsymbol{\mu}_j)\right)$$

with mean vector $\boldsymbol{\mu}_j$ and covariance matrix $\boldsymbol{\Sigma}_j$. Given a set of observed data points $\mathbf{x}_1, \ldots \mathbf{x}_n$ the complete set of parameters $\boldsymbol{\lambda} = \{w_j, \mu_j, \Sigma_j | 1 \leq j \leq m\}$ can be estimated by maximizing the log likelihood function:

$$L(\boldsymbol{\lambda}) = \sum_{i=1}^{n} \ln \left[\sum_{j=1}^{m} w_j \mathcal{N}(\mathbf{x}_i, \boldsymbol{\mu}_j, \boldsymbol{\Sigma}_j) \right] \tag{13.1}$$

Due to the summation over j inside the logarithm in (13.1), the maximization is not analytically traceable inducing the need for a numerical algorithm as the expectation-maximization (EM) algorithm [6].

Classification with GMMs. The generative approach for classification consists of first solving the inference problem of determining the class conditional densities $p(\mathbf{x}|t)$ for each class individually. In this way a GMM is obtained for each class that is governed by a set of parameters $\boldsymbol{\lambda}_t = \{w_{tj}, \boldsymbol{\mu}_{tj}, \boldsymbol{\Sigma}_{tj} | 1 \leq j \leq m_t\}$ where the set of parameters and the number of mixture components all depend on the class described by the target variable t. The goal is then to find the maximum a posteriori (MAP) estimate $\hat{t}_{MAP}$ of the class t to which a given data point $\mathbf{x}$ belongs. Using Bayes' theorem the posterior class probabilities can be found by:

$$p(t|\mathbf{x}) = \frac{p(\mathbf{x}|t)p(t)}{p(\mathbf{x})}$$

such that:

$$\hat{t}_{MAP} := \underset{1 \le t \le C}{\arg\max}\{p(t|\mathbf{x})\} = \underset{1 \le t \le C}{\arg\max}\{p(\mathbf{x}|t)p(t)\} \tag{13.2}$$

One can take into account some prior belief about the class to which $\mathbf{x}$ belongs by means of the *prior distribution* $p(t)$ on the classes. Alternatively one can assume equal prior probabilities for each class reducing the estimation in (13.2) to $\hat{t}_{MAP} = \arg\max_{1 \le t \le C}\{p(\mathbf{x}|t)\}$.

Choosing the number of components. When estimating a GMM, the number of classes has to be chosen which is not a trivial problem [6]. In a supervised setting one way to proceed is to use some of the available training data $\mathscr{D}$ to train the model with a range of values for this *hyper-parameter*. The rest of the data is split into a validation and a test set. The validation set is used to maximize performance scores (e.g. classification accuracy), whereas the test set is used to obtain an independent performance score to avoid over-fitting on the validation set [6]. Generally data is not abundant available inducing larger variances on the scores obtained from the validation and test data. Therefore the procedure is repeated in a K-fold cross-validation experiment where training data is partitioned into K-folds and each fold is held-out exactly once while the remaining $K - 1$ folds are used for training. For a discussion on the choice of K we refer to Reference 7. In many applications cross validations of at least fourfolds are valid choices.

13.2.2 Support Vector Machines

In this section the SVM classifier is treated which is fundamentally a *two-class classifier* that assigns a data instance $\mathbf{x}$ to one of the two classes presented by a target variable $t \in \{-1, 1\}$. There are multiple ways to extend to multi-class SVMs. For example an *one-versus-one approach* applies a two-class SVM on all possible pairs of classes. A test instance is then assigned to that class that has the highest number of 'votes' among the classifiers [8].

The optimization problem of SVMs. The geometric problem of separation can mathematically be translated into an optimization problem minimizing the cost described by some *cost function*. In order to find this optimal separation between the two classes a feature map $\boldsymbol{\phi} : \mathbb{R}^d \mapsto \mathbb{R}^p$ is used in an attempt to transform the geometric boundary (which is often non-linear) between the two classes in data space $\mathbb{R}^d$ to a linear boundary L in feature space (see Figure 13.1):

$$L : y(\mathbf{x}) = 0 \quad \text{with} \quad y(\mathbf{x}) = \mathbf{w}^T\boldsymbol{\phi}(\mathbf{x}) + b \quad (\mathbf{w} \in \mathbb{R}^{p \times 1}, b \in \mathbb{R}) \tag{13.3}$$

The estimation of the linear boundary is performed based on a set of training examples $\mathbf{x}_i$ with corresponding target values $t_i \in \{-1, 1\}$. In the ideal case this training set is linearly separable after transformation to the feature space, meaning that there exists constants $\mathbf{w} \in \mathbb{R}^{p \times 1}, b \in \mathbb{R}$ such that each training instance can be assigned to exactly one class according to the sign of $y(\mathbf{x})$ defined in (13.3). In other words one assumes that:

$$\forall 1 \le i \le n : t_i y(\mathbf{x}_i) > 0 \tag{13.4}$$

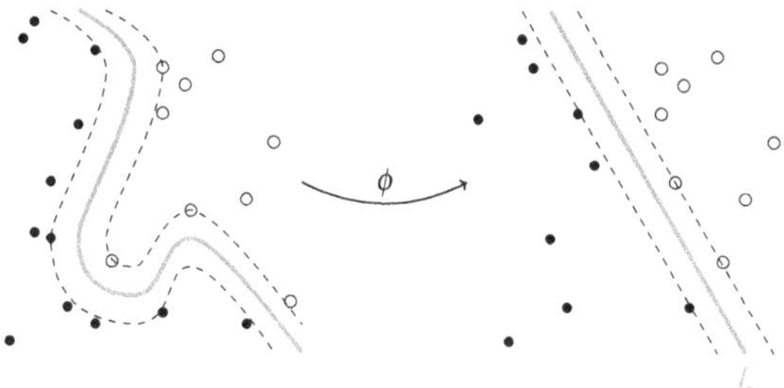

Figure 13.1 Linearisation of the decision boundary of SVMs using a feature map $\boldsymbol{\phi}$*. The dashed lines indicate the hyperplanes where the margin is maximized*

for some $\mathbf{w} \in \mathbb{R}^{p \times 1}, b \in \mathbb{R}$. In SVMs the *decision boundary* $L : y(\mathbf{x}) = 0$ is chosen to maximize the *margin* that is given by the smallest distance between L and any of the training instances $\mathbf{x}_i$ (Figure 13.1). In particular one is interested in constants $\mathbf{w}$ and b given by:

$$\underset{\mathbf{w},b}{\arg\max}\left[\min_i\left\{\frac{|y(\mathbf{x}_i)|}{||\mathbf{w}||}\right\}\right] \quad \text{or} \quad \underset{\mathbf{w},b}{\arg\max}\left[\min_i\left\{\frac{t_i(\mathbf{w}^T\boldsymbol{\phi}(\mathbf{x}_i)+b)}{||\mathbf{w}||}\right\}\right] \tag{13.5}$$

subject to the constraints (13.4). The constants $\mathbf{w}$ and $\mathbf{b}$ in (13.5) can be rescaled without changing the decision boundary $y(\mathbf{x}) = 0$ such that:

$$t_i(\mathbf{w}^T\boldsymbol{\phi}(\mathbf{x}_i) + b) = 1$$

for those instances that are closest to the decision boundary. This reduces the optimization in (13.5) to:[2]

$$\begin{aligned} &\underset{\mathbf{w},b}{\arg\max}\ \frac{1}{||\mathbf{w}||} \ \text{or} \ \underset{\mathbf{w},b}{\arg\min}\ \frac{1}{2}||\mathbf{w}||^2 \\ &\text{subject to } t_i y(\mathbf{x}_i) = t_i(\mathbf{w}^T\boldsymbol{\phi}(\mathbf{x}_i) + b) \geq 1, \quad i = 1, \ldots, n \end{aligned} \tag{13.6}$$

Once the margin has been maximized there will be at least two instances, so-called *support vectors*, $\widetilde{\mathbf{x}}_i$ that minimize the distance to L and therefore satisfy $|y(x)| = 1$. These support vectors are lying on the *maximum margin boundaries* given by hyperplanes in feature space where the margin is geometrically maximized (see Figure 13.2(a)).

In practice however a solution of (13.6) cannot always be guaranteed as training data can be overlapping such that data points can lie at the 'wrong side' of the decision boundary. Therefore the constraints in (13.6) are weakened allowing data instances to be inside the margins using *slack variables* ξ_i. Moreover points that lie on

[2]The factor $\frac{1}{2}$ is not necessarily but chosen for convenience when calculating derivatives of the Lagrangian in (13.11).

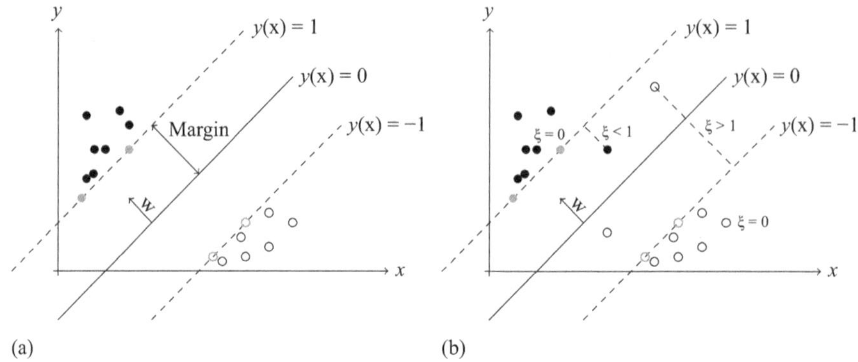

Figure 13.2 *(a) Illustration of the margin of an SVM with linearly separable data. The grey points are the* support vectors *lying on the* maximum margin boundaries. *(b) Illustration of the slack variables that are introduced when data is not linearly separable*

the wrong side of the boundary are penalized in the cost function, yielding the following optimization problem which is known as the C-SVM:

$$\underset{\mathbf{w},b}{\arg\min}\left\{\frac{1}{2}||\mathbf{w}||^2+\frac{C}{n}\sum_{i=1}^{n}\xi_i\right\} \tag{13.7}$$
$$\text{subject to } t_i y(\mathbf{x}_i)\geq 1-\xi_i \quad \text{and} \quad \xi_i\geq 0, \quad i=1,\ldots,n$$

The slack variables ξ_i determine the error on the initial conditions $t_i y(\mathbf{x}_i) \geq 1, (1 \leq i \leq n)$ in (13.6). They are defined by $\xi_i = 0$ for support vectors or data points that are on the correct side of the margin boundaries (see Figure 13.2). For so-called *margin errors* lying inside the margin boundaries or at the wrong side of L one defines $\xi_i = |t_i - y(\mathbf{x}_i)|$. When $0 < \xi < 1$ they are lying inside the margin boundaries but at the correct side of L. When $\xi > 1$ the points are at the wrong side of L (see Figure 13.2). The parameter $C > 0$ in (13.7) determines the penalty that is put on margin errors. A lower C allows a 'softer margin', while in the limit as $C \to +\infty$ one recovers the solution for separable data as before.

From *C*-SVM to ν-SVM. The parameter C is rather unintuitive and there is no *a priori* way to select it. However, a modification called the ν-SVM is often chosen that replaces the parameter C with a parameter ν that controls the number of margin errors and support vectors as will be shown in a moment. Moreover this parametrization provides a direct link with the OCSVM that will be introduced in Section 13.3.1.

In a ν-SVM the following constrained optimization problem is solved:

$$\underset{\mathbf{w},b,\rho}{\arg\min}\left\{\frac{1}{2}||\mathbf{w}||^2-\rho\nu+\frac{1}{n}\sum_{i=1}^{n}\xi_i\right\} \tag{13.8}$$
$$\text{subject to } \xi_i\geq 0, \rho\geq 0 \quad \text{and} \quad t_i y(\mathbf{x}_i)\geq \rho-\xi_i, \quad i=1,\ldots,n$$

The maximum margin boundaries are determined by $t_i(\mathbf{w}^T\boldsymbol{\phi}(\mathbf{x}_i)+b)=\rho$ and the slack variables ξ_i determine the margin errors as before. It's not hard to realize that when ν-SVM leads to an optimum $(\mathbf{w}_0, b_0, \rho_0)$, the decision surface with coefficients $(\mathbf{w}_0, b_0)$ can equally be obtained from an optimum of the C-SVM by setting $C=\frac{1}{\rho_0}$. To see this a rescaling in the parameters $(\mathbf{w}, b, \xi_i)$ in (13.8) is needed while setting $\rho=\rho_0$:

$$\overline{\mathbf{w}}=\frac{\mathbf{w}}{\rho_0}, \overline{b}=\frac{b}{\rho_0}, \overline{\xi_i}=\frac{\xi_i}{\rho_0} \tag{13.9}$$

such that:

$$\begin{aligned}\min_{\mathbf{w},b}\left\{\frac{1}{2}||\mathbf{w}||^2-\rho_0\nu+\frac{1}{n}\sum_{i=1}^{n}\xi_i\right\} &= \min_{\mathbf{w},b}\left\{\frac{1}{2}||\mathbf{w}||^2+\frac{1}{n}\sum_{i=1}^{n}\xi_i\right\}\\ &= \min_{\mathbf{w},b}\left\{\frac{1}{2}||\frac{\mathbf{w}}{\rho_0}||^2+\frac{1}{n\rho_0}\sum_{i=1}^{n}\frac{\xi_i}{\rho_0}\right\}\\ &= \min_{\overline{\mathbf{w}},\overline{\mathbf{b}}}\left\{\frac{1}{2}||\overline{\mathbf{w}}||^2+\frac{1}{n\rho_0}\sum_{i=1}^{n}\overline{\xi}_i\right\}\end{aligned}$$

while the constraints on $(\mathbf{w}, \mathbf{b})$ in (13.8) imply the constraints (13.7) on $(\overline{\mathbf{w}}, \overline{\mathbf{b}})$.

The solution of the ν-SVM optimization problem. To optimize the constraint optimization problem (13.8) the method of Lagrange multiplier is used [6]. The corresponding Lagrangian function is given by:

$$\begin{aligned}F(\mathbf{w},b,\boldsymbol{\xi},\rho) = &\frac{1}{2}||\mathbf{w}||^2-\nu\rho+\frac{1}{n}\sum_{i=1}^{n}\xi_i-\sum_{i=1}^{n}\alpha_i\Big(t_i(\mathbf{w}^T\boldsymbol{\phi}(\mathbf{x}_i)+b)-\rho+\xi_i\Big)\\ &-\sum_{i=1}^{n}\beta_i\xi_i-\delta\rho\end{aligned}$$

using multipliers $\alpha_i, \beta_i \geq 0, \delta \geq 0$ subject to the conditions ('The Karush–Kuhn–Tucker' conditions):

$$\alpha_i\Big(t_i(\mathbf{w}^T\boldsymbol{\phi}(\mathbf{x}_i)+b)-\rho+\xi_i\Big)=0, \quad \beta_i\xi_i=0 \tag{13.10}$$

This Lagrangian F is maximized setting the first-order partial derivatives to zero:

$$
\begin{aligned}
\frac{\partial F}{\partial w_k} &= w_k - \sum_{i=1}^{n} \alpha_i t_i \boldsymbol{\phi}_k(\mathbf{x}_i) = 0 \Leftrightarrow w_k = \sum_{i=1}^{n} \alpha_i t_i \boldsymbol{\phi}_k(\mathbf{x}_i) \\
\frac{\partial F}{\partial b} &= \sum_{i=1}^{n} \alpha_i t_i = 0 \\
\frac{\partial F}{\partial \xi_k} &= \frac{1}{n} - \alpha_k - \beta_k = 0 \Leftrightarrow \alpha_k = \frac{1}{n} - \beta_k \\
\frac{\partial F}{\partial \rho} &= -\nu + \sum_{i=1}^{n} \alpha_i - \delta = 0 \Leftrightarrow \nu = \sum_{i=1}^{n} \alpha_i - \delta
\end{aligned}
\tag{13.11}
$$

for $1 \leq k \leq n$. Substitution in F leads to the so-called *dual representation* of the ν-SVM optimization problem:

$$
\begin{aligned}
&F = -\frac{1}{2} \sum_{i=1}^{n} \sum_{j=1}^{n} \alpha_i \alpha_j t_i t_j (\boldsymbol{\phi}(\mathbf{x}_i) \bullet \boldsymbol{\phi}(\mathbf{x}_j)) \\
&\text{subject to} \quad 0 \leq \alpha_i \leq \frac{1}{n}, \quad \sum_{i=1}^{n} \alpha_i t_i = 0, \quad \sum_{i=1}^{n} \alpha_i \geq \nu
\end{aligned}
\tag{13.12}
$$

In particular from (13.11), it follows that the decision function $y(\mathbf{x}) = \mathbf{w}^T \boldsymbol{\phi}(\mathbf{x}) + b$ can be written in terms of a kernel function $k(\mathbf{x}, \mathbf{x}') = \boldsymbol{\phi}(\mathbf{x}) \bullet \boldsymbol{\phi}(\mathbf{x}')$:

$$
y(\mathbf{x}) = \sum_{i=1}^{n} \alpha_i t_i k(\mathbf{x}, \mathbf{x}_i) + b
$$

Due to the conditions in (13.10) only the support vectors $\widetilde{\mathbf{x}}_i$ satisfy $\alpha_i \neq 0$ and contribute to this sum. For this reason SVMs are also called *sparse kernel machines* as the kernel function $k(\mathbf{x}, \mathbf{x}')$ only has to be evaluated at a subset of the training data points reducing computation times for large datasets. Furthermore margin errors are characterised by $\xi_i > 0$ such that from (13.10) it follows that $\beta_i = 0$ and thus $\alpha_i = \frac{1}{n}$ from (13.11). As $\sum_{i=1}^{n} \alpha_i \geq \nu$ only a fraction ν of the α_i can equal $\frac{1}{n}$ such that ν is an upperbound on the fraction of margin errors as previously announced.

Kernel substitution. The dual representation (13.12) enables to work directly in terms of kernels and avoids the explicit introduction of a feature map $\boldsymbol{\phi}$, also known as the *'kernel trick'*. This allows implicitly to use feature spaces of infinite dimensionality. A commonly used kernel is given by the *Gaussian kernel*:

$$
k(\mathbf{x}, \mathbf{x}') = \exp\left(-\frac{||\mathbf{x} - \mathbf{x}'||^2}{2\sigma^2} \right) \tag{13.13}
$$

which corresponds to the choice of a feature vector with infinite dimensionality and σ denotes the so-called *kernel width*. Both σ and ν (or C) can be optimized as hyperparameters in a cross-validation experiment similar to the procedure introduced in Section 13.2.1 for choosing the number of components in a GMM.

13.2.3 Classification of activities of daily living

In this section a supervised GMM and SVM are applied on the classification of activities of daily living from acoustic sensor data. Data is recorded in a real-life home environment equipped with seven microphone nodes. Fig. 13.3(a) shows the floor plan of the home environment together with the microphone positions. In total 10 different activities of daily living were recorded during a period of three days and labelled as: 1, '*Brushing teeth*'; 2, '*Dishes*'; 3, '*Dressing*'; 4, '*Eating*'; 5, '*Preparing food*'; 6, '*Setting table*'; 7, '*Showering*'; 8, '*Sleeping*'; 9, '*Toileting*' and 10, '*Washing hands*'.

In Fig. 13.3(b) the system architecture that was used for the classification task is presented. Acoustic information is processed in blocks of 30s. Such block size corresponds to the minimal duration of activities that were observed in the data. Each block is further partitioned into frames of 25ms that overlap with 15ms. A frame is either (dominantly) generated by an 'interesting' sound source or background noise sources. For each block an averaged signal-to-noise ratio (SNR) is computed as the ratio between the average energy in the interesting frames and that in the noise related frames. Hence, each 30s all nodes capture a block of data of which only that block with the highest SNR is retained and used for further processing.

Although they were initially developed for speaker and speech application Mel-Frequency Cepstral Coefficients (MFCCs) are also popular features for audio classification. They were therefore adopted in this work to form a basis on which the classifier models can work. In the setting used in this work a block contains 300 frames of 25ms. For each frame a d-dimensional MFCC feature vector $\mathbf{x}_f \in \mathbb{R}^d$ $(1 \le f \le 300)$ is computed by retaining the d first coefficients from a cosine transformation of the log-power spectrum filtered by n_{mel} mel-filter banks [9]. In this way

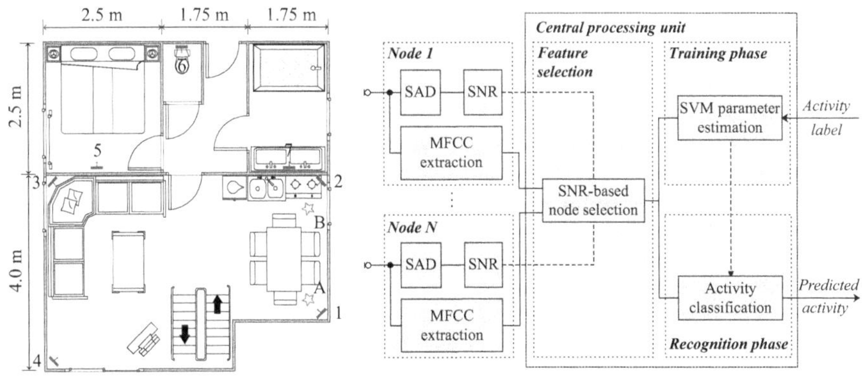

(a) (b)

Figure 13.3 (a) Floor plan of the home environment indicating the microphone positions 1–7. (b) The proposed system architecture for the classification of activities of daily living from each block a set of $q \leq 300$ feature vectors $\{\mathbf{x}_1, \ldots, \mathbf{x}_q\} \subset \mathbb{R}^d$ is extracted by using an energy threshold.

Both classifier models that were described in Sections 13.2.1 and 13.2.2 were validated for this task. Previous research indicated that a GMM of 10 Gaussian components with full covariance matrix is an appropriate choice for classifying activities of daily living [10]. To this end, for each frame a class-dependent GMM with conditional density $p(\mathbf{x}_f|t)$ is fitted on the MFCCs' feature vectors. Then, the probability that a block consisting of q frames is generated by a certain sound class is obtained as $p(\mathbf{x}_1, \ldots, \mathbf{x}_q|t) = \prod_{f=1}^{q} p(\mathbf{x}_f|t)$. Classification of blocks could then be based on an MAP estimation as in (13.2) assuming an uniform prior on the classes.

To apply a SVM classifier the different feature vectors of the block are described by the one so-called MFCC super vector $\tilde{\mathbf{x}}_{SuVe} \in \mathbb{R}^{2d}$ defined as the first and second-order statistics computed among the different feature vectors of a block, i.e.

$$\tilde{\mathbf{x}}_{SuVe} = \left(\frac{1}{q} \sum_{f=1}^{q} \mathbf{x}_f, \sqrt{\frac{1}{q} \sum_{f=1}^{q} (\mathbf{x}_f - \overline{\mathbf{x}}_f)^2} \right)$$

where sums and squares are component-wise defined. Also a GMM was trained using these super vectors (referred to as SuVe-GMM) in order to compare the performance of SVM and GMM when both are based on this type of feature vectors.

In Table 13.1 the mean and standard deviation of the classification accuracies (the percentage of blocks that are correctly classified) among the different type of classifiers are shown. The hyper-parameters of the GMMs and SVM are optimized in a fourfold cross-validation procedure. An one-versus-one coding scheme was used to extend the binary SVM formulation to the multi-class case.

During the experiments, the influence of the sampling frequency, the number of mel-filters n_{mel}, and the number of feature dimensions d on the performance are examined. As one can see, these results indicate that GMM and SVM models obtain equivalent classification accuracies and that they both outperform the SuVe-GMM set-up by 20% in terms of classification accuracy. Such behaviour is typically seen when comparing generative models to discriminative functions. Given the same amount of data discriminative functions behave more robust in higher dimensional input spaces. The large difference in scores between SuVe-GMM and GMM is due to the reduction in the amount of training data while doubling the feature dimensions when using the super vector set-up. In addition, these results also indicate that a sampling frequency of 16 kHz is appropriate for activity classification since lowering the sampling frequency to 8 kHz yields a decrease in accuracy while increasing to 32 kHz does not improve the accuracy significantly. Therefore, SVM with a sampling frequency of 16 kHz is the preferred alternative explored in this work on this task of ADL classification.

Table 13.2 shows the confusion matrix of SVM with a sample frequency of 16 kHz, 15 mel-filters and a feature dimension of 14. Most of the confusion occurs for the activities 'dishes', 'eating', 'preparing food' and 'setting table'. This seems

Table 13.1 *Mean and standard deviation computed using fourfold cross validation of the ADL classification accuracies for GMM, SuVe-GMM and SVM set-ups with different feature parameter settings. The highest obtained classification scores are marked in boldface*

n_{mel}	d	GMM			SuVe-GMM			SVM		
		8 kHz	**16 kHz**	**32 kHz**	**8 kHz**	**16 kHz**	**32 kHz**	**8 kHz**	**16 kHz**	**32 kHz**
10	7	69.6 ± 3.3%	73.3 ± 4.4%	73.6 ± 5.2%	46.7 ± 3.5%	48.3 ± 2.6%	46.4 ± 4.3%	68.5 ± 5.5%	72.9 ± 1.7%	71.4 ± 2.8%
15	7	70.4 ± 4.2%	73.4 ± 4.8%	74.2 ± 5.3%	48.0 ± 2.2%	**52.7 ± 4.2%**	48.2 ± 2.0%	69.3 ± 5.9%	72.8 ± 4.0%	73.5±2.0%
15	14	72.8 ± 4.8%	75.1 ± 4.5%	**76.5 ± 4.8%**	47.9 ± 5.4%	50.5 ± 5.7%	49.4 ± 3.5%	72.8 ± 5.1%	78.0 ± 2.8%	76.9 ± 2.8%
20	7	70.2 ± 3.1%	72.8 ± 4.9%	74.2 ± 5.3%	47.6 ± 8.3%	47.0 ± 2.7%	49.5 ± 3.5%	70.2 ± 7.4%	72.7 ± 0.7%	71.3 ± 2.4%
20	14	72.7 ± 4.4%	75.5 ± 5.1%	73.0 ± 4.7%	50.2 ± 3.6%	50.0 ± 3.1%	52.4 ± 5.3%	69.3 ± 2.7%	75.3 ± 4.3%	**78.2 ± 4.1%**

Table 13.2 SVM confusion matrix for a sample frequency of 16 kHz, 15 mel-filters and a feature dimension of 14. A classification score of 78.0 ± 2.8% is obtained

	Classified label									
Ground truth	**1**	**2**	**3**	**4**	**5**	**6**	**7**	**8**	**9**	**10**
1	**97.9%**	2.1%	–	–	–	–	–	–	–	–
2	1.7%	**58.6%**	6.9%	16.4%	8.6%	6.9%	–	–	–	0.9%
3	–	0.7%	**93.5%**	3.6%	–	2.2%	–	–	–	–
4	–	8.3%	2.9%	**77.2%**	4.9%	4.4%	1.5%	1.0%	–	–
5	–	19.0%	3.5%	6.3%	**55.6%**	9.2%	0.7%	4.9%	0.7%	–
6	–	6.6%	9.0%	4.1%	6.6%	**73.8%**	–	–	–	–
7	3.1%	–	–	–	–	–	**96.9%**	–	–	–
8	–	–	10.0%	12.5%	5.0%	–	–	**72.5%**	–	–
9	–	–	–	–	–	–	–	–	**100%**	–
10	4.2%	–	4.2%	–	–	–	–	–	–	**91.7%**

plausible as these activities contain joint acoustic information such as scraping cutlery. In a similar way 'brushing teeth', 'dishes', 'showering', 'toileting', and 'washing hands' are often confused as they contain the joint acoustic signal of running water.

13.3 Novelty detection

Novelty detection is a particular example of pattern recognition that attacks the problem of identifying patterns in data that are previously unseen. It shares many similarities with anomaly detection where one also wishes to detect abnormalities, but where these may not necessarily be entirely novel, i.e. a small amount of the training data can contain outliers or anomalies. The novelty detection paradigm provides an alternative approach to strong *class imbalance* that starts from a model of normal behaviour and detects deviations from this model [4]. It is for this reason that novelty detection is also termed one-class classification where there is no explicit model for 'abnormal behaviour'. Thus in this section we start from d-dimensional training data from one class only $\mathcal{D} = \{\mathbf{x}_1, \ldots \mathbf{x}_n\} \subset \mathbb{R}^d$. Statistically, the vectors $\mathbf{x} \in \mathcal{D}$ are assumed to be independent realizations of a stochastic variable X that is distributed according to a probability density function $y = p(\mathbf{x})$.

13.3.1 One-class support vector machines

A OCSVM solves an unsupervised learning problem related to a probability density estimation [8]. Instead of modelling the density of data, however, these methods aim to find a smooth boundary enclosing a region of high density. The strategy of an

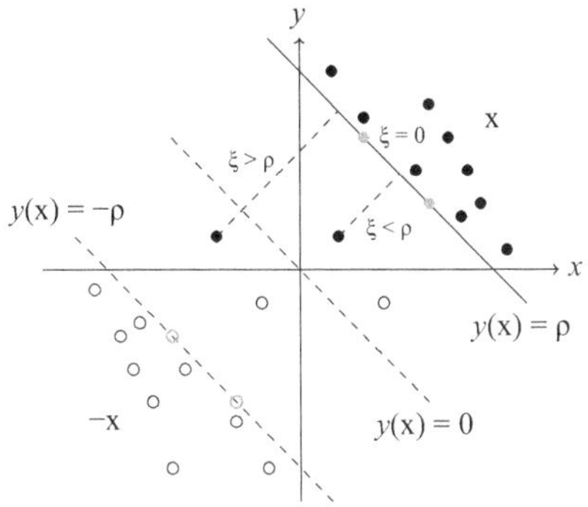

Figure 13.4 An one-class SVM pictured as a two-class SVM on the training data and the reflected data through the origin

OCSVM is to map the training data $\{\mathbf{x}_1, \ldots \mathbf{x}_n\}$ into a feature space where it can be separated from the origin with a maximal margin ρ. For this purpose the following constrained optimization problem is considered:

$$\arg\min_{\mathbf{w},\rho} \left\{ \frac{1}{2}||\mathbf{w}||^2 - \rho + \frac{1}{n\nu}\sum_{i=1}^{n} \xi_i \right\} \tag{13.14}$$
$$\text{subject to } \xi_i \geq 0 \quad \text{and} \quad y(\mathbf{x}_i) \geq \rho - \xi_i, \quad i = 1, \ldots, n$$

where $y(\mathbf{x}) = \mathbf{w}^T \boldsymbol{\phi}(x)$. A new instance $\mathbf{x}$ is then classified as being outside the support of the training data when $\mathbf{w}^T \boldsymbol{\phi}(\mathbf{x}_i) - \rho \leq 0$. The optimization problem in (13.14) is very similar to the one of the ν-SVM in (13.8). In fact, rescaling the parameters in (13.14) as:

$$\mathbf{w} = \frac{\overline{\mathbf{w}}}{\nu}, \quad \rho = \frac{\overline{\rho}}{\nu}, \quad \xi_i = \frac{\overline{\xi_i}}{\nu}$$

one obtains the cost function of the ν-SVM in (13.8) where the data $\{\boldsymbol{\phi}(\mathbf{x}_1), \ldots, \boldsymbol{\phi}(\mathbf{x}_n)\}$ is separated from $\{-\boldsymbol{\phi}(\mathbf{x}_1), \ldots, -\boldsymbol{\phi}(\mathbf{x}_n)\}$ by the hyperplane $\mathbf{w}^T \boldsymbol{\phi}(\mathbf{x}_i) = 0$ that passes through the origin in feature space. However, OCSVMs use the maximum margin boundary $\mathbf{w}^T \boldsymbol{\phi}(\mathbf{x}_i) = \rho$ to separate the support of the data from the rest of data space (see Figure 13.4).

Completely similar as in Section 13.2.2 the dual form can be derived by introducing the Lagrangian of the constrained optimization problem (13.14) and setting the derivatives with respect to w_i, ξ_i and ρ to zero:

$$L = -\frac{1}{2}\sum_{i=1}^{n}\sum_{j=1}^{n} \alpha_i \alpha_j t_i t_j (\boldsymbol{\phi}(\mathbf{x}_i) \bullet \boldsymbol{\phi}(\mathbf{x}_j))$$
$$\text{subject to} \quad 0 \leq \alpha_i \leq \frac{1}{\nu n}, \quad \sum_{i=1} \alpha_i = 1$$

The decision function in terms of the kernel function $k(\mathbf{x}, \mathbf{x}') = \boldsymbol{\phi}(\mathbf{x}) \bullet \boldsymbol{\phi}(\mathbf{x}')$ is now given as $y(\mathbf{x}) - \rho = \sum_{i=1}^{n} \alpha_i k(\mathbf{x}, \mathbf{x}_i) - \rho$. As before only the support vectors contribute to the sum. Margin errors are in this case termed outliers and the parameter ν is an upper bound on the fraction of outliers. In particular an OCSVM linearly separates the data in feature space from the origin, and the choice of a Gaussian kernel (13.13) (corresponding to the choice of an infinite dimensional feature vector) ensures that this is feasible [8].

13.3.2 Extreme value theory

A main drawback of OCSVMs is the need for a choice of the parameters ν and σ. The optimal values of these parameters are depending heavily on the application such that existing rule of thumbs generally perform suboptimal [11]. Only when examples of outliers are available the parameters can be optimized in a cross-validation experiment.

In many applications however outliers present some 'extreme' and rare behaviour. The use of EVT enables to fit a model on this class even when examples are completely absent circumventing the optimization procedure which is commonly used in SVMs. In this section we review the recent methodologies of the use of EVT for novelty detection and illustrate the methods on the detection of epileptic seizures [5, 12].

Point classification. Firstly the question is addressed whether a data point $\mathbf{x}$ is drawn from a distribution X or not. For this purpose a method is proposed that applies univariate EVT on the univariate distribution over the probability density values $p(\mathbf{x})$. The distribution Y of densities $y = p(\mathbf{x})$ is strongly related to that of X with a density function defined by:

$$q(y) = \frac{dQ}{dy}(y) \quad \text{where} \quad Q(y) = \int_{p^{-1}([0,y])} p(\mathbf{x}) d\mathbf{x} \tag{13.15}$$

Univariate EVT can be used to describe sets: $S_k = \{\mathbf{x}_1, \ldots, \mathbf{x}_k\}$ which have a typical minimal density with respect to $y = p(\mathbf{x})$. In order to avoid skewness near zero of such minimal densities, the maxima of transformed sequences $-\log(p(S_k))$ are considered:

$$m_k := \max\{-\log p(\mathbf{x}_1), \ldots - \log p(\mathbf{x}_k)\} = \max\{-\log(p(S_k))\} \tag{13.16}$$

which corresponds to the *'extreme' vectors* with respect to X and are seen as realizations of a stochastic variable M_k. For large k, M_k follows approximately a *Gumbel distribution* with cumulative distribution function:

$$G_k(m_k) \approx \exp\left(-\exp\left(-\frac{m_k - \alpha_k}{\beta_k}\right)\right) \tag{13.17}$$

where (α_k, β_k) describe, respectively, location and scale of the maxima related to sets S_k drawn from X. The choice of k implies a trade-off between bias and variance. A large k results in few maxima m_k that can be extracted from the training set and thus in a large estimation variance on M_k. A too small block size results in a poor estimation of the model of M_k as the approximation in (13.17) is only valid for larger k. A good compromise in our application is given by $k = 50$ [13]. In any case the validity of the approximation can visually be checked by a quantile–quantile (Q–Q)

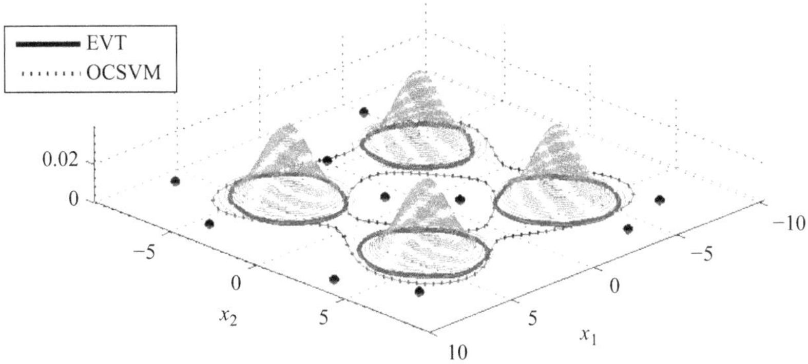

Figure 13.5 Density of a Gaussian mixture X of standard normal distributions centered at (±4,±4). The training instances in the abnormal class are indicated by a dot. Estimation of the support using OCSVMs and EVT is shown

plot, graphing the empirical quantiles against the theoretical quantiles obtained from the Gumbel distribution [14].

From the training set $\mathscr{D}$ a corresponding Gumbel distribution $\hat{G}_k$ of extremes can be estimated by simulating sets S_k of length k from a kernel density estimation $y = \hat{p}(\mathbf{x})$ of $y = p(\mathbf{x})$ and obtaining the estimations $\hat{\alpha}_k$ and $\hat{\beta}_k$ of the Gumbel parameters by maximum likelihood estimation from the simulated maxima $m_k = \max\{-\log(\hat{p}(S_k)\}$ [15]. By setting a threshold on $\hat{G}_k$ a point $\mathbf{x}$ can be termed a novelty when $\hat{G}(-\log \hat{p}(\mathbf{x}))$ exceeds the threshold.[3] From a probabilistic point of view a threshold of 95% can be chosen corresponding to a type-I error of 5% in the classification of extremes of sets of length k.

Figure 13.5 illustrates the estimation of the support of a Gaussian mixture of standard normal distributions centered at $(\pm 4, \pm 4)$. The choice of the parameters (ν, σ) of the OCSVM is based on a cross-validation experiment using unbalanced training data consisting of 10^3 instances from the normal class and 10 instances lying in the tail of the distribution. The lack of examples from the abnormal class makes it hard for the OCSVM to estimate the correct boundary. However, EVT provides a class of models for the tail region where training data is sparse and is able to estimate the boundary better by means of extrapolation from the normal class where data is abundantly available. The support of the data then corresponds to the density contour of $\hat{p}(\mathbf{x})$ at the 95% quantile of the Gumbel distribution.

Classification of sets. We address the question of novelty detection applied on complete sets $S_k = \{\mathbf{x}_1, \ldots, \mathbf{x}_k\} \subset \mathbb{R}^d$ of a specified number of k data instances that are independently drawn from some distribution. Novelty detection addresses the question whether such a set S_k of vectors is drawn from a distribution X or not. In practice

[3]A point $\mathbf{x}$ is considered as corresponding to an extreme vector of some set S_k of length k [16].

S_k can, for example present the last vector and the $k-1$ vectors observed before it such that information of the last k measurements can be combined using EVT.

In terms of statistical hypothesis testing the problem setting can be stated as:

$$H_0 \ : \ S_k \text{ is a set of vectors drawn from the population } X$$
$$H_1 \ : \ S_k \text{ is a novel set with respect to } X$$

From the point of view of hypothesis testing, it is clear that for $k > 1$ the problem is related to one of multiple testing. Indeed, for $k > 1$ the probability to make at least one false positive when testing each $\mathbf{x}_i \in S$ is given by:

$$P(\text{false positive}) = 1 - (1-\alpha)^k > \alpha$$

where α denotes the probability on a false positive when testing a single $\mathbf{x}_i$. As k gets larger the probability of a false alarm drastically increases. When, for example $k = 5$ and $\alpha = 5\%$, then P(false positive)=26%. The use of EVT enables to obtain the correct boundary of normality corresponding with the significance level α.

In order to classify such sets it is desired to fuse different types of information of S_k in order to build a classification model. The use of Poisson point processes (PPPs) allows us to do this in a very natural way as these models will allow us to fuse three different types of information of S_k given some threshold u: (i) the maximal exceedance m_k of $-\log p(S_k)$ above u (ii) the mean exceedance v_k of $-\log p(S_k)$ above u, and (iii) the number of exceedances n_k of $-\log p(S_k)$ above u. The distributions of the corresponding random variables M_k, V_k and N_k can be obtained by applying the PPP approach.

This approach of EVT states that the number of exceedances in $-\log p(S_k)$ above some high threshold u can be approximated by a *Poisson distribution* for large k, with a rate λ_k that can be parametrised in terms of the Gumbel parameters (α_k, β_k):

$$\lambda_k = \exp\left(\frac{u-\alpha_k}{\beta_k}\right) \tag{13.18}$$

The choice of u implies the same trade-off as the choice of k, a too large u results in a large estimation variance on the parameters $(\lambda_k, \alpha_k, \beta_k)$ while a too low u implies a poor approximation by the Poisson distribution. Compromises are described by rule of thumbs such as *Van Kerm's rule* stating that $u \approx \min\{\max\{2.5\bar{x}, q_{98}\}, q_{97}\}$ where $\bar{x}, q_{98}, q_{97}$ denote empirical estimates of mean and quantiles at 0.98, 0.97, respectively, using a sample drawn from $-\log p(X)$ [17]. As before, a kernel density estimation $y = \hat{p}(\mathbf{x})$ of $y = p(\mathbf{x})$ can be obtained from the training set $\mathscr{D}$ from which a number of n_b sets S can be simulated. When one observes m exceedances $z_i - u$, $z_i = -\log \hat{p}(\mathbf{x}_i)$ among these sets, the EVT parameters λ_k, α_k and β_k can be estimated by maximizing the Poisson process log-likelihood [14]:

$$-n_b \exp\left(\frac{u-\alpha_k}{\beta_k}\right) - m\log\beta_k - \sum_{i=1}^{m}\left(\frac{z_i - u}{\beta_k}\right) \tag{13.19}$$

Now, according to EVT, M_k (13.16) follows a Gumbel distribution with location α_k and scale β_k, N_k a Poisson distribution with rate λ_k and the exceedances $-\log(p(S_k)) - u$ an exponential distribution with scale β_k. The latter implies that given a number of exceedances n_k the variable V_k follows an *Erlang distribution* with shape parameter n_k and rate parameter $\frac{n_k}{\beta_k}$. With respect to each of the distributions M_k, N_k and V_k, a set S_k can be evaluated by means of a cumulative probability score that we, respectively, denotes as $\chi_g(S_k)$, $\chi_p(S_k)$ and $\chi_e(S_k)$ (the sub-indices refer to the underlying distributions: Gumbel, Poisson, and Erlang). These scores can be combined into one *novelty score* of S_k using a generalized mean:

$$\overline{\chi}_r(S_k) = \left(\frac{1}{3}(\chi_p(S_k)^r + \chi_e(S_k)^r + \chi_g(S_k)^r)\right)^{1/r} \tag{13.20}$$

Depending on the application one can choose an appropriate r. When $r \mapsto 0$ one obtains a geometric mean while for $r \mapsto -\infty$ and $r \mapsto +\infty$ one gets the minimal and maximal score, respectively. Furthermore $\overline{\chi}_r(S_k)$ is increasing as a function of r such that depending on the choice of r the sensitivity of the algorithm is influenced. A choice of $r = +\infty$ leads to a novelty system that gives an alarm when at least one cumulative probability exceeds a threshold and therefore implies maximal sensitivity but possible higher false alarm rates. For $r = -\infty$ all cumulative probabilities have to exceed a threshold implying less false alarms and thus generally lower sensitivity. All other choices are situated between these two extremes.

13.3.3 Epileptic seizure detection

In this section a case study in healthcare is considered using a dataset of acceleration data collected from movements of patients suffering from epilepsy [18]. The acceleration data was recorded during several nights using four 3D acceleration sensors that are attached to the extremities of seven patients with hypermotor seizures, all between the age of 5 and 16 years. Hypermotor seizures are epileptic convulsions that are marked by a strong and uncontrolled movement of the arms and legs that can last from a couple of seconds to some minutes. Due to the heavy movement, the patient can injure himself during the seizure, which increases the need for an alarm system, with a high detection rate.

Movement events E_s are extracted from the dataset using an energy threshold. Denote the acceleration vectors in these events as $E_s = \{\mathbf{a}_{tl} | 1 \leq t \leq T, 1 \leq l \leq 4\}$ where the indices refer to the time index and the limb, respectively (1=left arm, 2=right arm, 3=left leg, 4=right leg). A feature analysis [18] identifies three important features: (i) the movement length $f_1 = |E_s| = T$, (ii) the average energy in a movement:

$$f_2 = \frac{1}{T} \sum_{t,l} \|\mathbf{a}_{tl}\|^2$$

and (iii) the average of the maximal energy in an arm movement:

$$f_3 = \frac{1}{T} \sum_{t} \max\{\|\mathbf{a}_{t1}\|^2, \|\mathbf{a}_{t2}\|^2\}$$

The features are calculated on 50% overlapping sliding windows containing 125 samples [13] which are randomly subsampled to obtain sets S_k of fixed length $k = 50$

Table 13.3 Means and standard deviations of SS and PPV in a 10-fold cross-validation experiment for patients 1–7 based on an OCSVM and an EVT classifier

	OCSVM			EVT	
Pat.	**SS**	**PPV**	σ	**SS**	**PPV**
1	100.0 ± 0.0	31.66 ± 16.08	0.01	100.0 ± 0.0	52.8 ± 35.9
2	100.0 ± 0.0	37.90 ± 10.22	0.01	100.0 ± 0.0	71.8 ± 18.9
3	100.0 ± 0.0	40.19 ± 11.17	0.14	100.0 ± 0.0	64.7 ± 21.5
4	100.0 ± 0.0	17.62 ± 5.33	0.56	70.0 ± 25.8	40.5 ± 32.2
5	64.44 ± 10.21	19.12 ± 36.94	0.81	13.3 ± 11.5	15.8 ± 13.1
6	100.0 ± 0.0	39.04 ± 24.40	0.01	100.0 ± 0.0	69.6 ± 24.6
7	100.0 ± 0.0	40.07 ± 17.03	0.09	100.0 ± 0.0	52.6 ± 12.4

containing three-dimensional data instances $\mathbf{x}_i = (f_1^i, f_2^i, f_3^i)$, $1 \leq i \leq 50$ on which the EVT algorithm for the classification of sets can be applied. The validity of the Gumbel model for $k = 50$ can be assessed by means of quantile–quantile (Q–Q) plots [13].

In an EVT approach a kernel density estimation is performed to estimate the distribution X representing non-seizure movements and the related EVT parameters α_k, β_k, and λ_k for $k = 50$. The kernel width is set to $H = n^{-2/7}\,\hat{\Sigma} \in \mathbb{R}^{3\times 3}$ according to Scott's rule of thumb [15], where n denotes the number of data points in the training set and $\hat{\Sigma}$ the sample covariance matrix. Sets are classified by using the novelty score (13.20), while setting $r = -\infty$ and thresholding at 95%. This allows to minimize the false alarm rate in a 10-fold cross-validation experiment while the detection rate stayed at a high level. To evaluate our method the sensitivity (SS) and positive predictive value (PPV) is used:

$$SS = \frac{TP}{FP + FN}, \qquad PPV = \frac{TP}{TP + FN}$$

where the number of seizures that is detected is denoted as TP ('true positive') and the number that are not detected as FN ('false negatives'), while FP ('false positives') denotes the number of normal movements that triggered an alarm (see Table 13.3).

The use of PPPs for epileptic seizure detection seems appropriate as it is indeed plausible that a typical epileptic convulsion does not result in one very high excess in the acceleration data but to multiple exceedances with a high mean excess. Only for patient 5 a low PPV score was obtained due to the fact that for this patient seizures seemed less 'extreme' and thus less excesses were observed [18]. To illustrate this fact, consider the two movements of patient 2 shown in Fig. 13.6. As well the normal movement as the seizure contain extremes that exceed the threshold t determined by the 95% quantile of the Gumbel distribution of M_k. However, the movements in the seizure are clearly more violent than the normal movement. Because the number

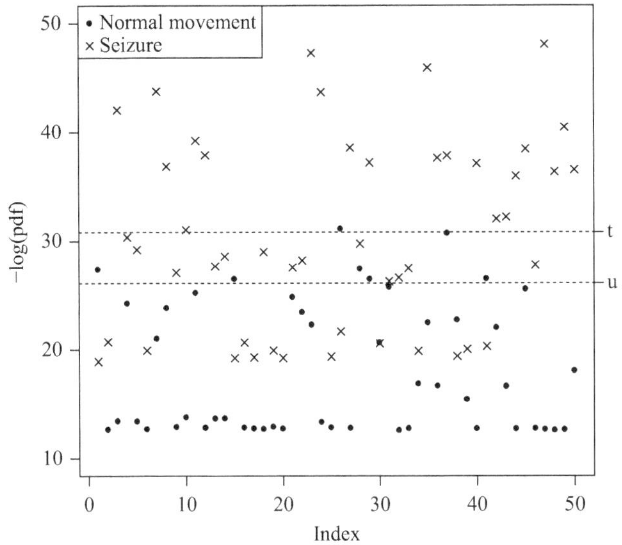

Figure 13.6 Plot of the log-densities $-\log(p(\mathbf{x}_i)), 1 \leq i \leq 50$ *of a normal movement and a seizure. The threshold t corresponds to the 95% quantile of the Gumbel distribution on* M_k *and u denotes the threshold as in (13.18) estimated by Van Kerm's rule of thumb*

of exceedances above u is high for each movement the scores $\chi_p(S_k)$ exceed 99% for both movements. However, there is a clear difference between the scores $\chi_e(S_k)$ that describe the mean excesses that are given by 80.47% and 99.99% for the normal movement and seizure, respectively.

As discussed in Section 13.3.1 an alternative approach to this novelty detection problem is an OCSVM classifier. To this end, features are extracted from complete movements such that each movement is represented by 1 feature vector. To make a consistent comparison with the EVT-method the same features and randomizations during the 10-fold cross validation are chosen. The parameter ν was set to 0.05 in accordance with the 95% threshold on the novelty scores based on the EVT-method and performance scores were optimized with respect to the kernel width σ varying over the range [0, 10] with a step size of 0.01. Results are shown in Table 13.3. The PPV scores of patients 1–4 and 6–7 are maximized while the SS scores are kept at 100%. The EVT-method is able to outperform the SVM approach in 5 of the 7 patients with a mean increase in PPV of 24.5%. For patient 5 it is possible to obtain a higher SS score and PPV score in comparison with our EVT-method by setting $\sigma = 0.81$. For this patient the SVM method was able to outperform the EVT method, although in contrast to the EVT approach the hyper-parameters of SVM were tuned using data from the seizures.

13.4 Conclusion

The focus in this chapter was on activity recognition and novelty detection that are at the core of HMS technologies.

Short tutorials were provided on GMMs and SVMs for supervised classification tasks. When applying these methods on a real-life application of classifying activities of daily living, it was found that the discriminative approach of SVM outperformed the GMM. The use of these supervised methods require expert interaction for labelling and therefore result in a substantial cost in practice. This implies the need for semi-supervised methods, where as well labelled as unlabelled data is used. Existing attempts are not adapted for their use in HMS environments where scalability (being able to roll-out a system with a high number of users) and re-usability (being able to apply the same model on different persons) are ongoing challenges [19,20].

For novelty detection OCSVMs and EVT are applied on the detection of epileptic seizures using accelerometer data. OCSVMs have the disadvantage to depend on several hyper-parameters that need to be tuned in a cross-validation experiment requiring data from the abnormal class. However, EVT is a field in statistics that is especially developed to form models of data that are situated away from the modes of a distribution and which can be adapted to circumvent the tuning of several parameters. The scarcity of the occurrence of abnormalities in many applications of HMSs requires an unusual high accuracy of novelty detection algorithms to overcome a high false alarm rate. Therefore combining several types of information using rich models (as, e.g. PPPs) is required in order to limit the number of false alarms.

References

[1] Acampora, G., Cook, D., Rashidi, P., and Vasilakos, A. A survey on ambient intelligence in healthcare. *Proceedings of the IEEE 101*, 12 (2013), 2470–2494.

[2] Paré, G., Jaana, M., and Sicotte, C. Systematic review of home telemonitoring for chronic diseases: The evidence base. *Journal of the American Medical Informatics Association 14*, 3 (2007), 269–277.

[3] Croonenborghs, T., Luca, S., Karsmakers, P., and Vanrumste, B. Healthcare decision support systems at home. In *Artificial Intelligence Applied to Assistive Technologies and Smart Environments: Papers from the AAAI-14 Workshop* (2014), B. Bouchard, A. Bouzouane, S. Giroux, A. Mihailidis, and S. Guillet, Eds., pp. 9–10.

[4] Pimentel, M. A. F., Clifton, D., Clifton, L., and Tarassenko, L. A review of novelty detection. *Signal Processing 99* (2014), 215–249.

[5] Clifton, D., Hugueny, S., and Tarassenko, L. Novelty detection with multivariate extreme value statistics. *Journal of Signal Processing Systems 65* (2011), 371–389.

[6] Bishop, C. *Pattern Recognition and Machine Learning*. Springer, New York, 2006.

[7] Hastie, T., Tibshirani, R., and Friedman, J. *The Elements of Statistical Learning*. Springer, New York, 2001.

[8] Schölkopf, B., and Smola, A. *Learning with Kernels: Support Vector Machines, Regularization, Optimization, and Beyond*. The MIT Press, London, 2002.

[9] Huang, X., Acero, A., and Hon, H.-W. *Spoken Language Processing: A Guide to Theory, Algorithm, and System Development*, 1st ed. Prentice Hall PTR, Upper Saddle River, NJ, USA, 2001.

[10] Vuegen, L., Van, B., Broeck, D., Karsmakers, P., Hamme, H. V., and Vanrumste, B. Automatic monitoring of activities of daily living based on real-life acoustic sensor data: A preliminary study. In *Workshop on Speech and Language Processing for Assistive Technologies* (2013), Association for Computational Linguistics (ACL), pp. 113–118.

[11] Jaakkola, T., Diekhans, M., and Haussler, D. Using the fisher kernel method to detect remote protein homologies. In *Proceedings of the Seventh International Conference on Intelligent Systems for Molecular Biology* (1999), AAAI Press, pp. 149–158.

[12] Luca, S., Karsmakers, P., and Vanrumste, B. Anomaly detection using the Poisson process limit for extremes. In *IEEE International Conference on Data Mining* (2014), R. Kumar, H. Toivonen, J. Pei, Z. H., and X. Wu, Eds., pp. 370–379.

[13] Luca, S., Karsmakers, P., Cuppens, K., *et al.* Detecting rare events using extreme value statistics applied to epileptic convulsions in children. *Journal of Artificial Intelligence in Medicine 60*, 2 (2014), 89–96.

[14] Embrechts, P., Klüppelberg, C., and Mikosch, T. *Modelling Extremal Events for Insurance and Finance*. Springer, Berlin, 1997.

[15] Scott, D. W. *Multivariate Density Estimation: Theory, Practice, and Visualization*. Wiley and Sons, New York, 1992.

[16] Roberts, S. Novelty detection using extreme value statistics. *IEE Proceedings on Vision, Image and Signal Processing 146*, 3 (1999), 124–129.

[17] Alfons, A., and Templ, M. Estimation of social exclusion indicators from complex surveys: The R package laeken. *Journal of Statistical Software 54*, 15 (2013), 1–25.

[18] Cuppens, K., Karsmakers, P., Van de Vel, A., *et al.* Accelerometer based home monitoring for detection of nocturnal hypermotor seizures based on novelty detection. *IEEE Journal of Biomedical and Health Informatics 60*, 2 (2013), 89–96.

[19] Guan, D., Yuan, W., Lee, Y.-K., and Gavrilov, L. Activity recognition based on semisupervised learning. In *13th IEEE International Conference on Embedded and Real-Time Computing Systems and Applications* (2007), IEEE, pp. 469–475.

[20] Stikic, M., Larlus, D., Ebert, S., and Schiele, B. Weakly supervised recognition of daily life activities with wearable sensors. *IEEE Transactions on Patterns Analysis and Machine Intelligence 33*, 12 (2011), 2521–2537.

Index